A martial arts
expert, personal
trainer and TV personality,
TIFFINY HALL is one of
Australia's most trusted health
experts and founder of online
fitness programs.
She has coached everyone from
athletes, mums and CEOs to
Hollywood stars.
@tiffhall_xo

THIS BOOK IS
DEDICATED TO EVERYONE
WHO'S FEELING SNACKY.

FEEL SATISFIED,
FULL AND FIRED UP!

200 DELICIOUS SNACKS TO KEEP YOU HEALTHY, HAPPY & FULL OF ENERGY

POWER SNACKS

TIFFINY HALL

murdoch books

Sydney | London

CONTENTS

HI, I'M TIFF AND I'M SNACKY.

That's right, I'm always snacky. I've been through phases where I flat-out denied myself snacks and guess what? I was so miserable. I love eating; I know this and I'm not going to deprive myself. So, instead of banning snacks, I decided to snack *right*, and now I'm going to share the secrets that helped me hit my goals, stay lean and feel awesome.

This book shares the most delicious snacks you'll ever create, taste, share and enjoy. There is something here for all fitness goals and all occasions. You could say this is *the* snack bible. If you enjoy food, love eating and don't want to kill your social life by depriving yourself, then this delicious book is for you.

Let's be real, we're never going to stop snacking so we may as well learn how to do it properly and how to make them healthy. No matter the reason behind your snacking— whether it's to have more energy, build more lean muscle, or just because you need a snack pronto, there's always a smart way to satisfy that need.

WHAT CONSTITUTES A SNACK?

Traditionally, a snack counted for under 250 calories, but my approach to fitness has never been about restrictive calorie counting—my approach is more about creating a lifestyle that includes healthy snacks.

Sometimes you might feel like having a treat snack, other times you might only have time for a liquid snack (like a smoothie or juice). Maybe you're focused on a goal like toning up or building strength so you opt for high-protein snacks, or perhaps for you it's all about those occasions when you become a snack queen—the one wowing family and friends with something delicious at a gathering or to bring to a friend's place.

I prefer to look at the overall nutritional value of the foods I consume over the number of calories.

WHY WRITE A SNACK BOOK?

I launched my online community in 2016, and my community is an inspirational, passionate bunch who share every meal, moment and milestone of their fitness journeys. Without fail, there's one topic that always comes up: snacks! Month after month, my community members begged me for more snack recipes, swaps, tips and hacks.

So, after four years, I finally shared it all (including my 'snackology'); everything that keeps me lean, fit, energetic, less stressed and, most importantly, satisfied. The book's been a big success and now is having a new life in this edition; it's been a pleasure to share my snack journey with you all.

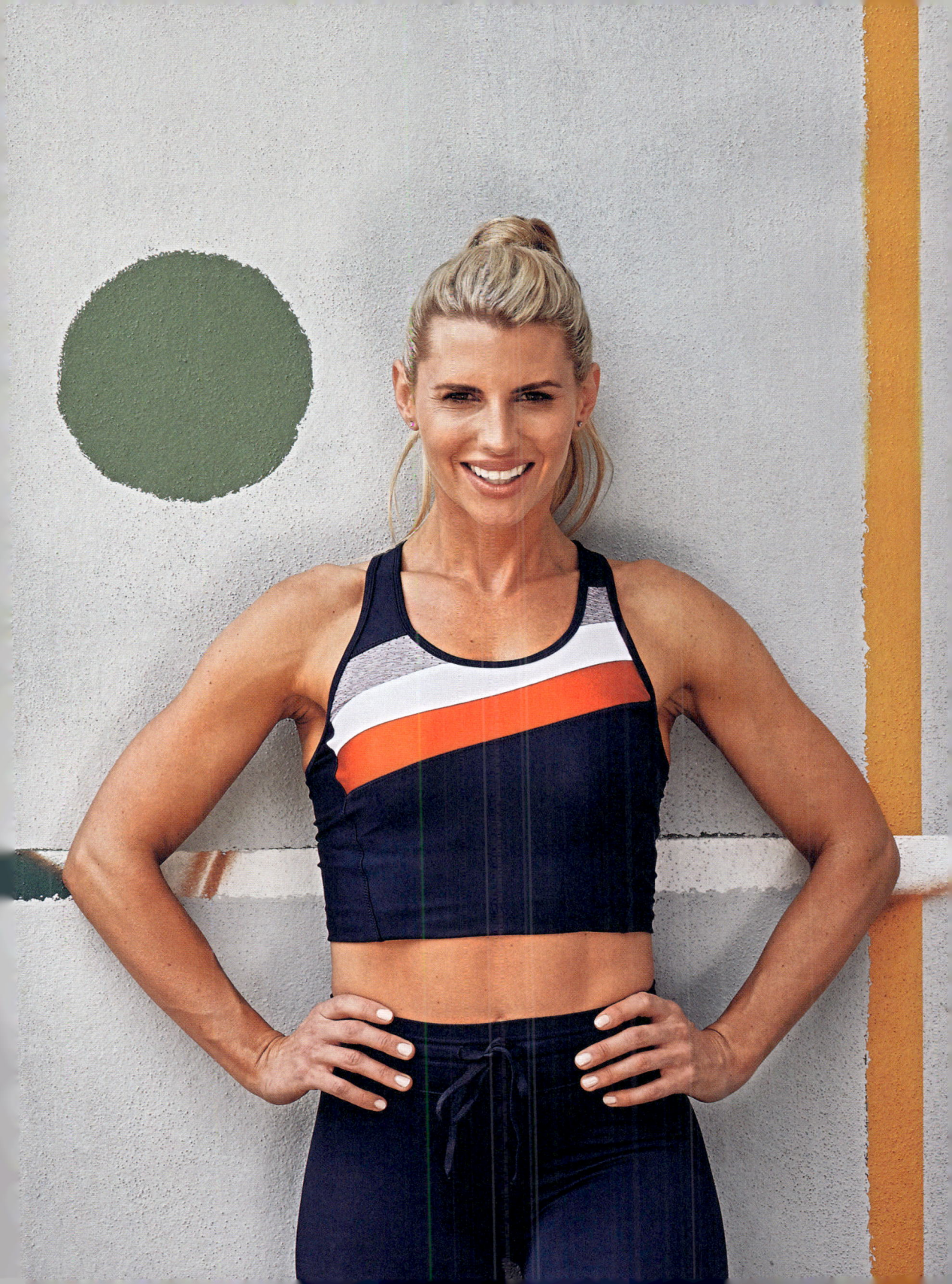

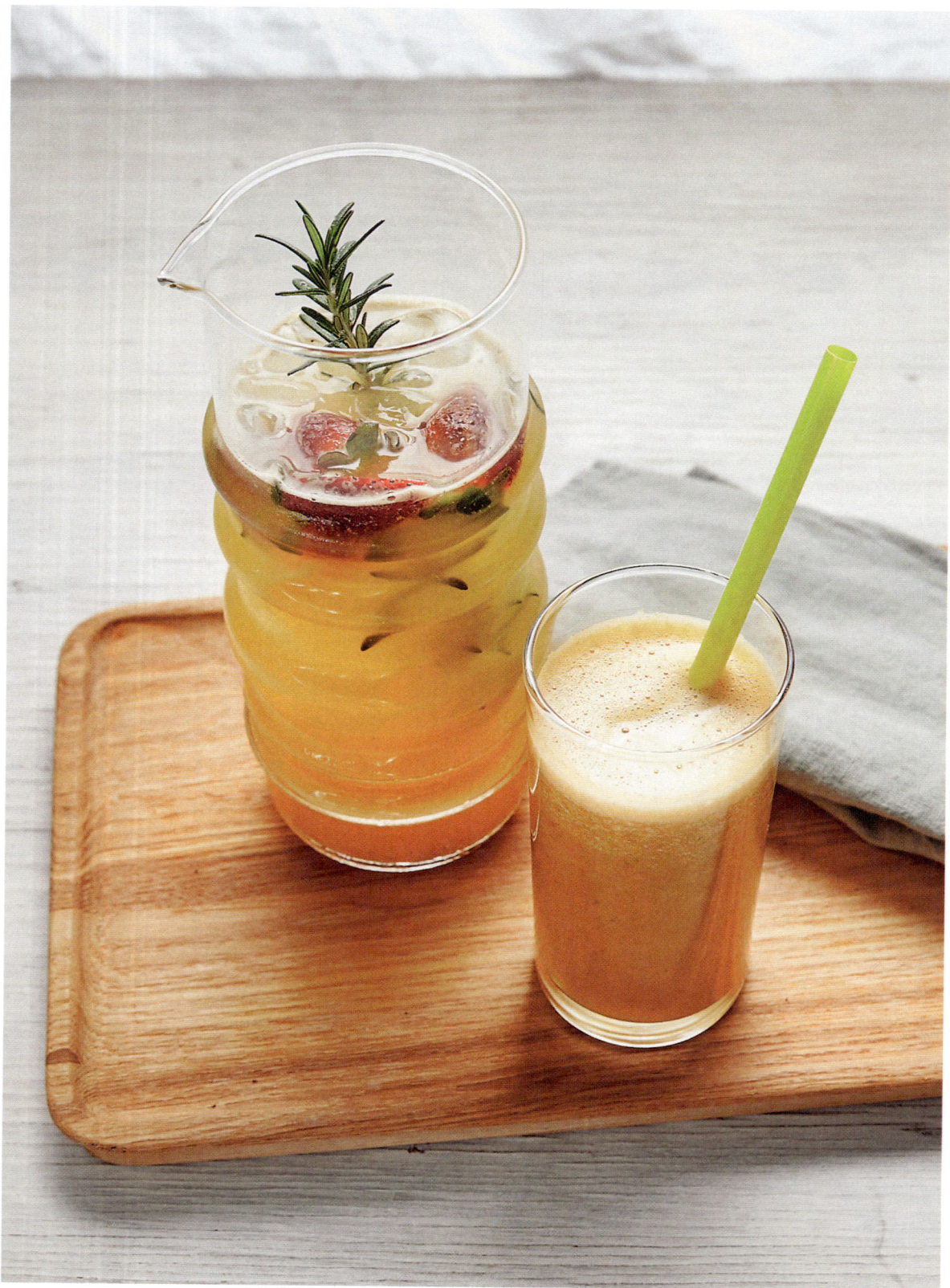

THE PROBLEM WITH FAD DIETS

At the moment, the pro-fasting movement and keto diet are extremely popular, and there's no doubt they're capable of getting results (for now). But do you want results **now** or do you want to keep getting results in the future? Often, these diets are not sustainable, they don't teach mindful eating and they're not social or kid-friendly.

Despite ketogenic diets causing initial weight loss due to changes in glycogen and water content (which I know can be motivating), they're too restrictive and can be hard to sustain in the long term. And, like the keto diet, fasting may work short term, but it's not optimal for athletes or those wishing to add muscle because of the long stretches of time without food and nutrients. In my mind, fasting is simply not a long-term lifestyle fix. In fact, for some people, the fasting window can increase appetite.

MY RELATIONSHIP WITH FOOD

Food, for me, has never been about over-indulging or deprivation; it's always been about performance and enjoyment.

From the homemade slices and protein balls Mum made us as kids (well before they were a thing in 'it' cafes) to the snack boxes I'd create for myself when I was working long hours or for my husband, who does shift work, snacks have always saved the day. They kept my brain sharp at university and helped keep me going when training, when building my business and when writing books—including this one.

Snacks have also taught me to be mindful with food: they help me hang in a few more hours until the main meal; they function as a reset when I need to refocus on my goals; they are concentration companions that carry me through big days at work; they are rejuvenation aids when I'm feeling flat, and energy boosters when I'm exhausted.

'THANKS, TIFF. BUT I JUST WANTED SOME RECIPES.' 'THEY'RE COMING, PROMISE!'

Training, being physically fit and performing at my optimum level is important for what I do. Not only is my job physically demanding, but my little boy, Arnold (Arnie), also happens to be a tornado of energy, which requires me to have oodles of high-voltage zing. But the main reason I snack is to feel satisfied. I hate feeling empty, hungry, hangry and fungry (as in really 'f-ing' hungry)!

It's pretty simple: if you don't eat, you get hungry. When you get hungry, you risk succumbing to emotional eating. Suddenly, food choices become about what you feel like rather than what you need. Who doesn't feel like chocolate at three o'clock in the afternoon? But a chocolate snack is going to zap your energy not replenish it—that sugar will stimulate your appetite and you'll want more of it. Everything we put into our bodies creates a reaction; it's nature. Holy moly, guacamole, I can't wait to give your afternoon snack a makeover.

Skipping meals also creates what I call a 'starving then stuffing' cycle. You feel that deprivation chemically in your brain, and when you allow yourself to eat again, it can be hard not to binge because those hormones mean business!

THE MAGIC OF (HEALTHY) SNACKING

I discovered the real power of snacks when I was pregnant and breastfeeding. I needed constant energy—the *right* energy—and although I was eating healthily for breakfast, lunch and dinner, healthy snacking helped me to stay on track and have enough beautiful energy to nurture Arnie. Psychologically, snacks help us to feel satiated, and therefore prevent us from emotionally eating when we are not hungry or feeling deprived, and completely bereft of yumminess. In fact, healthy snacking has many benefits—for the body, mind *and* the spirit.

Body benefits

Healthy snacking will improve your overall health, increase your energy levels and help you to lose weight and tone up. Eating nutritionally packed snacks also stabilises blood sugar levels, improves cholesterol levels and lowers your risks for certain diseases.

Mind magic

Healthy snacks can improve concentration, increase memory and enhance mental alertness and awareness. This makes it easier for us to learn in school, get sh*t done in the office, and be present and happy when we're out with friends and family.

If you have kids, think of their attitude towards food. Do they respect their snacks? Healthy snacks are good for children because the extra nutrients help promote growth and development. Healthy snacks will also increase your child's vitamin, protein and calorie intake and keep them healthy and strong. It will also encourage a healthy snack mindset, for life.

Emotional enhancement

Yummy snacks are a source of joy and inspiration. I feel my spirits soar when a fresh blondie slice comes cruising out of the oven! Whether you favour healthy sweet snacks, spicy snacks or savoury snacks, there's a lot to gain by feeding the soul, too. And although we've been told that less is more when it comes to losing stubborn weight, satisfying our bodies throughout the day (with a healthy snack) can do a lot more for us than denying them can.

MY 'SNACKOLOGY'

My 'snackology' (snacking philosophy) is this: healthy snacks such as the ones in this book won't hinder your progress or stop you from reaching your goals. In fact, they'll help you get there! A treat snack will never hurt your progress, but a binge will.

This is why I always include snack treats in my meal plans. I know that if I don't, that badass binge monster will come out and wreak havoc. I'm a big believer in the power of saying, 'I *am* allowed.' It stops that dangerous all-or-nothing mentality from taking hold.

How often you snack is a personal decision. I aim to stick to three main meals and two to three snacks a day (depending on my energy output). On high-energy days when I have a lot on, I find the right number of snacks for me is three: one mid-morning and one in the afternoon, plus a post-workout snack. This gets me through all the slumps. Three meals and three snacks; it's my perfect power source.

I believe that a balanced approach always wins—eating too much or too little can deplete your health, wellbeing and energy levels. So, listen to your body and stick with what works for you. Aim to eat every four to six hours, try not to go too long without protein and don't buy into any fads.

Previously, poor old snacks have only ever featured as a single chapter in my recipe books, or as a side note; but here, my friends—due to popular demand—they are the main event. Roll out the red carpet, we're celebrating them in all their delicious glory.

Let these recipes teach you how to eat mindfully, how to snack healthily and how good a treat every now and then is for the soul. My hope is that you enjoy every single bite. Now, enough from me. Let's snack!

TIFF XO

RECIPE KEY

Dairy Free	Gluten Free	Nut Free	Vegetarian	Vegan

You'll also find gluten-free and dairy-free labels on recipes in this book that can be easily adjusted to suit those styles of eating.

For recipes that stipulate the number of items made, unless otherwise specified these consist of individual servings.

CHAPTER I

PRE + POST WORKOUT SNACKS

It might seem strange to kick off a book about snacks with a whole lot of info on water, but hear me out. Whenever I work with a new client and they have a goal to lose weight, gain more lean muscle or tone up, I always start by asking them how much water they drink, rather than how often they snack because snackiness is often disguised as thirstiness.

As far as survival instincts go, thirst is one of the most important as our bodies are basically cucumbers—made almost entirely of water. If you're dehydrated you'll feel lethargic. In training, you'll lose speed and strength; you'll have constant brain farts and feel light-headed. And here's the lemon twist: when you are dehydrated you will feel MORE SNACKY!

This is because the part of the brain that regulates and triggers thirst in the body is the same part of the brain that motivates hunger and cravings. So, you may not need a snack right now, you may just be thirsty.

This thirst/hunger centre of the brain is called the hypothalamus, and it also regulates your body temperature and sleep (along with thirst and appetite). Sensors in the hypothalamus constantly monitor the blood's concentration of sodium and other substances. So after a big workout when you've sweated a lot, or after eating a lot of salt, your hypothalamus realises you're dehydrated and sends out a strong message: *Hey! Drink a glass of water, STAT!*

Try my Water Week to accelerate smart snacking

Try prioritising drinking only water for seven days. You can snack, eat meals and exercise as normal, this is just about what you're drinking. Think about all the calories and sugar you'll be saving: soft drinks, fruit juices, milkshakes, tea and coffee and alcohol can really up your daily calories and dehydrate you. Just one can of soft drink can have more than 15 teaspoons of sugar.

ALLOWED ON THE WATER WEEK

- Espresso coffees are sanctioned. (I would NEVER take your morning coffee away.)
- Herbal teas, black teas and black coffee.
- Mineral water is a go.
- Smoothies and juices that are snacks worked into your mealplan for the day are just fine.
- Feel free to add flavour to your water with cucumber, lemon, lime, mint or berries.

LIMIT ON THE WATER WEEK

- Milky coffees with added sugar and syrups
- Alcohol
- Soft drinks
- Diet soft drinks
- Fruit juices
- Milkshakes
- Sports drinks
- Energy drinks
- Anything that isn't H₂0!

Fail to plan, plan to graze

Planning your snacks and sticking to regular snack times that work for you is very important. I've included more snack prep ideas and tips on page 166.

I love eating frequently. Fuelling the muscles that work as my fat-burning factories keeps my metabolism strong and my body lean. In fact, did you know that for every 0.5–1 kilogram of lean muscle you gain, your body can burn extra calories at rest? Feeding that muscle and keeping my energy levels stable have always been my top priorities.

In contrast, grazing around the clock prevents your body from burning fat efficiently. When you're constantly eating, you're constantly releasing more insulin, the storage hormone. This means the insulin is helping your body to convert and store more fat, rather than use the fat from your energy stores as fuel.

ALL HAIL THE PROTEIN-DENSE SNACK!

When it comes to healthy snacks, not all are created equal; protein-dense foods are some of the best snacks around because they fire up powerful physical responses in your body. They can help you reach your health goals, and keep you out of the kitchen and the pantry for longer stretches of time.

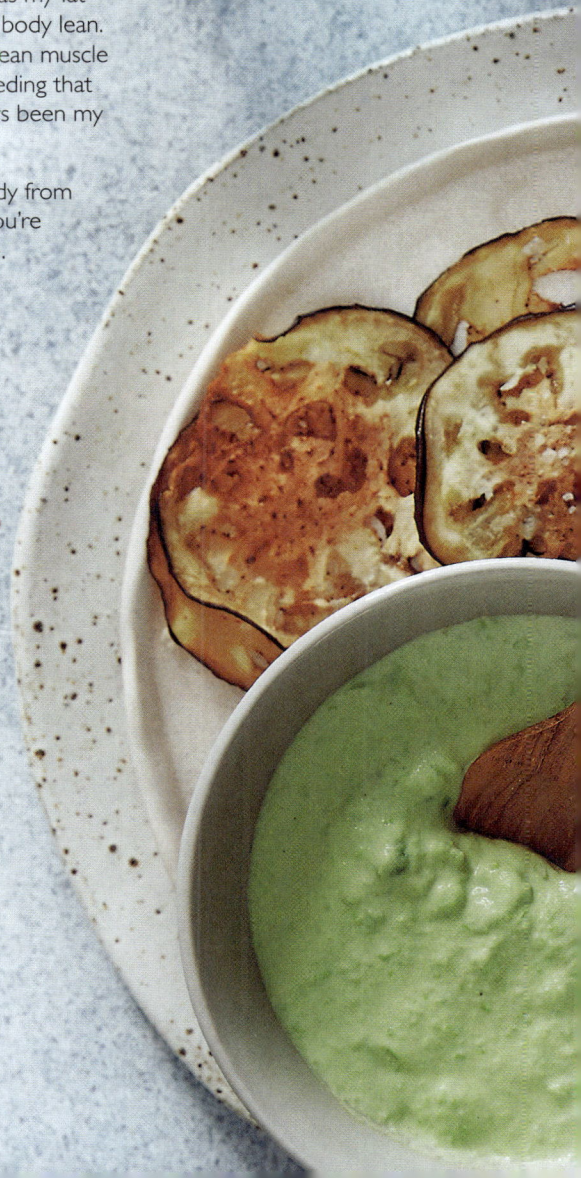

ALMOND AND CRANBERRY GRANOLA BARS

MAKES 16
PREP TIME 5 minutes
COOK TIME 22 minutes

200 g (7 oz/2 cups) rolled (porridge) oats
140 g (5 oz/1 cup) dried cranberries, finely
   chopped
160 g (5⅔ oz/1 cup) almonds, chopped
1 tablespoon chia seeds
¼ teaspoon sea salt
40 g (1½ oz/¼ cup) pepitas (pumpkin seeds)
175 g (6 oz/½ cup) honey
55 g (2 oz/¼ cup) coconut oil
2 teaspoons natural vanilla extract

Preheat the oven to 150°C (300°F), and line a
20 cm (8 inch) baking tin with baking paper.

Combine all of the dry ingredients in a medium
bowl.

Heat the honey and coconut oil in a small
saucepan over medium heat until just melted. Add
the vanilla, then pour the mixture into the bowl of
dry ingredients and stir through.

Spread the mixture into the prepared tray,
pressing firmly into an even layer.

Bake for 20–25 minutes and remove from oven.
Allow to cool on a wire rack for 1 hour, then
chill in the fridge for 2 hours before slicing into
16 bars.

Store in an airtight container in the cupboard for
1 week or refrigerate for up to 2 weeks. These
are also great to freeze.

QUINOA FRUIT AND NUT BARS

MAKES 12
PREP TIME 15 minutes
COOK TIME 12 minutes

90 g (3¼ oz/½ cup) quinoa flakes
80 g (2¾ oz/½ cup) almonds
2 tablespoons shredded coconut
1½ tablespoons honey
2 tablespoons coconut oil
70 g (2½ oz/½ cup) dried cranberries,
   plus 1 tablespoon
60 g (2¼ oz/½ cup) dried apricots,
   coarsely chopped
40 g (1½ oz/¼ cup) pepitas (pumpkin seeds)
75 g (2⅔ oz/½ cup) sunflower seeds
1 tablespoon chopped pistachio nut kernels
1 tablespoon chia seeds

Preheat the oven to 180°C (350°F) and line a
square 20 cm (8 inch) baking tin with baking paper.

Spread the quinoa flakes, almonds and
coconut evenly on a baking tray and bake for
8–10 minutes, or until lightly golden.

Warm the honey and coconut oil in a small
saucepan over medium–low heat until combined.

Blitz the toasted ingredients in a food processor
with half of the cranberries and the apricots,
pepitas and sunflower seeds until everything is
finely chopped.

Add the honey mixture and blitz again to
combine.

Press the mixture into the prepared tin,
pressing down firmly. Scatter over the remaining
cranberries and the pistachios and chia seeds,
then gently press these into the mixture.

Cover with plastic wrap and refrigerate for 1 hour
before slicing into 12. These will keep in an airtight
container for up to 5 days.

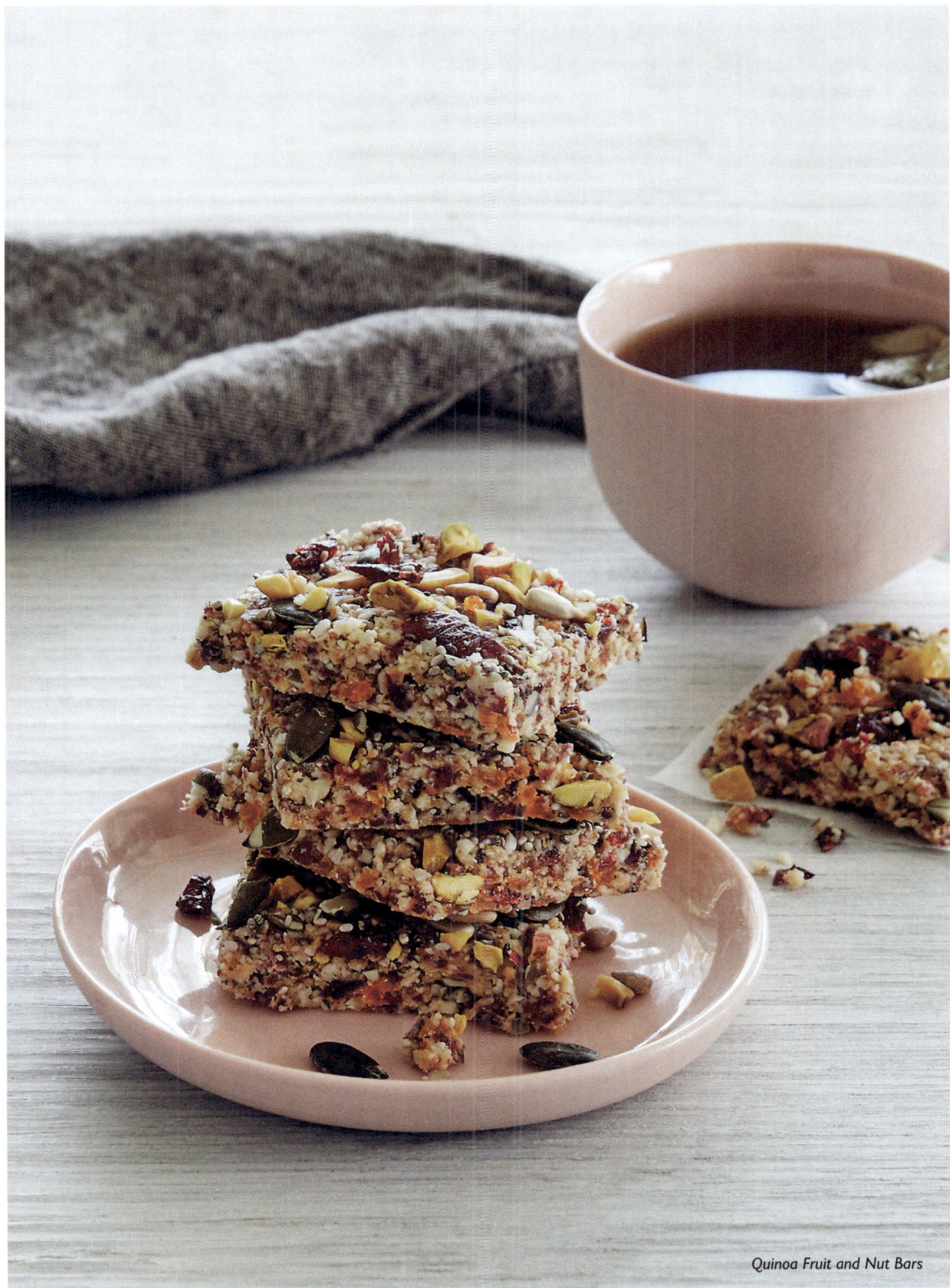

Quinoa Fruit and Nut Bars

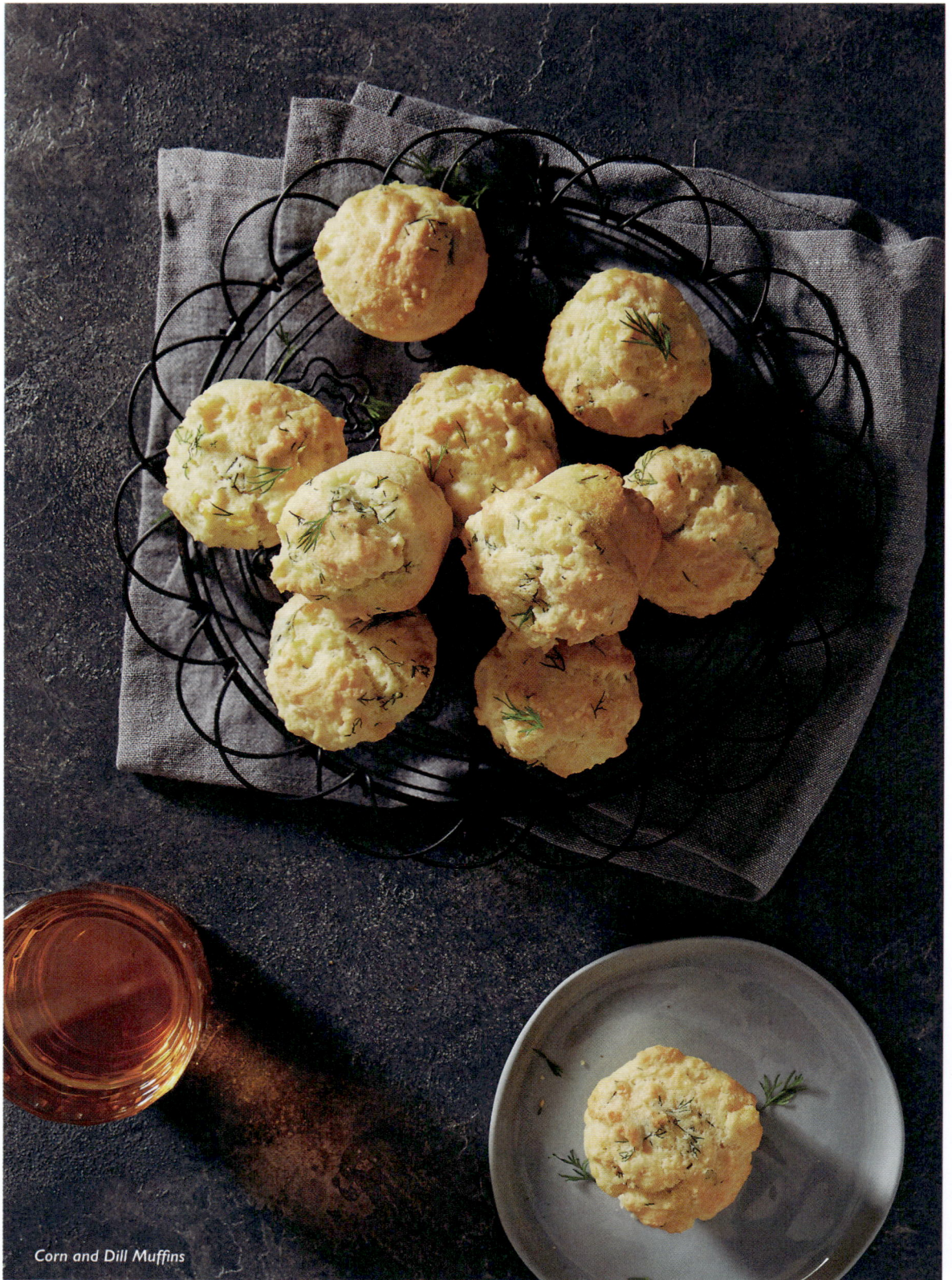

Corn and Dill Muffins

CORN AND DILL MUFFINS

MAKES 12
PREP TIME 5 minutes
COOK TIME 15 minutes

300 g (10½ oz/2 cups) self-raising wholemeal
   (whole-wheat) flour (or gluten-free if needed)
200 g (7 oz) tinned corn kernels, drained
salt and pepper
80 ml (2½ fl oz/⅓ cup) olive oil
260 g (9¼ oz/1 cup) Greek-style yoghurt
2 eggs
3 tablespoons chopped dill

Preheat the oven to 180°C (350°F) and grease a 12-hole standard (60 ml/2 fl oz/¼ cup) muffin tin.

Combine the flour, corn and salt and pepper in a mixing bowl.

In another mixing bowl, whisk the olive oil, yoghurt, eggs and dill together, then gently stir into the flour mixture until just combined.

Spoon the batter into the prepared tin and bake for 15–20 minutes, or until a toothpick inserted into one of the muffins comes out clean.

Allow to cool in the tin for 5 minutes before turning onto a wire rack. Serve warm or cold. Serve right away, or store in an airtight container for up to 3 days.

PUMPKIN FALAFEL BITES

MAKES 14 (2 per snack)
PREP TIME 20 minutes
COOK TIME 45 minutes

500 g (1 lb 2 oz) pumpkin, peeled and diced
2 teaspoons olive oil
1 teaspoon coriander seeds
1 teaspoon cumin seeds
½ teaspoon dried chilli flakes
400 g (14 oz) tinned chickpeas, drained and
   rinsed
60 g (2¼ oz) rice flour
2 garlic cloves
¼ bunch coriander (cilantro), coarsely chopped
1 tablespoon lemon juice
100 g (3½ oz) feta cheese, crumbled
salt and pepper
1 tablespoon Greek-style yoghurt, to serve

Preheat the oven to 200°C (400°F) and line two baking trays with baking paper.

Toss the pumpkin with the oil and spices, spread around the trays and roast for 20 minutes, or until tender.

Put the roasted pumpkin into a food processor with the chickpeas, flour, garlic, coriander and lemon juice, and blitz to combine. Transfer to a bowl and fold through the feta. Taste, and season with salt and pepper as needed. Cover and refrigerate for 1 hour to firm up.

Roll heaped tablespoons of the mixture into 14 balls, arrange on a lined tray and bake for 25–30 minutes, or until lightly golden brown.

Serve 2 falafel bites dipped in the yoghurt for a snack. Any leftovers can be refrigerated in an airtight container for up to 5 days, or can be frozen for up to 3 months.

MINI TACO WITH HUMMUS AND AVO

SERVES 4
PREP TIME 5 minutes
COOK TIME 3 minutes

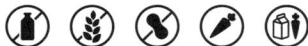

4 × 25 g (1 oz) wholegrain (or gluten-free)
  pitta breads, warmed
½ avocado, quartered
75 g (2⅔ oz/⅓ cup) hummus
2 flat-leaf (Italian) parsley sprigs, chopped
½ lemon
salt and pepper

Top one side of each pitta bread with avocado, hummus and parsley.

Squeeze over some lemon, season with salt and pepper and fold in half to serve.

BEETROOT HUMMUS AND FETA CORN THINS

SERVES 1
PREP TIME 5 minutes

2 Corn Thins
2 tablespoons beetroot (beet) hummus
1 radish, thinly sliced
20 g (¾ oz) feta cheese, crumbled
1 sprig flat-leaf (Italian) parsley, leaves picked

Top each Corn Thin with hummus and a few radish slices, then sprinkle over some feta and parsley leaves.

MY THREE LAWS OF SNACKING

1. **DON'T snack on empty calories.** Processed junk foods only stimulate your appetite and make you eat more.

2. **DON'T skip snacks!** Don't let yourself get too hungry or you'll find yourself lost in the pantry feasting on high-energy foods.

3. **DON'T abuse snacks.** They're not meals; they're designed to keep you ticking over between the main events.

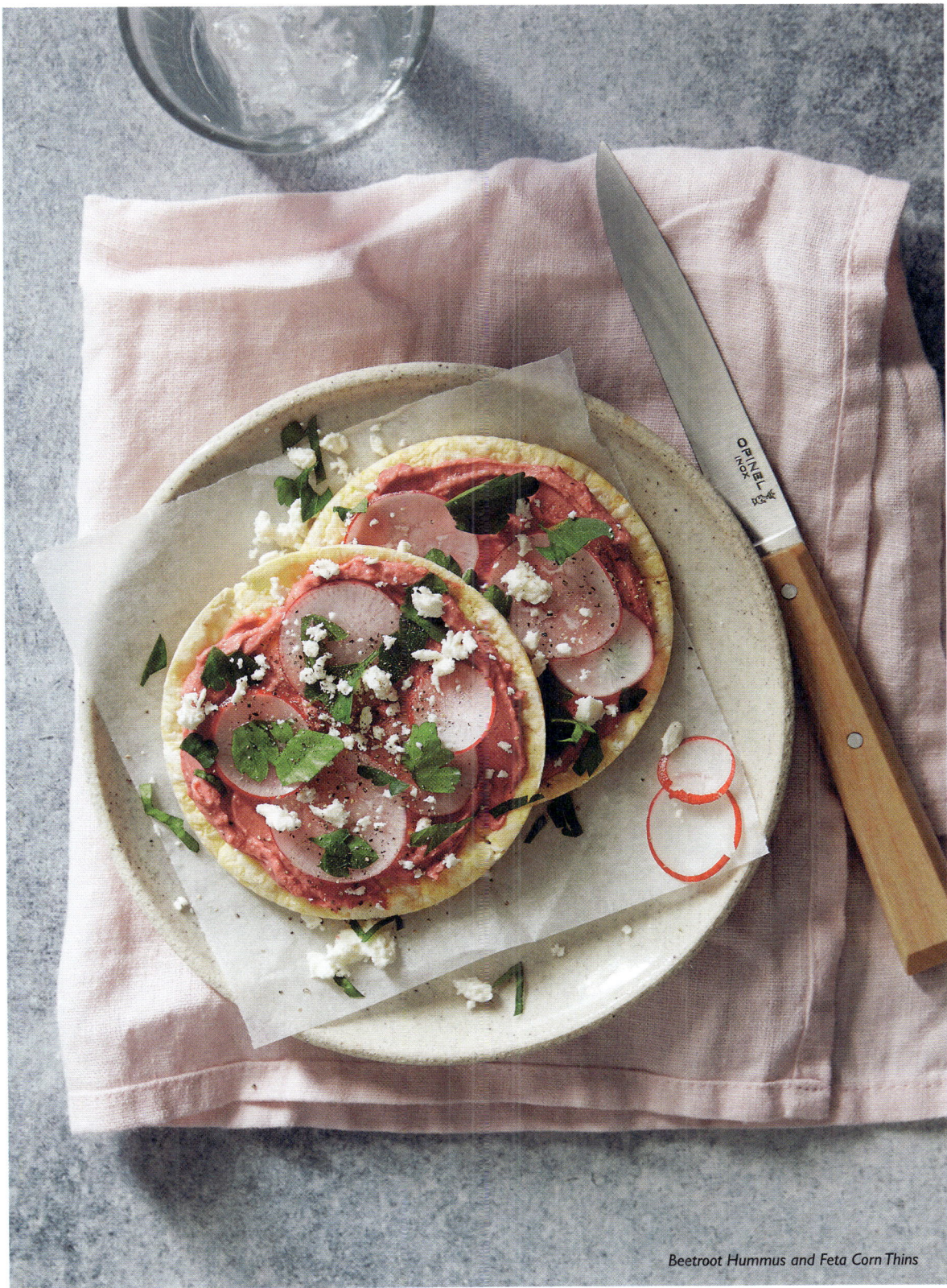

Beetroot Hummus and Feta Corn Thins

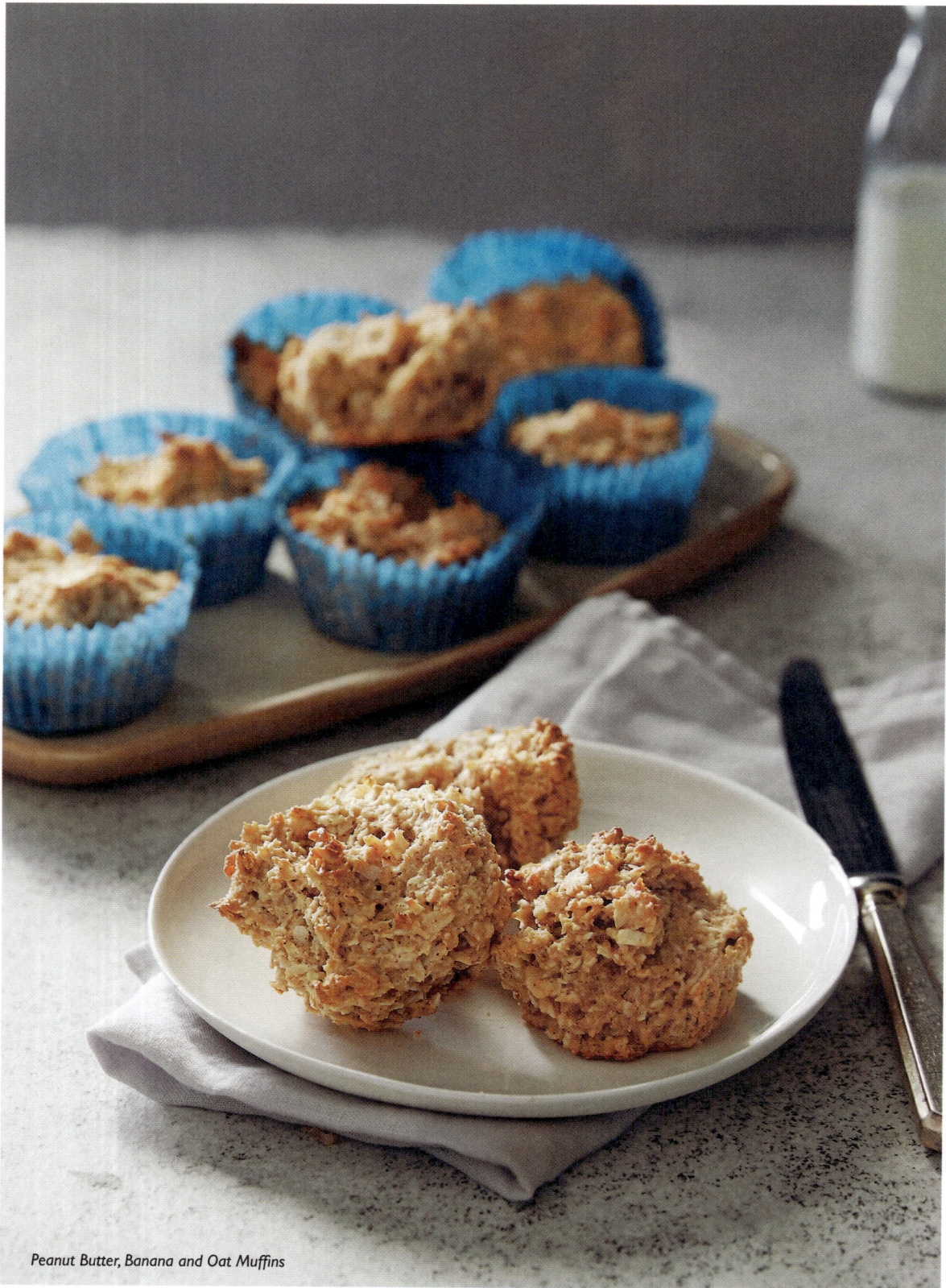

Peanut Butter, Banana and Oat Muffins

PEANUT BUTTER, BANANA AND OAT MUFFINS

MAKES 6
PREP TIME 10 minutes
COOK TIME 15 minutes

150 g (5½ oz/1½ cups) rolled (porridge) oats
3 tablespoons desiccated coconut
2 ripe bananas
190 g (6¾ oz/⅔ cup) Greek-style yoghurt
1 tablespoon honey
1 teaspoon baking powder
1 tablespoon crunchy peanut butter
1 teaspoon ground cinnamon

Preheat the oven to 180°C (350°F) and line six holes of a standard (60 ml/¼ cup) muffin tin with paper cases.

Blitz the oats in a food processor until they resemble flour. Add all of the remaining ingredients and pulse until just combined.

Spoon the mixture into the paper cases.

Bake for 15 minutes, or until a toothpick inserted into one of the muffins comes out clean.

Cool completely on a wire rack, and store in an airtight container for up to 3 days.

RASPBERRY PROTEIN POT

SERVES 1
PREP TIME 5 minutes

110 g (3¾ oz/½ cup) frozen raspberries
75 g (2⅔ oz/¼ cup) cottage cheese
70 g (2½ oz/¼ cup) Greek-style yoghurt
1 teaspoon natural vanilla extract
3 ice cubes

Combine three-quarters of the raspberries with the other ingredients in a food processor and blend until smooth.

Serve topped with the remaining berries.

COCONUT AND DATE POWER BARS

MAKES 16
PREP TIME 10 minutes

2 teaspoons coconut oil
3 tablespoons rolled (porridge) oats
35 g (1¼ oz/½ cup) shredded coconut
65 g (2⅓ oz/½ cup) slivered almonds
70 g (2½ oz/½ cup) peanuts
60 g (2¼ oz) medjool dates, pitted

Line a small rectangular dish with baking paper.

Heat the oil in a frying pan over medium–low heat and toast the oats and 2 tablespoons of the shredded coconut until golden. Set aside to cool.

Put the almonds, peanuts and the remaining shredded coconut in a food processor and pulse until combined.

Add the dates and continue to pulse until the mixture sticks together. Spoon into the prepared dish, spread evenly and press down gently.

Scatter over the toasted coconut mix, cover with baking paper and press into the top.

Place in the freezer for 15 minutes, then cut into 16 bars. Store in an airtight container for up to 3 days. Any extras can be frozen for up to 3 months.

PEANUT BUTTER AND HONEY OAT COOKIES

MAKES 12
PREP TIME 5 minutes
COOK TIME 8 minutes

140 g (5 oz/½ cup) crunchy peanut butter
90 g (3¼ oz/¼ cup) honey
1 large egg
175 g (6 oz/1¾ cups) rolled (porridge) oats
½ teaspoon baking powder

Preheat the oven to 180°C (350°F). Line a baking tray with baking paper.

Place the peanut butter and honey in a small bowl and use a wooden spoon or a hand mixer to beat until whipped and fluffy. Beat in the egg.

Add the oats and baking powder to the mixture, and mix well until a dough forms.

Spoon tablespoon-sized balls of the mixture onto the baking tray and slightly flatten with the back of the spoon.

Bake for 8 minutes, or until the cookies are golden brown. Allow to cool on the tray for a few minutes before transferring to a wire rack to cool completely. Store in an airtight container for up to 5 days.

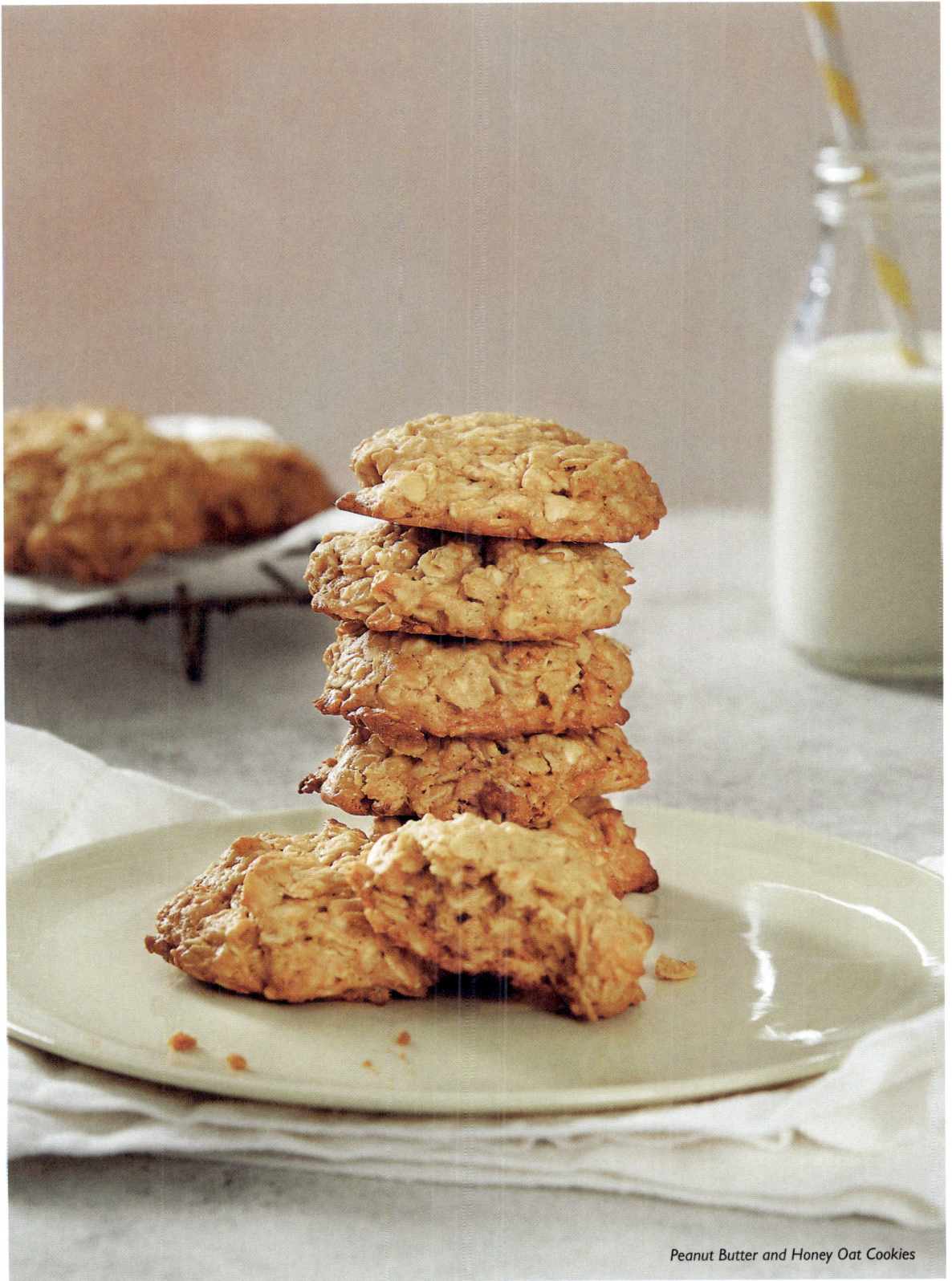

Peanut Butter and Honey Oat Cookies

REFUEL BARS

MAKES 24 **PREP TIME** 10 minutes **COOK TIME** 30 minutes

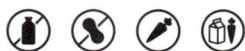

250 g (9 oz) medjool dates, pitted and coarsely chopped
125 g (4½ oz) dried figs, coarsely chopped
125 g (4½ oz) sultanas
zest of 1 orange
zest of 1 lemon
210 g (7½ oz/2 cups) quick oats
55 g (2 oz/⅓ cup) rice flour
75 g (2⅔ oz/½ cup) sunflower seeds
250 ml (9 fl oz/1 cup) orange juice
1 tablespoon lemon juice
235 g (8½ oz/⅔ cup) golden syrup
2 tablespoons sesame seeds

Preheat the oven to 180°C (350°F). Line a 33 × 15 cm (13 × 6 inch) baking tin with baking paper and lightly grease the sides.

Blend the dates, figs, sultanas and citrus zests in a food processor until well blended.

Add the oats, flour and sunflower seeds, and pulse for a few seconds until just combined. Transfer to a bowl.

Heat the citrus juices with the golden syrup in a small saucepan over low heat, stirring until the syrup has melted. Add to the dry mix and stir until combined.

Press firmly into the prepared tin, then cover with a sheet of baking paper and roll a glass over the top to smooth the surface. Bake for 25 minutes.

Remove from the oven, sprinkle with sesame seeds and leave in the tin to cool. Cut into 24 bars and store in an airtight container in the fridge for a week, or in the freezer for up to 3 months.

Tip:
Serve with some Greek-style yoghurt for an extra protein boost!

BANANA AND YOGHURT SNACK

SERVES 1
PREP TIME 2 minutes

70 g (2½ oz/¼ cup) Greek-style yoghurt
½ sliced banana
1 tablespoon chopped almonds (or other nut/
  seed mix)

Place the yoghurt in a small bowl and stir through
the banana. Top with the almonds.

BERRY YOGHURT SNACK

SERVES 1
PREP TIME 2 minutes

95 g (3¼ oz/⅓ cup) Greek-style yoghurt
35 g (1½ oz/¼ cup) frozen mixed berries
1 teaspoon slivered almonds
1 teaspoon pepitas (pumpkin seeds)
1 teaspoon sesame seeds

Place the yoghurt in a bowl and top with the
berries, nuts and seeds.

WHETHER YOU'RE ABOUT
TO HIT THE GYM OR NEED
TO REFUEL THE TANK
AFTER, THESE SNACKS ARE
DESIGNED TO HELP YOUR
BODY MAXIMISE YOUR
WORKOUT OR REPAIR
YOUR MUSCLES AFTER.

CHICKEN NOODLE AND SWEETCORN SNACK SOUP

SERVES 4 **PREP TIME** 10 minutes **COOK TIME** 30 minutes

½ onion, coarsely chopped
1 carrot, coarsely chopped
1 celery stalk, coarsely chopped
1 garlic clove, crushed
1 teaspoon olive oil
1 litre (35 fl oz/4 cups) chicken stock or water
200 g (7 oz) chicken breast, thicker parts scored for even cooking
100 g (3½ oz/⅔ cup) frozen corn kernels
40 g (1½ oz) dried rice noodles, broken into pieces
30 g (1 oz) baby spinach, coarsely chopped
1 teaspoon soy sauce (use tamari if gluten free), optional

Blend the onion, carrot, celery and garlic to a rough paste in a food processor.

Heat the oil in a non-stick saucepan over medium heat, add the vegetable paste and cook for a few minutes.

Add the stock (or water) and simmer gently for 10 minutes to allow the flavours to infuse.

Add the chicken and bring the soup back up to a gentle simmer. Cook for about 10 minutes, or until the chicken is cooked through.

Remove from the heat and stand, covered, for 10 minutes. Remove the chicken, allow to cool slightly, then shred the meat using two forks.

Add the corn and noodles to the pan then return to the heat and boil for a few minutes, or until the noodles are cooked. Taste and adjust the seasoning, if needed.

Add the spinach and shredded chicken to the soup, and stir through. Add a splash of soy sauce if you like, for extra flavour.

Serve right away, or freeze in individual portions for a quick grab-and-go snack.

STAY ON TRACK

Grazing can cause you to lose track of the calories you've consumed and the macronutrients you've missed out on. When you have three well-balanced meals a day and two or three snacks, it's much easier to eat mindfully and enjoy nutritionally balanced meals.

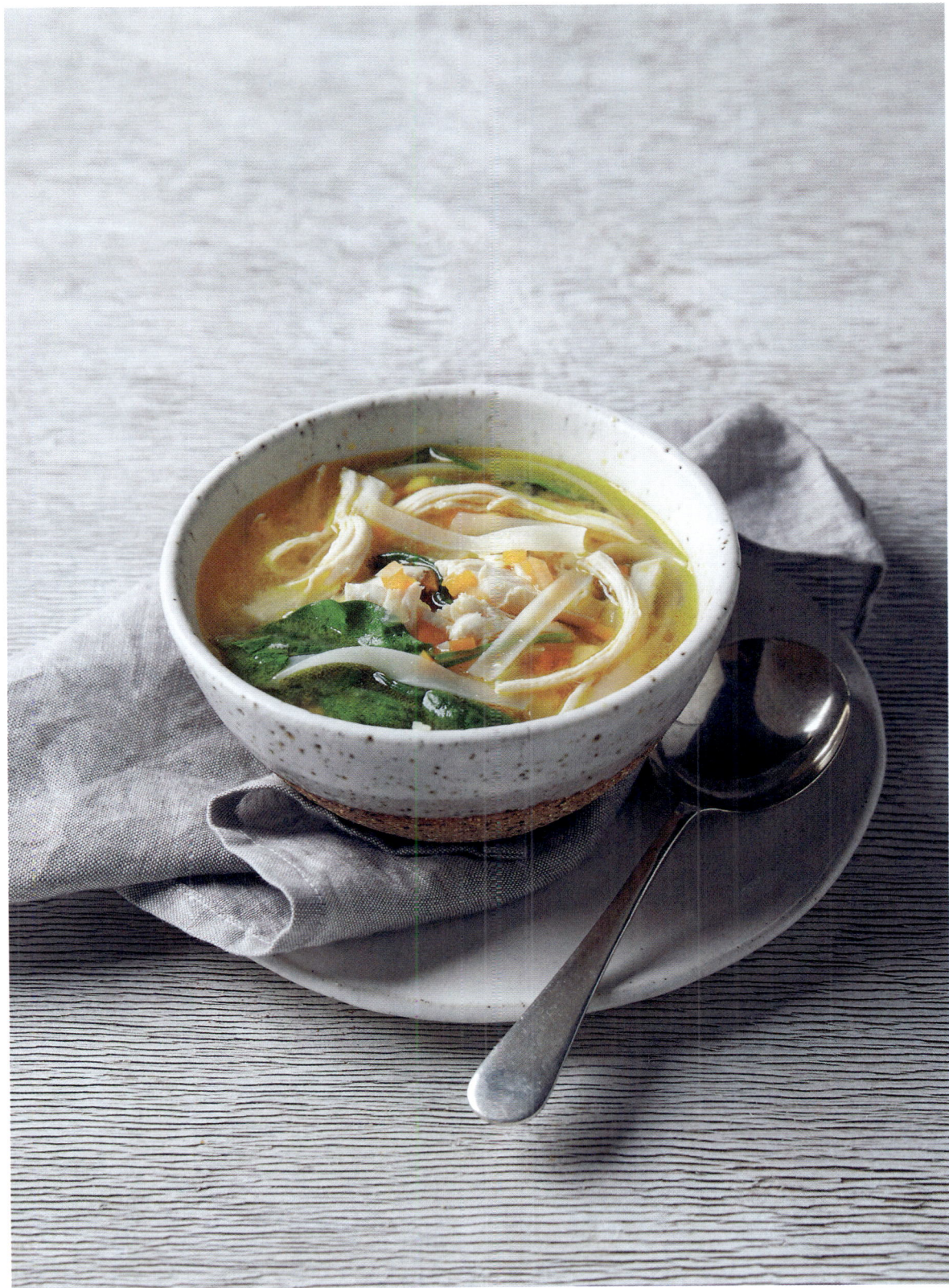

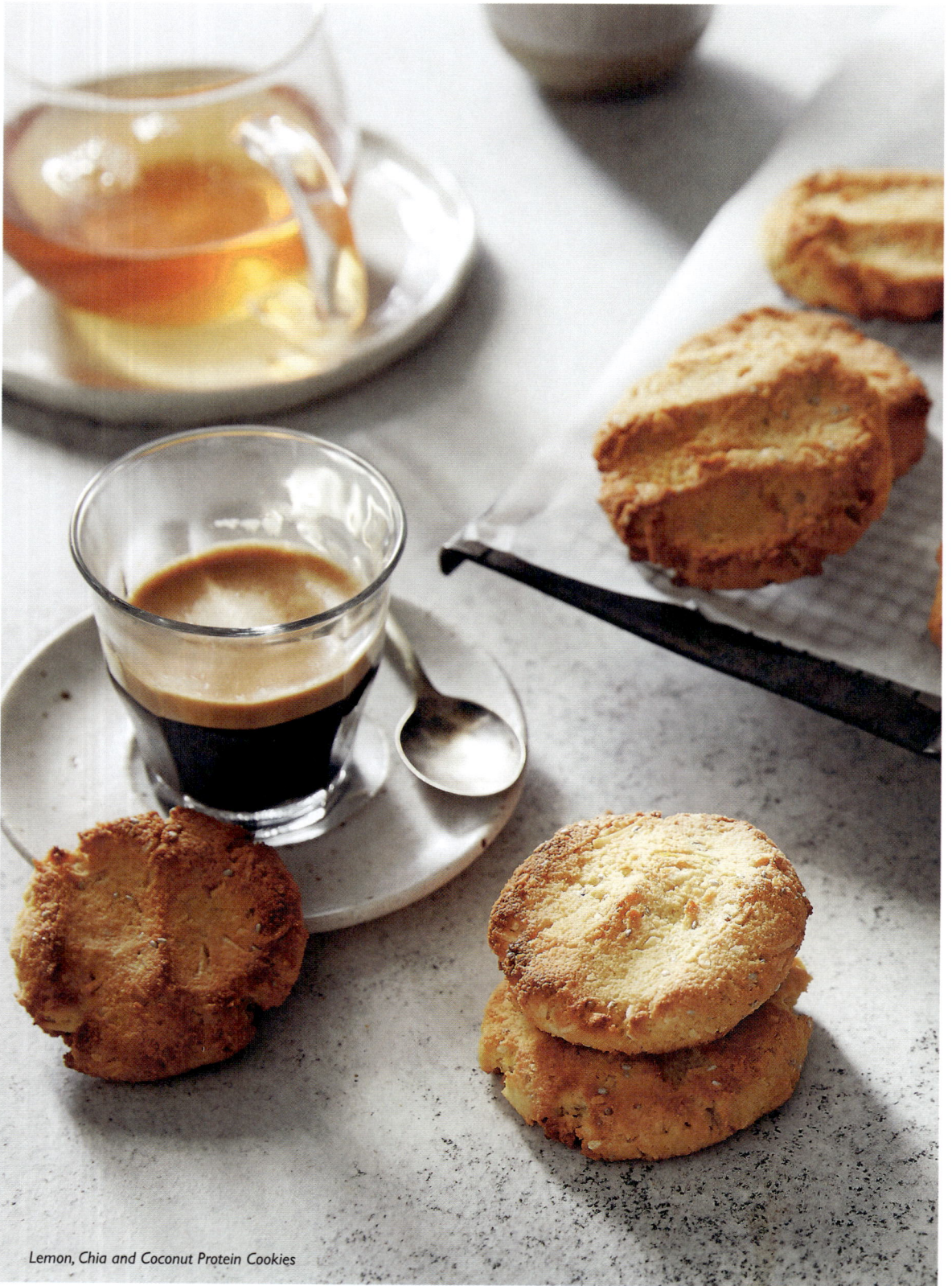

Lemon, Chia and Coconut Protein Cookies

LEMON, CHIA AND COCONUT PROTEIN COOKIES

MAKES 16
PREP TIME 10 minutes
COOK TIME 12 minutes

1 tablespoon chia seeds,
200 g (7 oz/2 cups) almond meal
45 g (1⅔ oz/½ cup) desiccated coconut
30 g (1 oz) vanilla protein powder
2 tablespoons coconut oil, melted
2 tablespoons honey
zest and juice of 1 lemon
2 large eggs, whisked

Place the chia seeds in a small bowl or jug with 3 tablespoons water and stir, then leave for 10 minutes.

Preheat the oven to 180°C (350°F) and line a baking tray with baking paper.

Combine the almond meal, coconut, protein powder and the soaked chia seeds in a bowl.

In a separate bowl, combine the melted coconut oil and honey, then mix in 1 tablespoon of zest and 1½ tablespoons lemon juice and the egg and combine thoroughly.

Add the wet ingredients to the dry ingredients and stir until combined.

Using a tablespoon, scoop out spoonfuls of the mixture and roll these into balls. Place onto the baking tray and gently press flat.

Bake for 10–12 minutes, or until golden.

Allow to cool on a wire rack. Store in an airtight container.

PEANUT BUTTER PROTEIN BARS

MAKES 16
PREP TIME 10 minutes

140 g (5 oz/½ cup) natural, crunchy peanut butter
90 g (3¼ oz/¼ cup) honey
1 teaspoon natural vanilla extract
150 g (5½ oz/1½ cups) rolled (porridge) oats, blitzed to flour
50 g (1¾ oz/½ cup) vegan protein powder
15 g (½ oz/½ cup) puffed rice
½ teaspoon salt

Line a 20 cm (8 inch) square baking tray with baking paper.

Warm the peanut butter, honey, vanilla and 60 ml (2 fl oz/¼ cup) water in a saucepan or microwave and stir until blended.

Combine the oat flour, protein powder, puffed rice and salt in a medium bowl and stir through the peanut butter mixture. (You may need to add a splash of water.)

Press this mixture into the lined tray, cover with more baking paper then smooth out and compress the top using a rolling pin or glass jar.

Freeze for 20 minutes before slicing into 16 pieces.

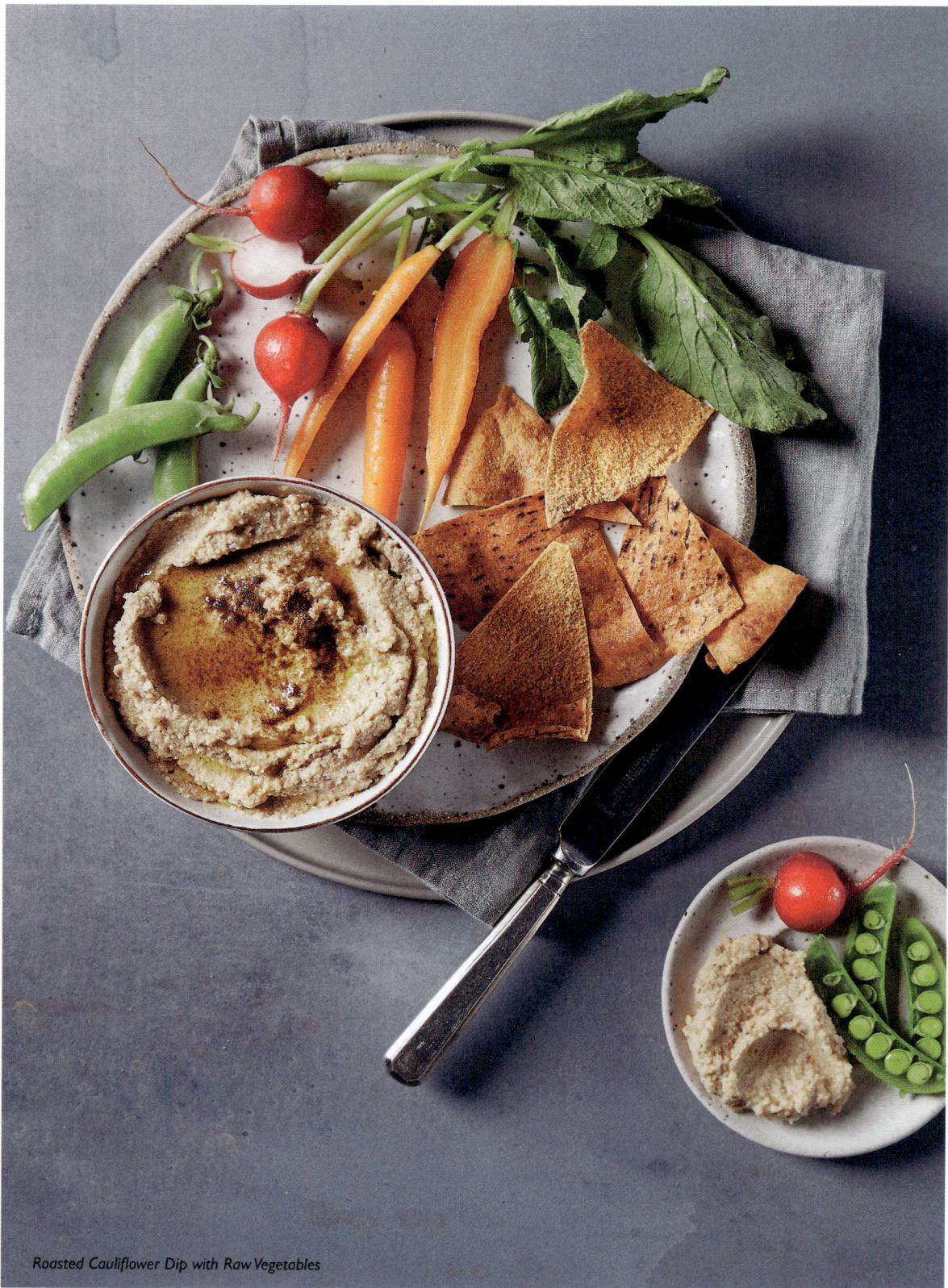

Roasted Cauliflower Dip with Raw Vegetables

ROASTED CAULIFLOWER DIP WITH RAW VEGETABLES

SERVES 4
PREP TIME 10 minutes
COOK TIME 25 minutes

1 head of cauliflower, cut into florets
2 teaspoons olive oil
1½ teaspoons ground cumin
salt and pepper
1 wholemeal (whole-wheat) (or gluten-free) pitta bread, cut into triangles
135 g (4¾ oz/½ cup) cottage cheese
juice of ½ lemon
½ bunch baby carrots, halved lengthways
4 radishes, cut in half
50 g (1¾ oz) sugar snap peas, ends trimmed

Preheat the oven to 180°C (350°F) and line two baking trays with baking paper.

Place the cauliflower on one of the prepared baking trays. In a bowl, mix together the oil and cumin, season well with salt and pepper then rub the mixture into the cauliflower florets. Transfer to the oven and roast for 25 minutes, or until caramelised and a knife passes easily through. Cool slightly.

Place the pitta triangles on the other prepared tray, place in the oven and bake for 4–5 minutes until crispy.

Transfer the cauliflower to a food processor and blend with the cottage cheese and lemon juice until smooth.

Serve the cauliflower dip with the vegetables and pitta chips.

HOMEMADE TUNA DIP AND PITTA CRISPS

SERVES 6
PREP TIME 10 minutes
COOK TIME 3 minutes

185 g (6½ oz) tinned tuna in olive oil, drained and oil reserved
3 anchovy fillets in oil, drained
40 g (1½ oz/¼ cup) raw cashews
1 garlic clove, coarsely chopped
3 tablespoons lemon juice
1–2 tablespoons hot water
salt and pepper
2 × 40 g (1½ oz) wholegrain (whole-wheat) (or gluten-free) pitta breads
⅛–¼ teaspoon chilli flakes, to serve

Put the tuna and 2 tablespoons of its reserved oil in a food processor with the anchovies, cashews, garlic, lemon juice and 1 tablespoon of hot water.

Blend to a smooth paste, adding more hot water, if necessary, then taste and adjust the seasoning. Spoon into a bowl, cover with plastic wrap then place in the fridge to chill for 10 minutes.

Toast the pitta bread and serve with the dip, sprinkled with chilli flakes.

JUICES, TONICS, BLENDS & SMOOTHIES

CHAPTER 2

Get familiar with the two types of snacking

Hungry snacking—also known as mindful eating or conscious eating—is the good kind of snacking. It's the opposite of zombie snacking, which is when you eat mindlessly or because of negative emotions rather than because your body is hungry. Snacking when hungry means you are responding to a physiological need to eat. The more you get to know the difference between these two types of snacking, the better you'll feel, in body and mind.

HUNGRY SNACKING

1. Breathing as you eat and paying attention to your body—like really, really tuning in—and stopping when you are full.

2. Snacking in response to your body's appetite cues: growling tummy, light-headedness, low energy, lack of motivation, poor concentration or fatigue.

3. Snacking because you know your body will be depleted before or after exercise, or because you're on the run and having a hectic day.

4. Preparing a snack and enjoying the process. You're respecting the snack.

VS.

ZOMBIE SNACKING

1. Not listening to your body or your body's appetite cues.

2. Snacking when you are thirsty and not hungry.

3. Snacking because your emotions are bullying you into it (you're sad, bored, frustrated, stressed, etc.).

4. Snacking on foods that are emotionally comforting. I call these 'stuffing foods' because they stuff down the emotions and make us not feel them as fiercely.

5. Snacking and multitasking—not focusing on the snack and therefore not focusing on what your body needs.

6. Snacking all the time—all-day grazing.

T-TOX VITAMIN ELIXIRS

Nourish your body and boost your immune system with the natural goodness of fruit and vegetables to detox your body. Detox is all about eliminating toxins from your body, and it can be effective for weight loss. But a Tiff-Tox (or 'T-Tox') is all about detoxifying your system while replenishing your energy levels and boosting your immune system with vitamins and antioxidants to leave your body smiling from the inside out.

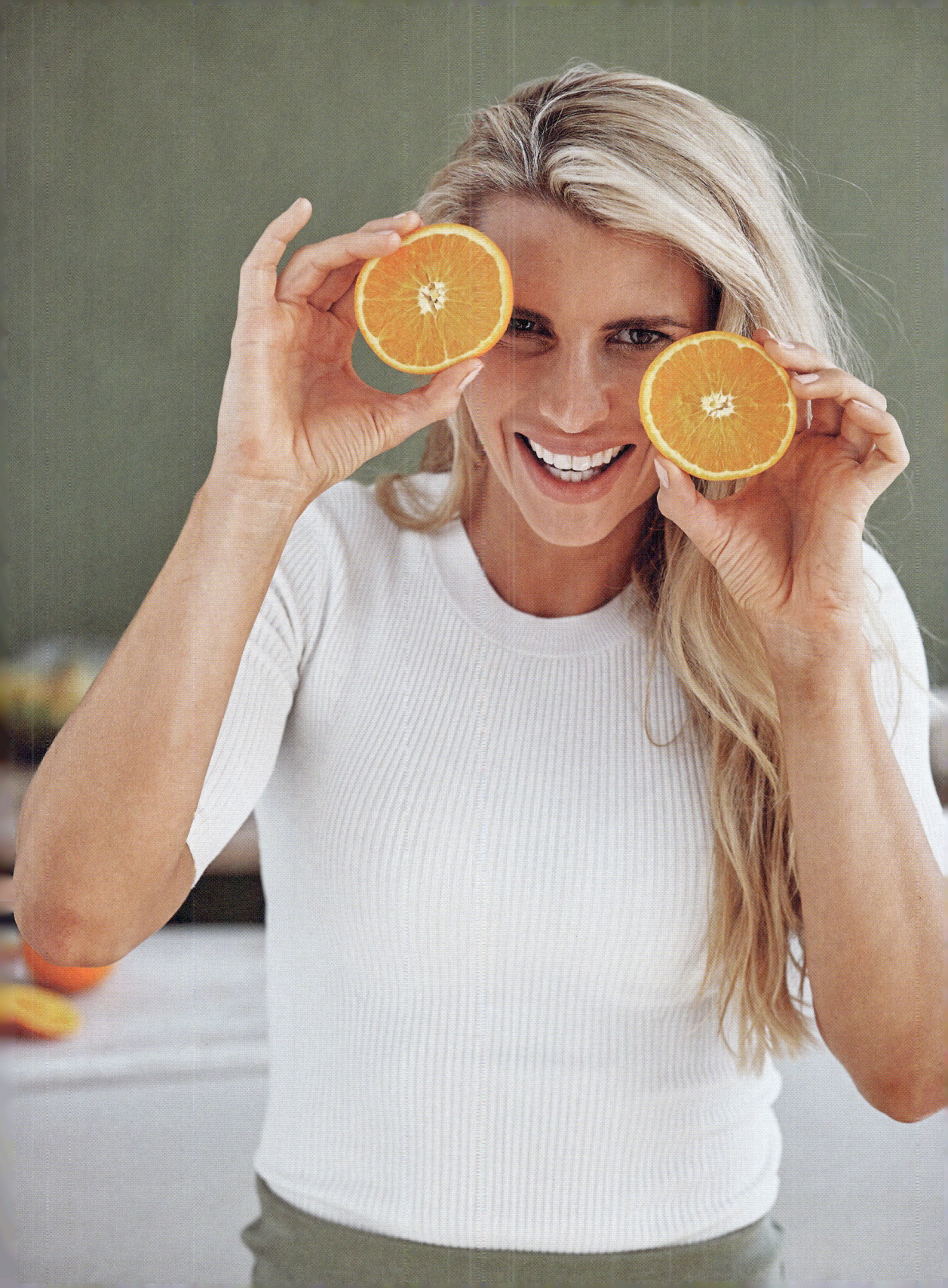

BEETROOT, CARROT AND GINGER JUICE

SERVES 1
PREP TIME 5 minutes

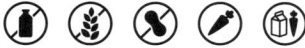

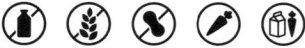

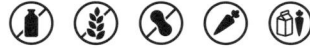

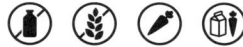

1 carrot
100 g (3½ oz) beetroot (beet), peeled and diced
1 lemon, peeled
250 ml (9 fl oz/1 cup) coconut water
1 teaspoon grated ginger
1 mint sprig, leaves picked

Place all of the ingredients except the mint in a blender and blitz on high until smooth. Pour into a glass to serve and garnish with the mint.

RUBY RADIANCE JUICE

SERVES 1
PREP TIME 5 minutes

250 ml (9 fl oz/1 cup) coconut water
1 carrot, cut in chunks
½ apple
1 lemon, peeled
2–3 ice cubes
40 g (1½ oz) peeled beetroot (beet)

Place all of the ingredients in a blender and blitz on high until smooth. Pour into a glass to serve.

CELERY, APPLE AND KIWI JUICE

SERVES 1
PREP TIME 5 minutes

1 celery stalk, coarsely chopped
½ granny smith apple, coarsely chopped
1 kiwi fruit, peeled
225 ml (7¾ fl oz) coconut water
1 teaspoon lime juice

Combine all of the ingredients in a blender, blend until smooth then pour into a glass and serve.

ORANGE, CARROT AND GINGER CLEANSING JUICE

SERVES 1
PREP TIME 5 minutes

1 carrot
1 orange, peeled
250 ml (9 fl oz/1 cup) coconut water
1 teaspoon finely grated ginger
1 tablespoon almonds

Place all of the ingredients in a blender and blitz on high until smooth. Pour into a glass to serve.

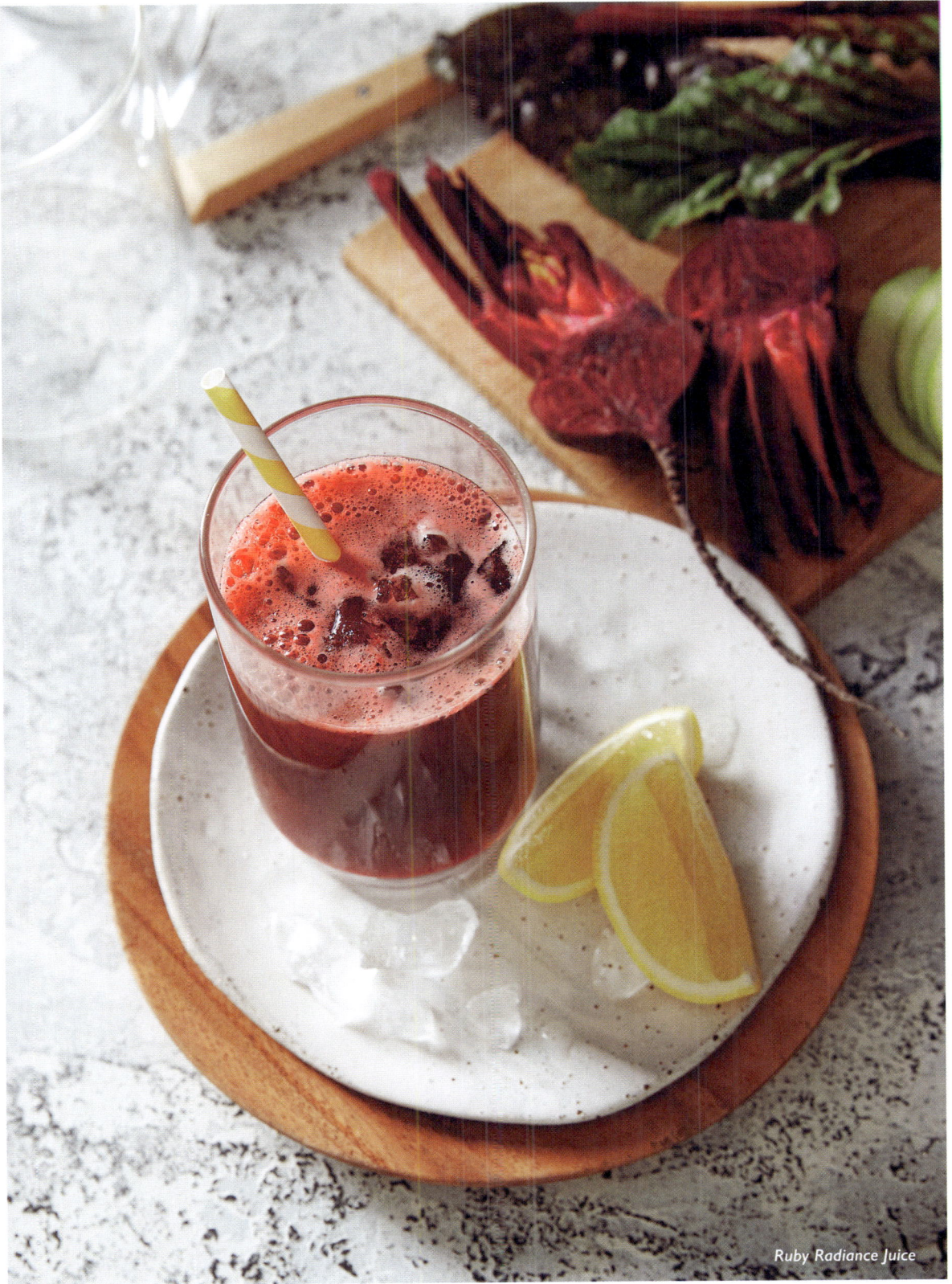

Ruby Radiance Juice

IMMUNE-BOOSTING JUICE

SERVES 1
PREP TIME 5 minutes

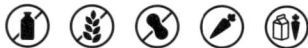

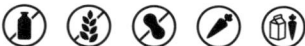

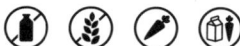

½ carrot
1 Lebanese (short) cucumber
juice of 1 orange
juice of ½ lemon
½ teaspoon ground ginger
¼ teaspoon ground turmeric
pinch of black pepper
4–6 ice cubes

Place all of the ingredients in a blender and blitz on high until smooth. Add some water, if preferred. Pour into a glass to serve.

DETOXIFYING SMOOTHIE

SERVES 1
PREP TIME 5 minutes

1 small granny smith apple, coarsely chopped
finely grated zest and flesh of ½ lemon
finely grated zest and flesh of ½ lime
1 large kale leaf, including stem, coarsely chopped
2 teaspoons rice malt syrup
1 mint sprig
3–4 ice cubes
125 ml (4 fl oz/½ cup) water

Place all of the ingredients in a blender and blitz on high until smooth. Pour into a glass to serve.

LEMON AND CAYENNE PEPPER TONIC

SERVES 1
PREP TIME 5 minutes
COOK TIME 5 minutes

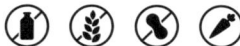

½ lemon
⅛ teaspoon cayenne pepper
⅛ teaspoon cracked black pepper
½ teaspoon honey
200 ml (7 fl oz) water

Squeeze the juice from the lemon half into a small saucepan. Add the lemon rind, cayenne pepper, cracked pepper, honey and water.

Bring to the boil over medium–high heat, then remove from the heat and strain into a cup.

Garnish with a slice of lemon.

INNER GOODNESS GREEN JUICE

SERVES 1
PREP TIME 5 minutes

1 granny smith apple, coarsely chopped
2 celery stalks, including leaves, coarsely chopped
1 Lebanese (short) cucumber
3 kale leaves, stems and spines removed, coarsely chopped
1 lime, peeled
100 ml (3½ fl oz) coconut water
20 g (¾ oz) almonds, coarsely chopped
25 g (¾ oz/½ cup) baby spinach leaves

Place all of the ingredients in a blender and blitz on high until smooth. Pour into a glass to serve.

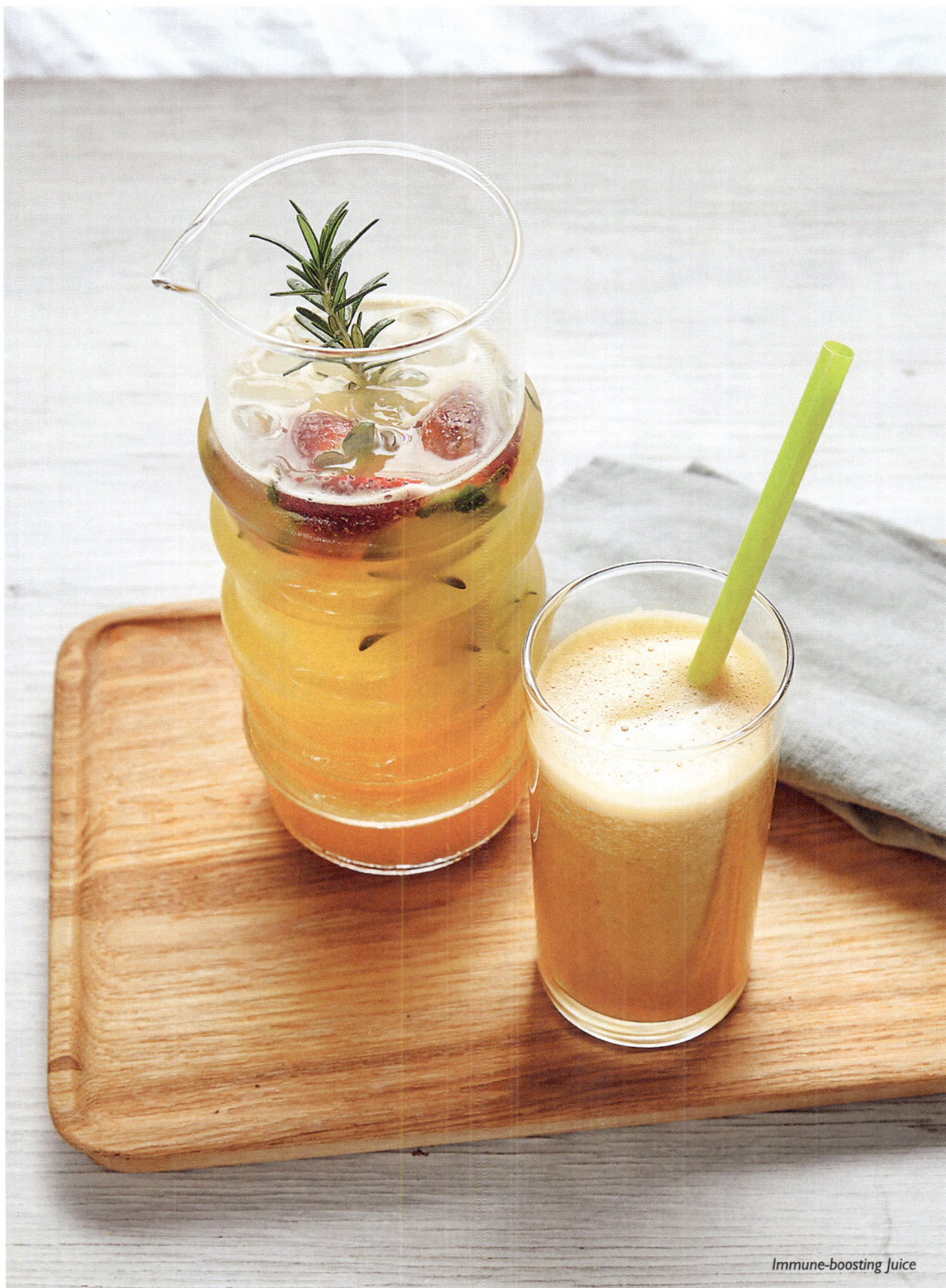

Immune-boosting Juice

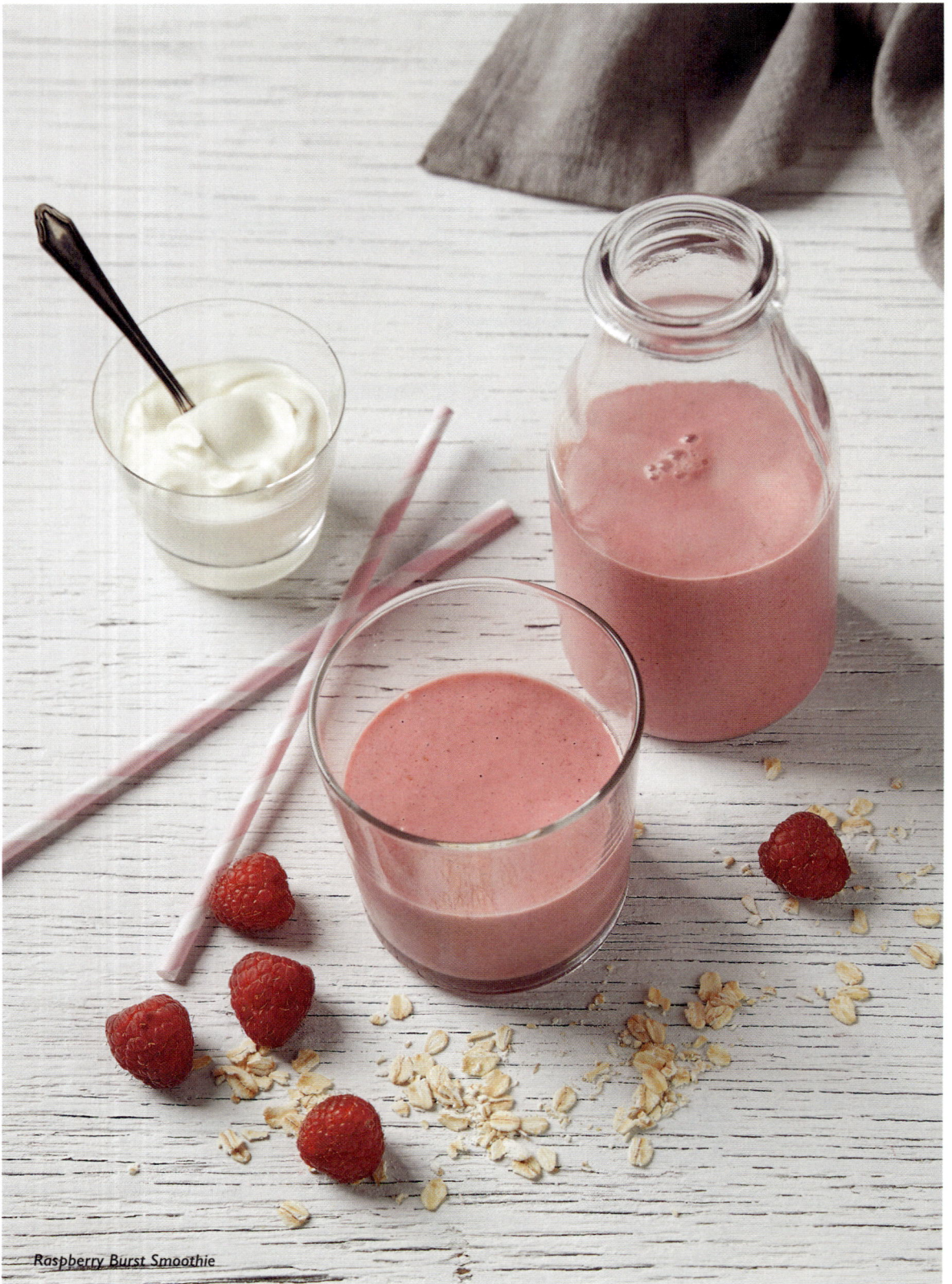

Raspberry Burst Smoothie

RASPBERRY BURST SMOOTHIE

SERVES 1 for breakfast/2 as a snack
PREP TIME 5 minutes

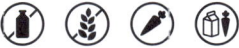

½ frozen banana
70 g (2½ oz /½ cup) frozen raspberries
3 tablespoons Greek-style yoghurt
30 g (1 oz) vanilla protein powder
1 tablespoon rolled (porridge) oats (use brown rice flakes or quinoa flakes if gluten free)
3–4 ice cubes

Place all of the ingredients in a blender with 250 ml (9 fl oz/1 cup) water and blitz on high until smooth. Pour into a glass to serve.

ALMOND HIT SMOOTHIE

SERVES 1 for breakfast/2 as a snack
PREP TIME 5 minutes

½ frozen banana
1 tablespoon almond butter
125 ml (4 fl oz/½ cup) milk of choice
4 almonds, coarsely chopped
2 teaspoons chia seeds
3–4 ice cubes

Place all of the ingredients in a blender and blitz on high until smooth. Pour into a glass to serve.

CHERRY BOMB SMOOTHIE

SERVES 1 for breakfast/2 as a snack
PREP TIME 5 minutes

125 g (4½ oz/½ cup) frozen pitted cherries
3 tablespoons Greek-style yoghurt
100 ml (3½ fl oz) coconut water
30 g (1 oz) protein powder
1 tablespoon cocoa powder
½ teaspoon natural vanilla extract
5 g (⅛ oz) coconut flakes
3–4 ice cubes
1 fresh cherry, to serve (optional)

Place all of the ingredients, reserving a few coconut flakes, in a blender and blitz on high until smooth.

Pour into a glass and top with the reserved coconut flakes and fresh cherry, if using, to serve.

If you're looking for a great complete breakfast, any of these breakfast smoothies will do the trick. Each recipe serves one as a meal, two as a snack.

LEAN GREEN SMOOTHIE

SERVES 1 for breakfast/2 as a snack
PREP TIME 5 minutes

185 ml (6 fl oz/¾ cup) coconut water
½ teaspoon chia seeds, plus extra to serve
25 g (1 oz/½ cup) baby spinach leaves
¼ avocado
¼ bunch mint, leaves picked, reserving some
    leaves to garnish
1 teaspoon almond butter
½ frozen banana
30 g (1 oz) vanilla vegan protein powder
3–4 ice cubes

Add the coconut water and chia seeds to a
blender and allow to stand for 2 minutes.

Add the remaining ingredients to the blender and
blitz on high until smooth.

Pour into a glass and garnish with a sprinkle of
chia seeds and a few mint leaves.

MANGO CHEESECAKE SMOOTHIE

SERVES 1 for breakfast/2 as a snack
PREP TIME 5 minutes

95 g (3¼ oz/⅓ cup) cottage cheese
2 tablespoons coconut milk
80 g (2¾ oz) frozen mango
10 g (¼ oz) macadamia nuts
1 teaspoon desiccated coconut
1 teaspoon honey
3–4 ice cubes

Place all of the ingredients in a blender with 170 ml
(5½ fl oz/⅔ cup) water and blitz on high until
smooth. (Add a little more water if the smoothie is
too thick.)

Pour into a glass to serve.

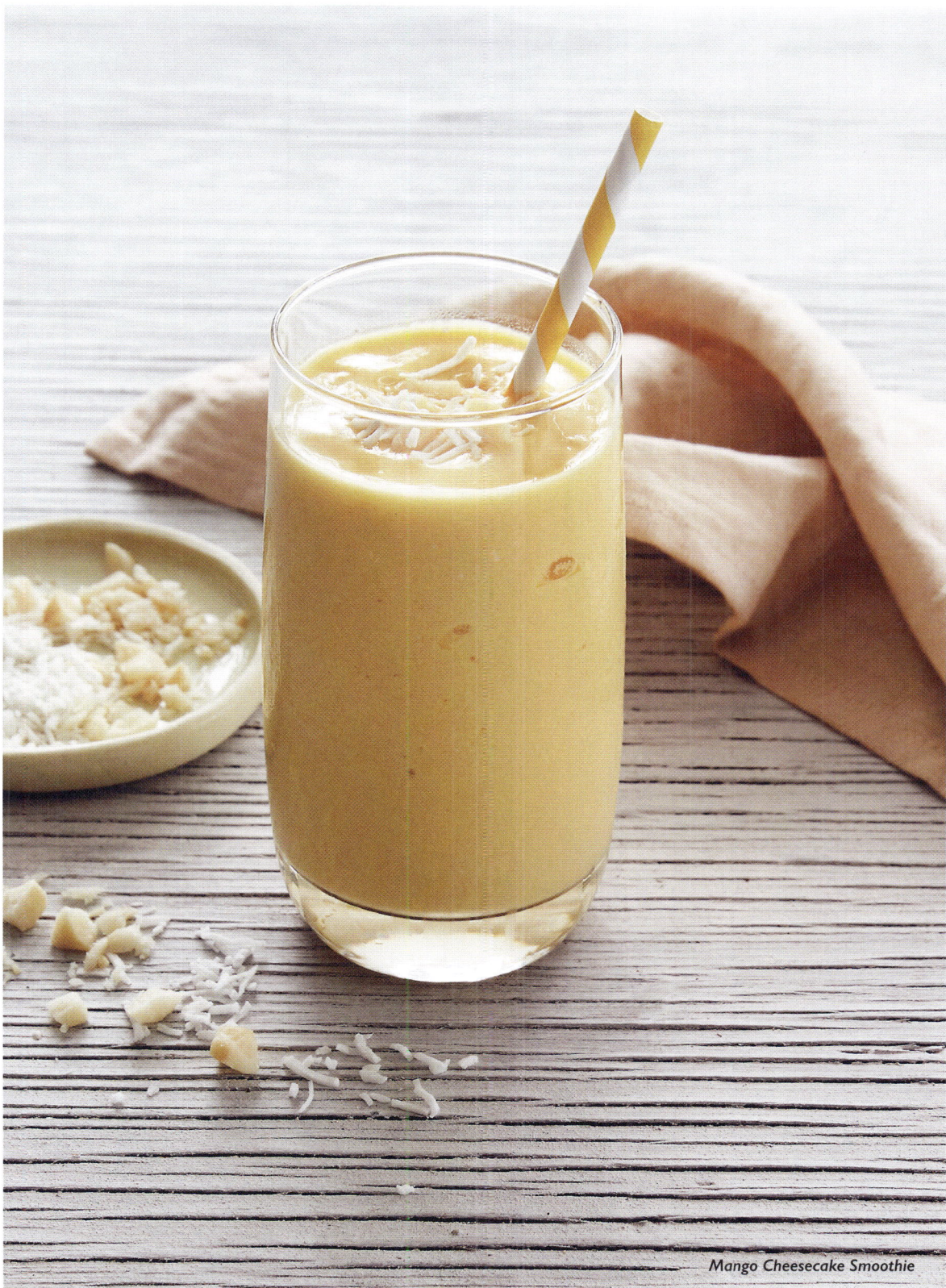

Mango Cheesecake Smoothie

PEACHES AND CREAM SMOOTHIE

SERVES 1 for breakfast/2 as a snack
PREP TIME 5 minutes

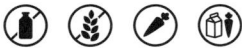

½ peach, stone removed
½ frozen banana
1 tablespoon Greek-style yoghurt
1 teaspoon honey
185 ml (6 fl oz/¾ cup) milk of your choice
30 g (1 oz) vanilla protein powder
3–4 ice cubes

Place all of the ingredients in a blender and blend until smooth and creamy.

Pour into a glass and serve.

CLEANSING BREAKFAST SMOOTHIE

SERVES 1 for breakfast/2 as a snack
PREP TIME 5 minutes

250 ml (9 fl oz/1 cup) coconut water
30 g (1 oz) vanilla vegan protein powder
15 g (½ oz) almonds
1 or 2 kale leaves, stems and spines removed, shredded
½ granny smith apple, cored
1 tablespoon lemon juice
3–4 ice cubes

Place all of the ingredients in a blender and blend until smooth.

Pour into a glass and serve.

PEANUT BUTTER CHOCOLATE SMOOTHIE

SERVES 1 for breakfast/2 as a snack
PREP TIME 5 minutes

125 ml (4 fl oz/½ cup) almond milk
135 g (4¾ oz/½ cup) cottage cheese
½ frozen banana
1 tablespoon rolled (porridge) oats (use brown rice or quinoa flakes if gluten free)
1 tablespoon cocoa powder
2 teaspoons natural peanut butter
3–4 ice cubes

Place all of the ingredients in a blender and blend until smooth.

Pour into a glass and serve.

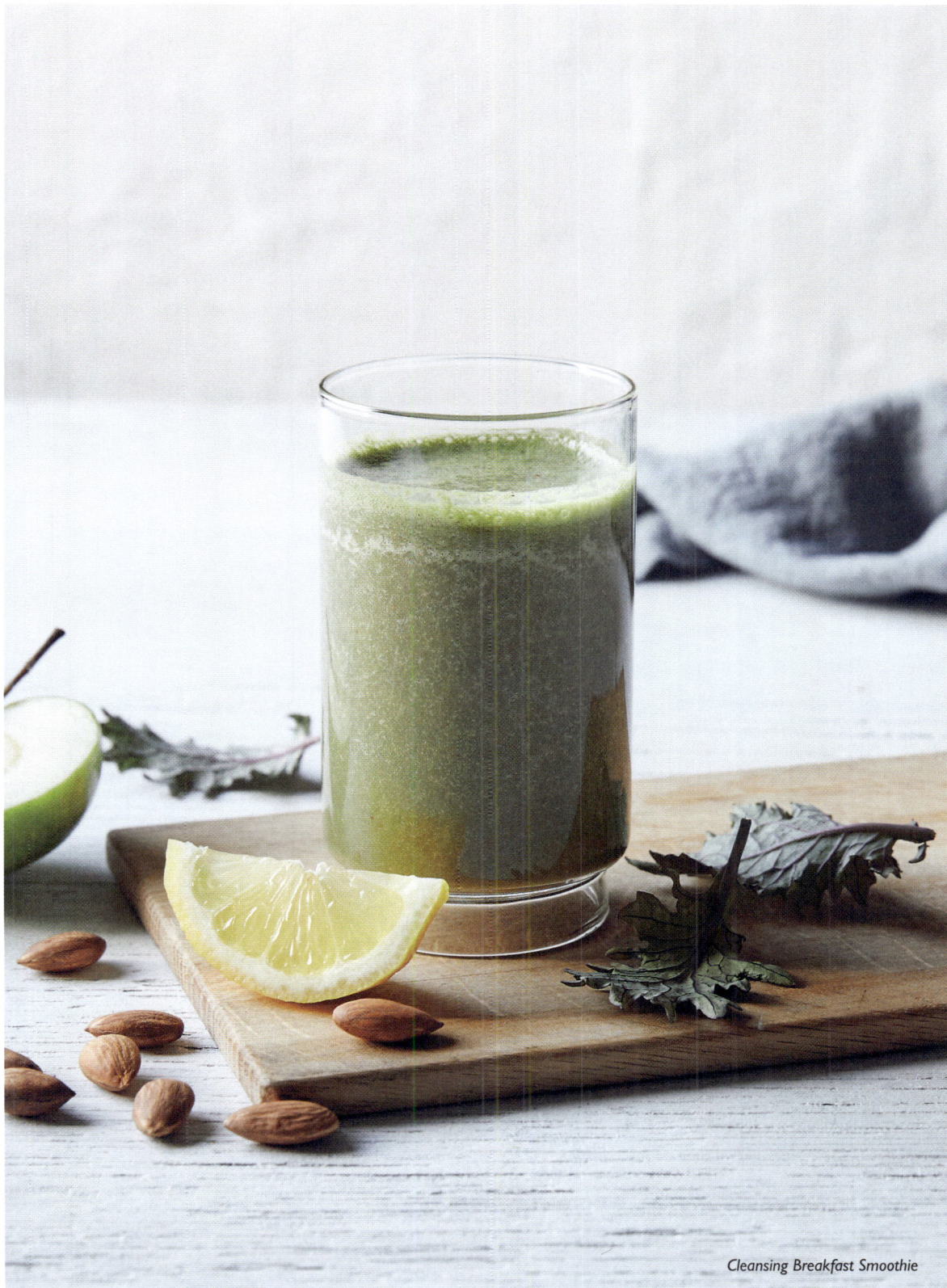

Cleansing Breakfast Smoothie

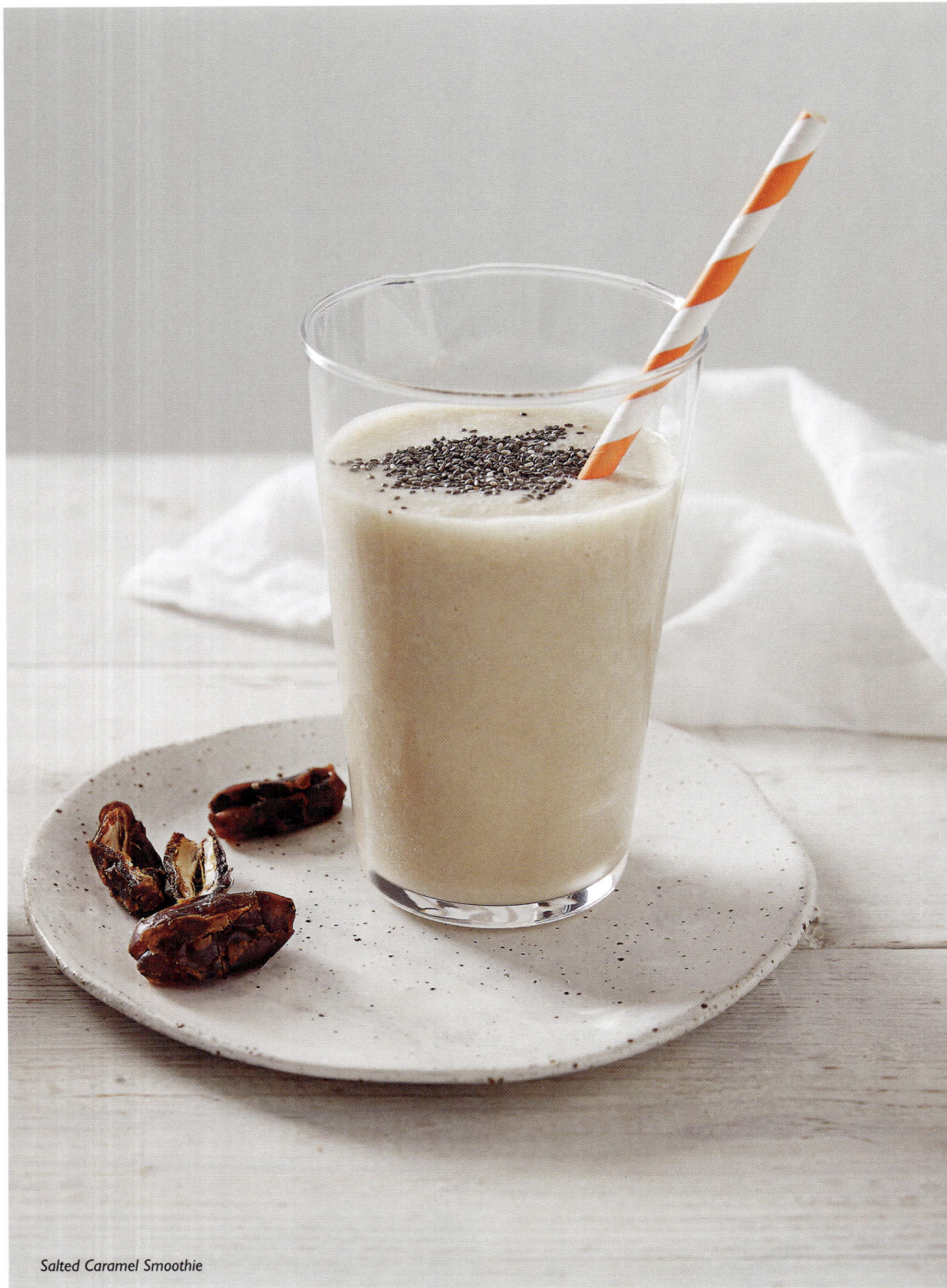

Salted Caramel Smoothie

SALTED CARAMEL SMOOTHIE

SERVES 1 for breakfast/2 as a snack
PREP TIME 5 minutes

250 ml (9 fl oz/1 cup) milk of your choice
2 tablespoons plain yoghurt
2 medjool dates, pitted
30 g (1 oz) vanilla protein powder
¼ teaspoon salt
3–4 ice cubes
1 teaspoon chia seeds

Place all of the ingredients except the chia seeds in a blender and blitz on high until smooth.

Pour into a glass and stir through the chia seeds to serve.

BERRY YOGHURT SMOOTHIE

SERVES 1
PREP TIME 5 minutes

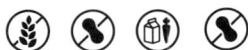

125 ml (4 fl oz/½ cup) milk of your choice
3 tablespoons plain yoghurt
70 g (2½ oz/½ cup) mixed frozen berries
3–4 ice cubes

Combine all of the ingredients in a blender and whizz until smooth. Pour into a glass and serve.

STRAWBERRY SNACK LASSI

SERVES 1
PREP TIME 5 minutes

95 g (3¼ oz/⅓ cup) Greek-style yoghurt
80 g (2¾ oz) strawberries, hulled
2 tablespoons cottage cheese
3–4 ice cubes

Combine all of the ingredients in a blender and whizz until smooth, then serve in a glass.

GO GREENER SMOOTHIE

SERVES 1
PREP TIME 5 minutes

¼ kiwi fruit
pulp from ½ passionfruit
1 kale leaf, stem removed
small handful of baby spinach leaves
1 teaspoon finely grated ginger
125 ml (4 fl oz/½ cup) coconut water
chia seeds, for sprinkling
3–4 ice cubes

Combine all of the ingredients except the chia seeds in a blender and whizz until smooth.

Pour into a glass then sprinkle with chia seeds to serve.

SENSATIONAL SMOOTHIES

Smoothies. Hello! No matter how busy you are, you are never too busy for a healthy snack. It couldn't be easier to chuck all the good stuff in a blender (a high-speed blender is a game changer) and press a button. Drink your snack if you're on the go, and go get 'em!

CHAI TEA LATTE

SERVES 1
PREP TIME 2 minutes
COOK TIME 3 minutes

1 chai tea bag
250 ml (9 fl oz/1 cup) almond milk
1 teaspoon honey
1 star anise
¼ teaspoon ground cinnamon, plus extra for sprinkling

Place the teabag and milk in a small saucepan over medium heat for 1–2 minutes.

Add the remaining ingredients and stir through. Continue to warm the mixture and allow the flavours to infuse for 5 minutes, then remove the star anise from the pan. Pour into a mug and sprinkle with extra cinnamon to serve.

CAFFEINE PICK-ME-UP SMOOTHIE

SERVES 1
PREP TIME 10 minutes

1 shot espresso
½ teaspoon raw cacao powder
¼ frozen banana
½ teaspoon natural vanilla extract
60 ml (2 fl oz/¼ cup) almond milk or nut milk of your choice
3–4 ice cubes

Combine all of the ingredients in a blender and blitz until smooth.

GOLDEN COCONUT MILK

SERVES 1
PREP TIME 5 minutes
COOK TIME 5 minutes

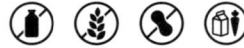

60 ml (2 fl oz/¼ cup) coconut milk
125 ml (4 fl oz/½ cup) coconut water
½ teaspoon honey
½ teaspoon natural vanilla extract
½ teaspoon ground cinnamon, plus extra to serve
½ teaspoon ground turmeric
¼ teaspoon ground ginger
⅛ teaspoon ground cardamom

Combine all of the ingredients in a blender and blitz for a minute until smooth.

Transfer to a microwave-safe mug and heat on medium–high for 1 minute, stirring halfway through. (Or heat in a saucepan over low heat for a few minutes.)

Serve with a sprinkle of cinnamon.

ANTIOXIDANT SMOOTHIE

SERVES 1
PREP TIME 5 minutes

60 ml (2 fl oz/¼ cup) almond milk, or nut milk of your choice
10 g (¼ oz/¼ cup) baby spinach leaves
20 g (¾ oz) frozen mango
¼ teaspoon matcha powder
½ teaspoon natural vanilla extract
3–4 ice cubes

Combine all of the ingredients in a blender and blend until smooth.

Pour into a glass and serve.

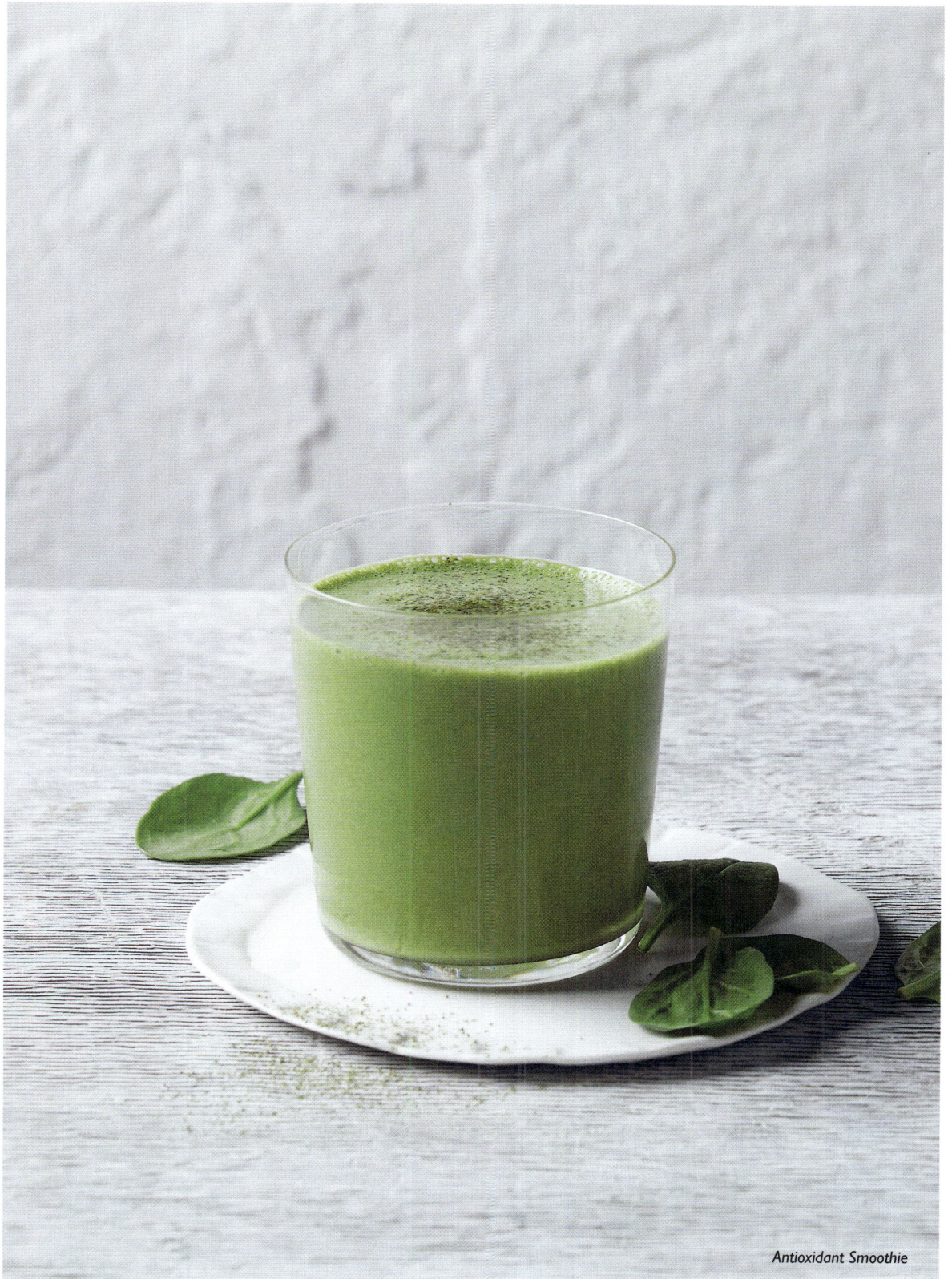

Antioxidant Smoothie

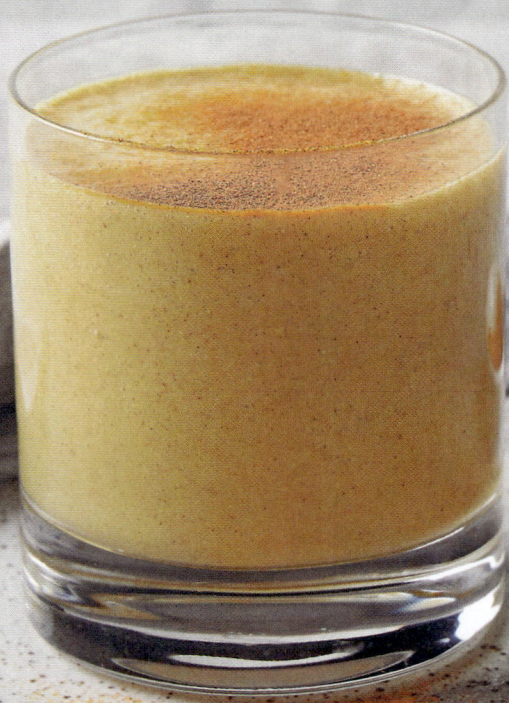

Turmeric Latte Smoothie

BANANA AND CHIA SNACK SMOOTHIE

SERVES 1
PREP TIME 5 minutes

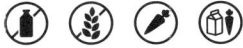

1 frozen banana
125 ml (4 fl oz/½ cup) almond milk or milk
    of choice if not dairy free
60 ml (2 fl oz/¼ cup) water
½ teaspoon chia seeds, plus ½ teaspoon to serve
¼ teaspoon ground cinnamon
1 teaspoon natural, crunchy peanut butter
3–4 ice cubes

Place all of the ingredients except the chia seeds for garnish into a blender and whizz until smooth.

Pour into a glass and garnish with the chia seeds.

TURMERIC LATTE SMOOTHIE

SERVES 1
PREP TIME 5 minutes

¼ frozen banana
1 teaspoon grated ginger
½ teaspoon ground cinnamon, plus extra to
    serve
¼ teaspoon ground turmeric
½ teaspoon natural vanilla extract
½ teaspoon chia seeds
60 ml (2 fl oz/¼ cup) almond milk or milk
    of choice if not dairy free
3–4 ice cubes

Combine all of the ingredients in a blender and whizz until smooth. Sprinkle with extra cinnamon to serve.

SUPER FOOD HOT CHOCOLATE

SERVES 1
PREP TIME 5 minutes
COOK TIME 5 minutes

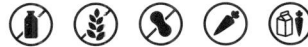

1 chai tea bag
170 ml (5½ fl oz/⅔ cup) boiling water
80 ml (2½ fl oz/⅓ cup) coconut milk or milk
    of choice if not dairy free
1 teaspoon maple syrup
1 tablespoon raw cacao powder or cocoa powder
⅛ teaspoon ground cinnamon

Steep the teabag in the boiling water for 5 minutes.

Remove the teabag and add the tea to a small saucepan with the milk and maple syrup, and gently heat over medium–low heat.

Mix the cacao and cinnamon with 1–2 tablespoons of the warm milk mixture until smooth, then add to the pan of warmed milk, stirring until thick and smooth. Serve warm in a mug.

POWER SMOOTHIE

SERVES 1
PREP TIME 10 minutes

¼ frozen banana
1 teaspoon rolled (porridge) oats, plus extra
    to serve
60 ml (2 fl oz/¼ cup) almond milk, or nut milk
    of your choice
½ teaspoon ground cinnamon, plus extra to
    serve
3–4 ice cubes

Combine all of the ingredients in a blender and blend until smooth. Sprinkle with extra cinnamon and rolled oats to serve.

IMMUNE-BOOSTING BEEF BONE BROTH

MAKES about 500 ml (17 fl oz/2 cups)
PREP TIME 30 minutes
COOK TIME 4 hours

1 kg (2 lb 4 oz) beef bones
2 tablespoons grated ginger
1 garlic bulb, halved horizontally
2 onions, coarsely chopped
   (skin on)
4 carrots, coarsely chopped
4 celery stalks, coarsely chopped
2 teaspoons salt
2 tablespoons apple cider vinegar
3.5 litres (122 fl oz/14 cups) water (preferably filtered)

Roast the beef bones in a lined tray for at least 30 minutes at 200°C (400°F). Combine the roasted bones with the rest of the ingredients in a very large saucepan over high heat. Bring to the boil and then lower to a simmer, covered, for 3–3½ hours. Alternatively, combine all of the ingredients in a slow-cooker and cook on low for 4–12 hours.

Cool slightly then strain into jars and chill in the fridge. Store in an airtight container for up to 5 days, or freeze for up to 6 months.

Reheat before serving, and add salt to taste. Enjoy a cup of hot broth on its own, as a snack, or use as a base for your favourite soups and stews.

Tip:

For chicken broth, swap a large chicken carcass (bones) for the beef bones – no roasting necessary – and cook for between 3 and 6 hours. I also like to add a tablespoon of grated turmeric and ½ tablespoon of peppercorns while cooking. Delicious on its own with a squeeze of lemon and a pinch of salt.

BANANA, OAT AND COCONUT SMOOTHIE

SERVES 1
PREP TIME 5 minutes

2 teaspoons shredded coconut
½ frozen banana
125 ml (4 fl oz/½ cup) milk
125 ml (4 fl oz/½ cup) water
1 teaspoon maple syrup
1 tablespoon rolled (porridge) oats (if gluten-free, use brown rice or quinoa flakes)

Place 1 teaspoon of the coconut, the banana, milk, water, syrup and oats (or gluten-free substitute) in a blender and blitz on high until smooth.

Pour into a glass and top with the remaining coconut to serve.

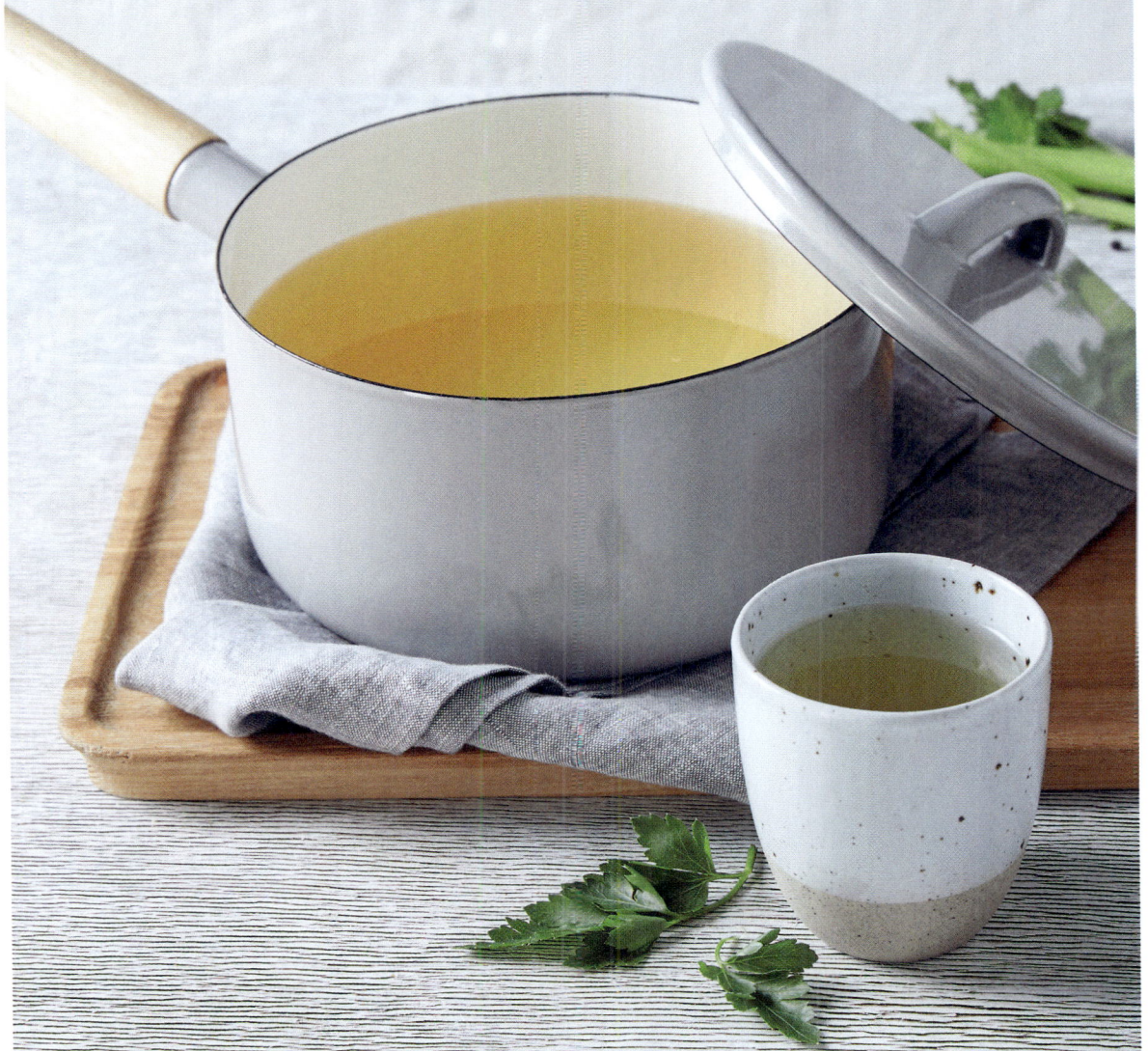

Immune-boosting Beef Bone Broth

GOAL-GETTER SNACKS

CHAPTER 3

FITNESS GOALS

We all have different fitness goals and whatever yours are, these snacks will fast-track you to success. There are low-carb and low-calorie snacks for weight loss, and higher protein and higher calorie snacks for sculpting muscle.

Protein keeps you feeling full for longer

Protein packs a punch because it helps to reduce hunger and increases satiety (that feeling of satisfaction). Yep, you'll feel fuller for longer, and will therefore eat less overall.

Protein helps reduce hunger via several mechanisms, including changes to our hunger hormones such as ghrelin. Protein also helps control blood sugar levels and digestion. And, because it's generally more filling, you don't need a big serve. Numerous studies have proven this when providing participants with an 'anything goes diet' with no restrictions. In one study, when participants consumed 30 per cent of their total intake from protein, they dropped their overall intake by over 400 calories per day.

A LITTLE MORE ABOUT MY SNACKOLOGY

If you're uncomfortable with the stigma around the word 'snack', think of it as a mini-meal or simply as a fuel stop—something to keep you going until you get to the main meal so you can stay on track and reach your goals. When the day drags on (and you're practically falling asleep at your desk) or when it's three o'clock and you still have the whole dinner-bath-bed routine to get through with the kids, you need a little something to sustain your mood and energy. And you know what? That's totally fine—more than fine. It's actually really important to refuel, as that improves performance, mood and concentration.

Mindful snacking

If you deprive yourself of something, you will crave it more. It's not rocket science, it's just human nature. Binges happen when we say, 'NO!' Snacks help feed the mind and help your mindset to carry you over to your next healthy meal.

If you are on a weight-loss mealplan, you need snacks to emotionally and mentally help you stay on track. When snacks are worked into your mealplan they pose no threat to your weight-loss progress. Managing your hunger between meals will help to keep your blood sugar levels stable.

Unfortunately, many people defer to sugar-stuffed packaged snacks, junk food and sodas for their in-between meal snacks. Such foods have little to no nutritional value. However, you can have delicious healthy alternatives. Yep, you can have healthy office snacks, healthy movie snacks, healthy party snacks, healthy school snacks and healthy bedtime snacks! I know what you're thinking: *Where has this snack Bible been all my life?*

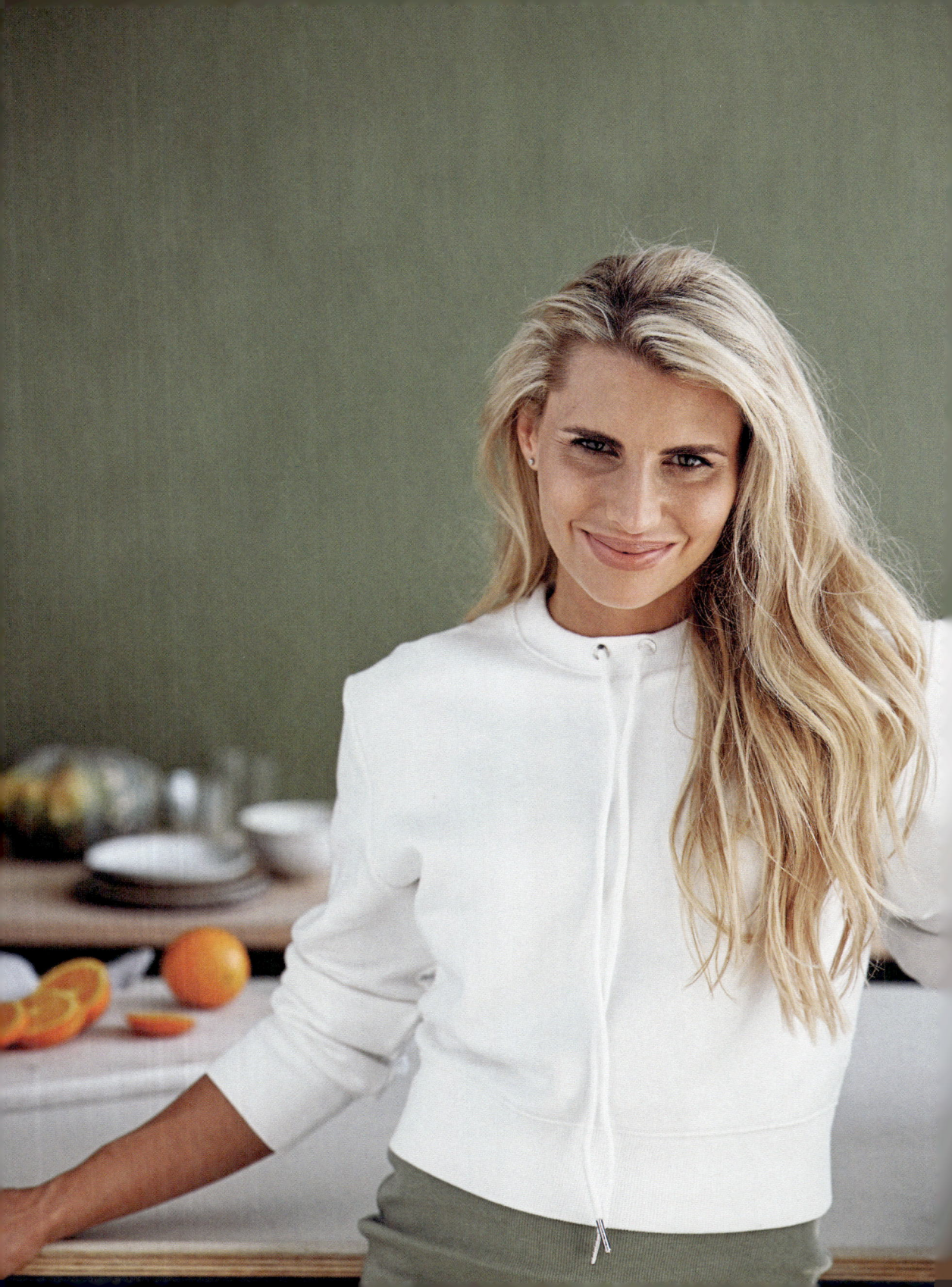

GIVE YOURSELF A BREAK
WITH MY THREE-HOUR RESET RULE

What is the three-hour reset rule?

It's when you reset your food intake (and attitude) every three hours. My rule treats every meal and every snack as a new event, so if you do slip up and eat a processed snack when you didn't plan to, you don't write the whole day off. Instead, you allow yourself to enjoy the treat (yep, you are allowed to enjoy it), then reset and start fresh.

People tell me all the time that one chocolate bar, one chip out of the bag can often make them feel like they failed and that their day (or week, or even month!) is blown. This all-or-nothing attitude is not sustainable—and it's not a healthy way to live.

My three-hour reset rule can help short circuit that attitude and help you to stay focused, balanced and enjoy life. Remember, there are going to be days where your snacks are not as healthy or you end up grazing. But applying this rule will help you to focus on the future and stop dwelling on the past.

YOU CAN APPLY MY THREE-HOUR RESET RULE TO ANYTHING! NOT JUST SNACKS.

It's true! My three-hour reset rule doesn't just apply to snacks and food. You can apply it to all aspects of your life. If your morning coffee spilled down your top on the train to work, your car broke down on the way to an important job interview, your toddler didn't go down for their nap so you couldn't get your workout in— don't let it ruin your day. Take a moment to be angry or frustrated, feel the feels, then reset. Who knows what the next three hours might bring—it could still end up being the best day of your life.

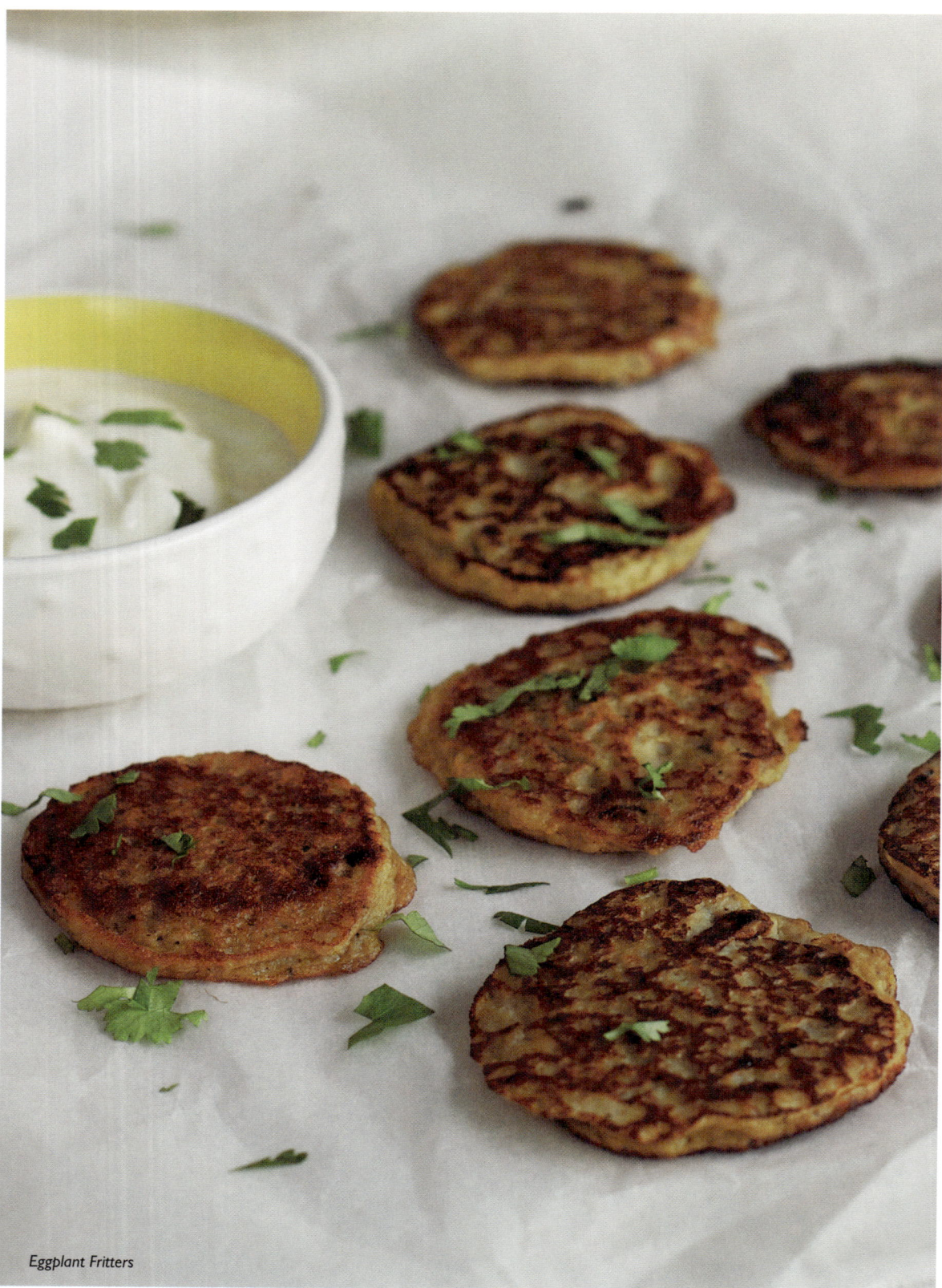

Eggplant Fritters

EGGPLANT FRITTERS

MAKES 20 (3–4 per snack)
PREP TIME 5 minutes
COOK TIME 40 minutes

2 eggplants (aubergines)
1 egg, lightly beaten
2 tablespoons cornflour (cornstarch)
salt and pepper
1 tablespoon olive oil
1 lemon
1 tablespoon chopped coriander (cilantro) leaves
70 g (2½ oz/¼ cup) tzatziki (see page 106)

Preheat the oven to 220°C (425°F). Line a baking tray with baking paper.

Prick the eggplants all over with a fork, place on the baking tray and cook for 30 minutes. Once cooked, allow to cool, then slice open and use a spoon to scoop out the flesh. Put the flesh in a bowl and combine with the egg and cornflour. Season with salt and pepper.

Heat the oil in a frying pan over medium heat and add tablespoon-sized dollops of the mixture to the pan, being careful not to overcrowd. Cook for a few minutes on each side until golden.

Squeeze over some lemon, scatter with coriander and serve with tzatziki.

KALE AND SEA SALT CRISPS

SERVES 2
PREP TIME 5 minutes
COOK TIME 10 minutes

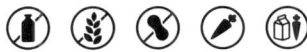

1 bunch curly kale, washed and dried
1 tablespoon olive oil
½ teaspoon sea salt

OPTIONAL TOPPINGS
½ teaspoon sesame seeds
½ teaspoon chilli flakes
½ teaspoon dukkah

Preheat the oven to 180°C (350°F).

Remove and discard the kale stems. Tear the leaves into pieces and place in a bowl.

Massage the leaves with the oil, then place on a baking tray. Sprinkle over sea salt and any other optional toppings and bake for 10 minutes, or until nice and crispy.

Allow to cool and then eat right away, or store in an airtight container.

CORN THINS WITH PROSCIUTTO, AVOCADO AND THYME

SERVES 1
PREP TIME 5 minutes

¼ avocado, mashed
2 Corn Thins
20 g (¾ oz) prosciutto
1 thyme sprig, leaves stripped
salt and pepper

Spread the avocado over the Corn Thins, top with prosciutto, then scatter over the thyme leaves and season with salt and pepper to serve.

CHEESY HAM CUCUMBER SUB

SERVES 1
PREP TIME 5 minutes

30 g (1 oz) cream cheese
1 tablespoon snipped chives
50 g (1¾ oz) sliced ham
½ telegraph (long) cucumber, halved lengthways and seeds scooped out

Place the cream cheese and chives into a small bowl and mix to combine.

Spread the cream cheese mixture onto the cucumber where seeds used to be. Place the ham on one side of the cucumber then place the other length of cucumber on top.

MINI MUSHROOM FRITTATAS

MAKES 12 (2 per snack)
PREP TIME 10 minutes
COOK TIME 15 minutes

2 teaspoons olive oil, plus extra for greasing
120 g (4¼ oz) button mushrooms, coarsely chopped
1 teaspoon dried thyme
200 g (7 oz/4 cups) baby spinach leaves
4 large eggs
2 tablespoons milk
130 g (4½ oz/½ cup) Greek-style yoghurt
salt and pepper
60 g (2¼ oz) feta cheese, crumbled

Preheat the oven to 180°C (350°F) and lightly grease 12 holes of a mini-muffin tin with oil.

Heat the olive oil in a frying pan over medium heat and sauté the mushrooms and thyme for 5 minutes. Stir through the spinach and continue to cook until the spinach has just wilted. Remove the pan from the heat.

Whisk the eggs, milk and yoghurt together in a bowl and season with salt and pepper.

Divide the spinach mixture between the muffin holes. Add the egg mixture, then top with the feta.

Bake for 10 minutes, or until just set. Stand for 10 minutes before removing from the tin. These will keep in an airtight container in the fridge for up to 3 days.

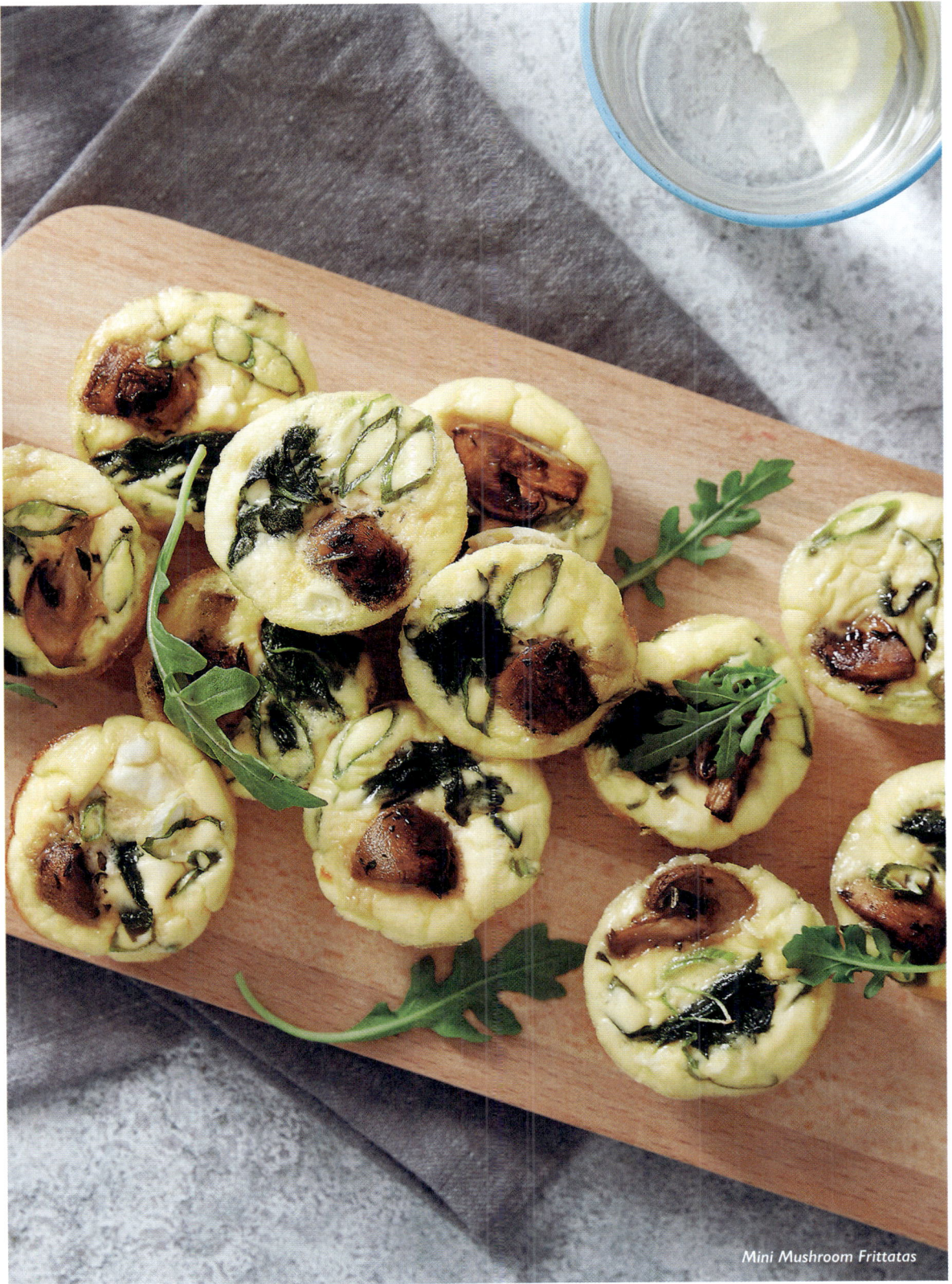

Mini Mushroom Frittatas

PEA DIP WITH CRACKERS AND VEGGIE STICKS

SERVES 15 **PREP TIME** 30 minutes

PEA DIP
2 tablespoons raw cashew nuts
140 g (5 oz/1 cup) frozen peas,
   defrosted
1 garlic clove, crushed
2 tablespoons lemon juice
½ tablespoon sunflower seeds
½ tablespoon pepitas (pumpkin
   seeds)

TO SERVE
1 carrot, cut into batons
8 asparagus spears, woody ends
   snapped off

CRACKERS
90 g (3¼ oz/½ cup) quinoa
   flakes
80 g (2¾ oz/¾ cup) almond
   meal
35 g (1¼ oz/¼ cup) chia seeds
80 g (2¾ oz/½ cup) pepitas
   (pumpkin seeds)
125 g (4½ oz) chickpeas, drained
   and rinsed
75 g (2⅔ oz/½ cup) sunflower
   seeds
95 g (3¼ oz/½ cup) coconut oil,
   melted
1 egg, lightly whisked
80 ml (2½ fl oz/⅓ cup) water

Preheat the oven to 180°C (350°F). Lightly grease and line two baking trays with baking paper.

Start by making the crackers. Place the quinoa flakes, almond meal, chia seeds, pepitas, chickpeas and sunflower seeds in a food processor. Pulse on high until the ingredients have broken down to a crumb consistency. Pour into a large mixing bowl.

Make a well in the centre of the mixture and pour the coconut oil, egg and water into it. Using a wooden spoon, start to mix the ingredients together to form a dough.

Place half of the dough on a sheet of baking paper and put another sheet of baking paper on top. Using a rolling pin, roll the dough out to 5 mm (¼ inch) thick.

Slide the baking paper with the dough onto one of the baking trays and, using a sharp knife, cut into 12 squares. Repeat with the other half of dough.

Place in the oven and bake for 15–17 minutes, or until golden. Cool on a wire rack.

Meanwhile, soak the cashews in warm water for 10 minutes.

Drain the cashews then add them to a food processor with the peas, garlic, lemon juice and 2 tablespoons of water and pulse to your desired dip consistency, then season with salt and pepper. You may need to add more water if it's too thick.

Heat a saucepan over medium heat and toast the seeds until golden then remove the seeds from the pan and set aside.

Fill the saucepan with salted water and bring to the boil. Add the asparagus, return to the boil, drain and refresh in cold water.

Sprinkle the seeds over the pea dip and serve with the crackers and veggie sticks.

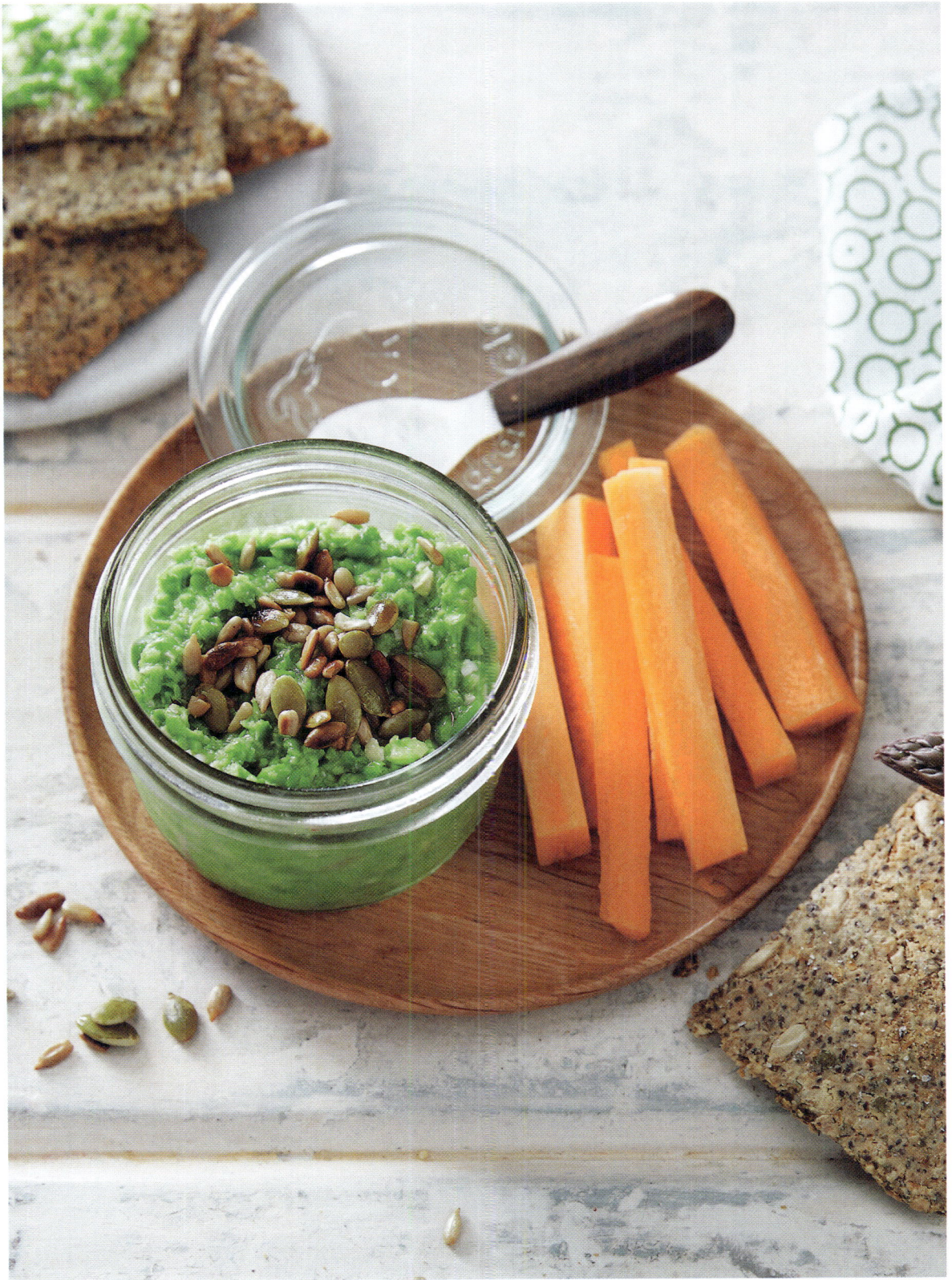

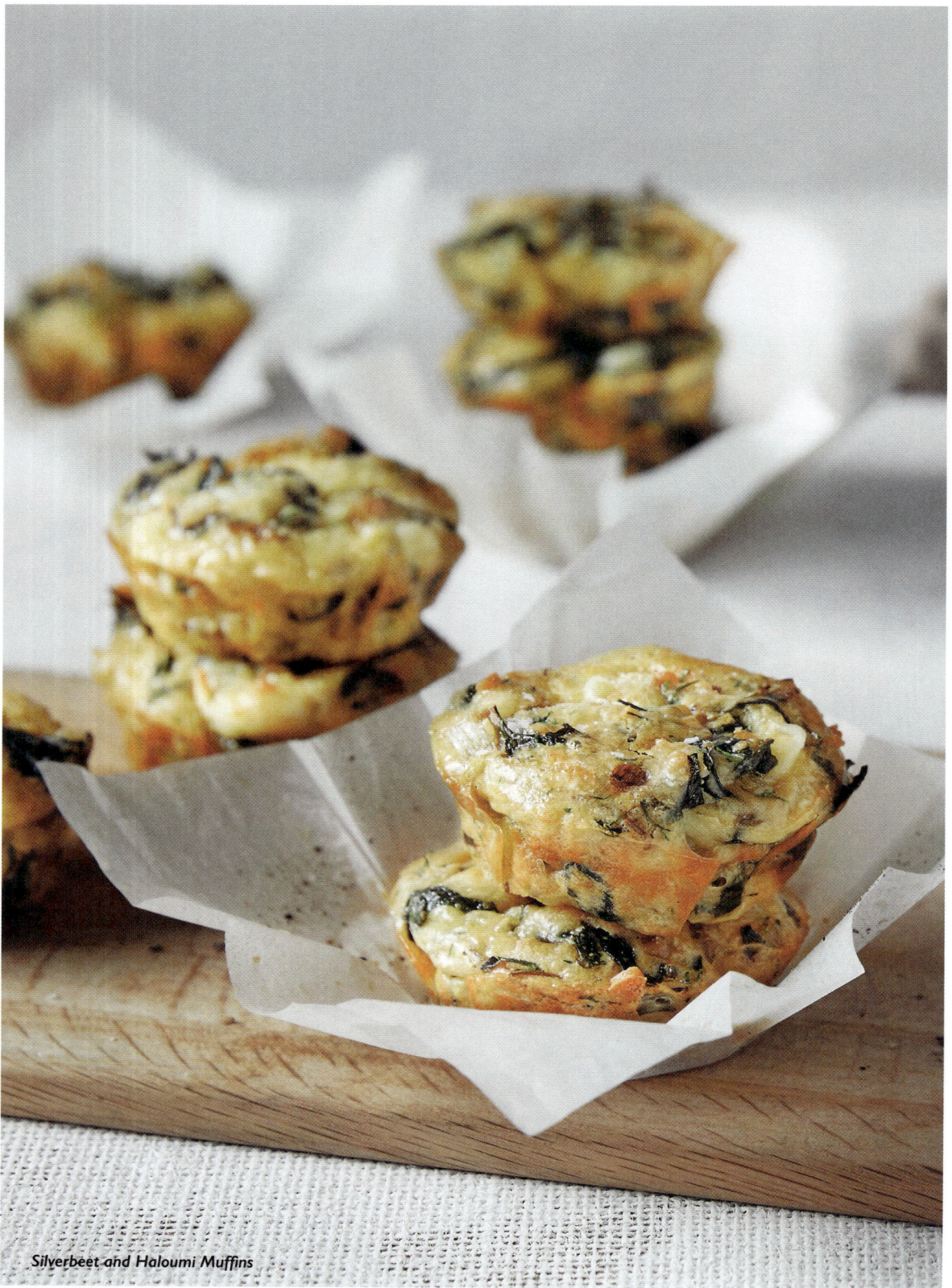

Silverbeet and Haloumi Muffins

SILVERBEET AND HALOUMI MUFFINS

MAKES 12
PREP TIME 15 minutes
COOK TIME 35 minutes

2 teaspoons olive oil
1 onion, finely diced
700 g (1 lb 9 oz/1 bunch) silverbeet, trimmed and washed, leaves shredded and stems chopped separately
2 garlic cloves, minced
225 g (8 oz) haloumi cheese, grated
6 large eggs, lightly beaten
4 dill sprigs, finely chopped
50 g (1¾ oz/⅓ cup) plain (all-purpose) flour (or gluten-free if required)
1 teaspoon baking powder
salt and pepper

Preheat the oven to 180°C (350°F) and line a 12-hole standard (60 ml/¼ cup) muffin tin with paper cases.

Heat the oil in a large non-stick frying pan over medium heat. Add the onion and silverbeet stems and cook for 10 minutes, or until soft. Add the garlic and cook for a further minute until fragrant. Add the silverbeet leaves and cook for 5 minutes more, or until the leaves are just wilting and the liquid has evaporated. Spread the mixture around a tray or a plate and leave to cool.

Put the haloumi in a large bowl with the eggs, dill, flour and baking powder, and season with salt and pepper. Mix to combine, then gently mix through the cooled silverbeet and divide the batter between the muffin holes.

Bake for 15–20 minutes, until puffed and golden.

Any remaining muffins can be stored in an airtight container in the fridge for 3 days or frozen for up to 3 months.

SWEET POTATO AND BEETROOT CRISPS WITH TZATZIKI

SERVES 4
PREP TIME 10 minutes
COOK TIME 20 minutes

1 sweet potato, thinly sliced on a mandoline
1 beetroot (beet), thinly sliced on a mandoline
2 teaspoons olive oil
salt and pepper
130 g (4½ oz/½ cup) tzatziki (see page 106)

Preheat the oven to 200°C (400°F) and line a baking tray with baking paper.

Place the sweet potato into one bowl and the beetroot slices in another. Add some oil, salt and pepper to each bowl, and toss well to coat the vegetables.

Spread the sweet potato slices on one side of the prepared tray and the beetroot on the other. Place in the oven to bake for 20 minutes, or until crispy. Remove from the oven and allow to cool.

Serve the crisps with tzatziki. Any leftovers can be stored in an airtight container so they remain crispy.

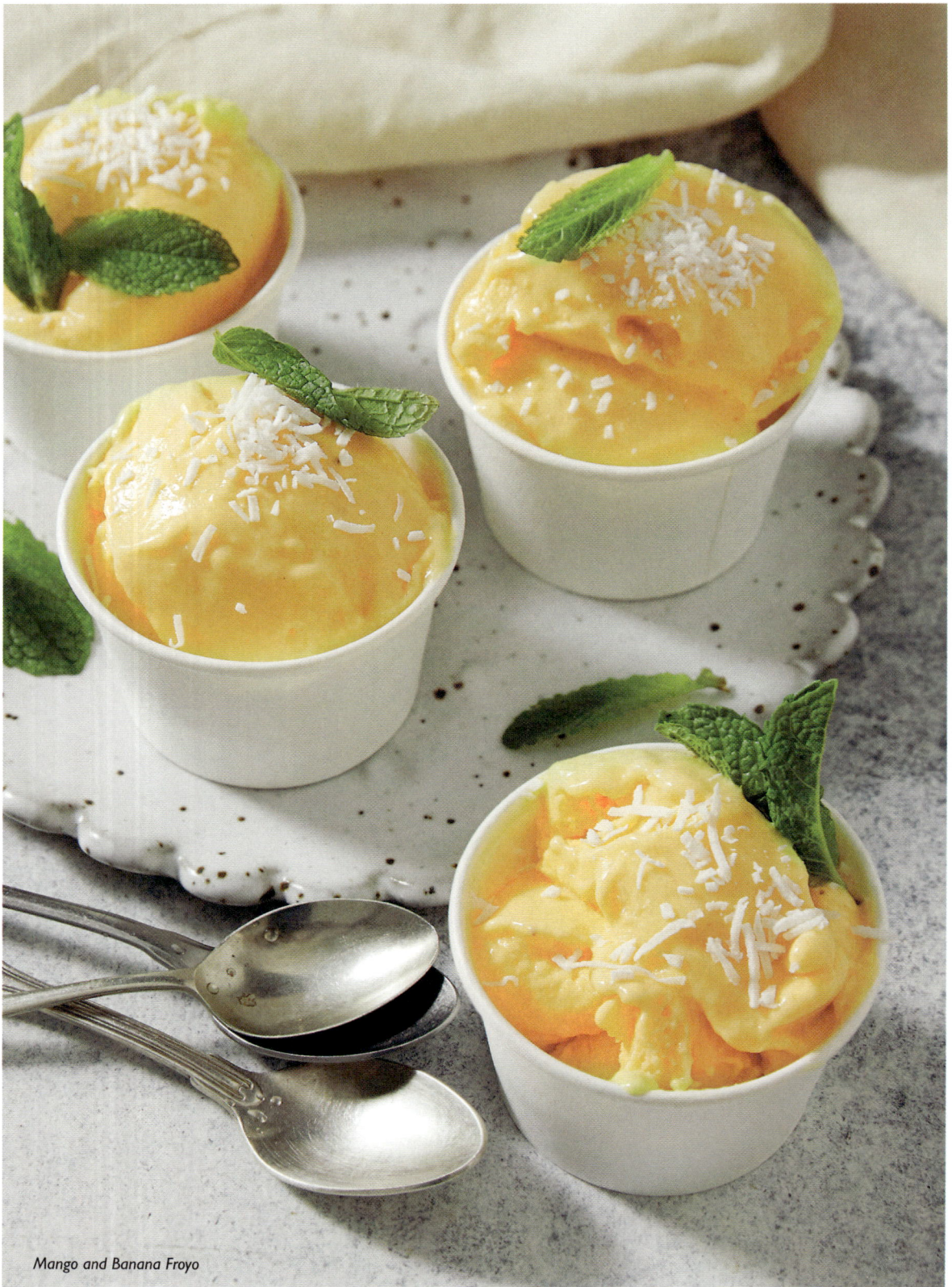

Mango and Banana Froyo

MANGO AND BANANA FROYO

SERVES 2
PREP TIME 5 minutes

250 g (9 oz) diced frozen mango
1 frozen banana
125 g (4½ oz/½ cup) Greek-style yoghurt
1 teaspoon shredded coconut
1 mint sprig, leaves picked (optional)

Place the mango, banana and yoghurt in a food processor or blender and blitz until smooth.

Divide between two bowls, then top with coconut and mint, if using, to serve.

FRUIT AND NUT SNACK CUP

SERVES 2
PREP TIME 5 minutes

½ banana, sliced
2 teaspoons almond butter
125 g (4½ oz/½ cup) Greek-style yoghurt
70 g (2½ oz/⅓ cup) mixed berries (fresh or frozen)
2 teaspoons slivered almonds

Divide the sliced banana between two small glass jars or bowls. Top with the almond butter, yoghurt, berries and slivered almonds to serve.

SPINACH AND WHITE BEAN DIP WITH VEGETABLE STICKS

SERVES 4
PREP TIME 10 minutes
COOK TIME 3 minutes

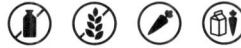

2 teaspoons olive oil
1 garlic clove, crushed
40 g (1½ oz/¼ cup) almonds, coarsely chopped
90 g (3¼ oz/2 cups) baby spinach leaves
400 g (14 oz) tinned white beans, drained and rinsed
1 bunch mint, leaves picked
2 tablespoons lemon juice

TO SERVE
1 cucumber, cut into sticks
1 carrot, cut into sticks

Heat the oil and garlic in a small saucepan over medium heat and cook for a few minutes until the garlic has softened.

Put the garlic into a food processor with 30 g (1 oz) of the almonds and the spinach, beans, mint and lemon juice then pulse until smooth.

Taste and adjust the flavours, if needed, then place in a serving bowl and top with the remaining almonds. Serve with the vegetables.

STRAWBERRY AND RICOTTA BRUSCHETTA

SERVES 1
PREP TIME 5 minutes

2 tablespoons ricotta cheese
3 Corn Thins
6 strawberries, hulled and sliced
1 basil sprig, leaves picked

Spread the ricotta over the Corn Thins and top with strawberries and basil leaves to serve.

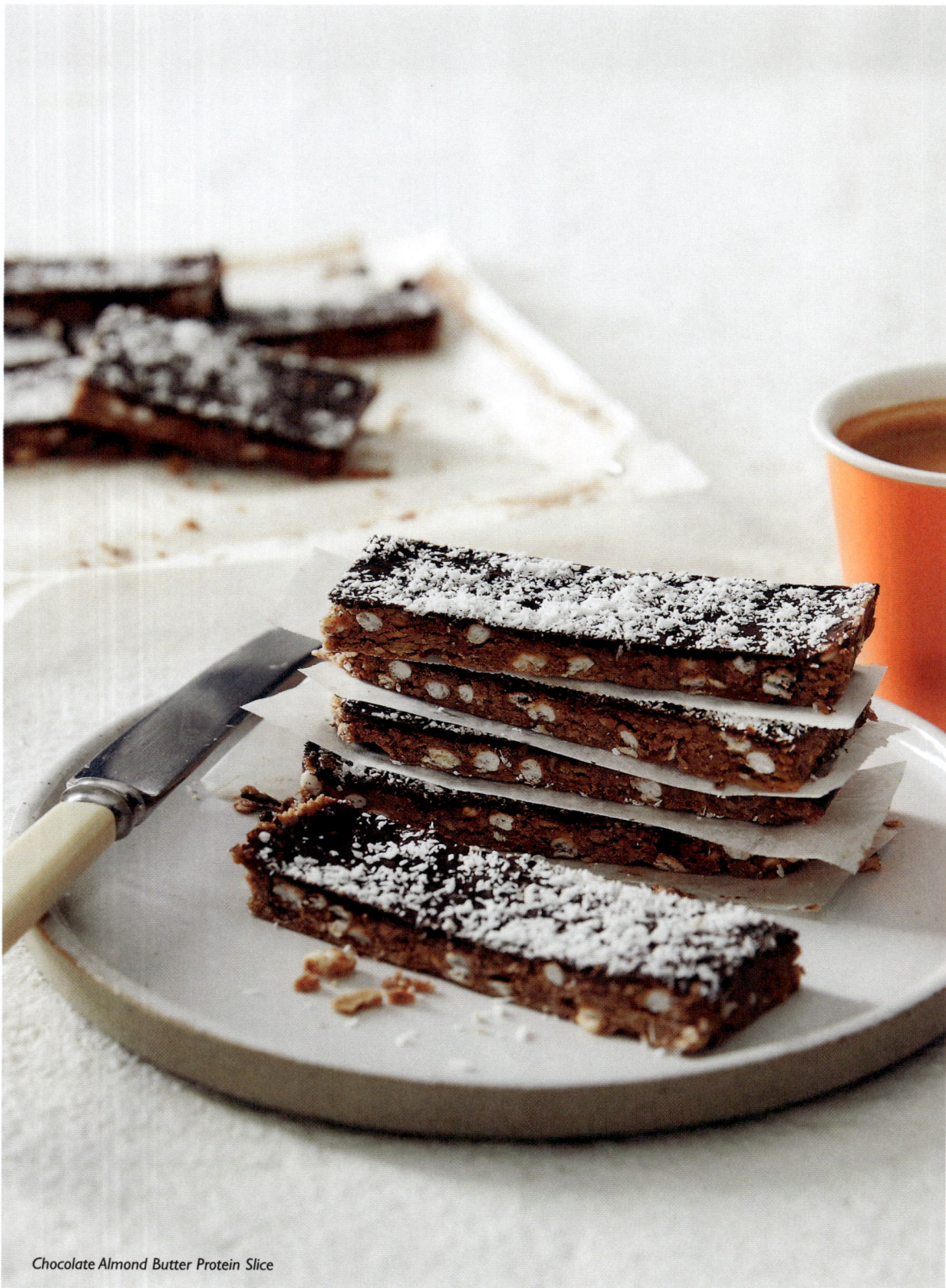

Chocolate Almond Butter Protein Slice

CHOCOLATE ALMOND BUTTER PROTEIN SLICE

MAKES 16
PREP TIME 15 minutes
COOK TIME 5 minutes

100 g (3½ oz/1 cup) rolled (porridge) oats
1 tablespoon cocoa powder
60 g (2¼ oz) protein powder
15 g (½ oz/½ cup) puffed rice
3 tablespoons coconut oil
135 g (4¾ oz/½ cup) almond butter
2 tablespoons maple syrup
40 g (1½ oz) dark chocolate (70%), coarsely chopped
2 tablespoons desiccated coconut

Line a square 20 cm (8 inch) baking tin with baking paper, leaving some paper overhanging at either end to make removing the slice easy. Lightly grease the areas of the tin on the sides not covered by the baking paper.

Blend half the oats with the cocoa and protein powders to a flour consistency. Transfer to a medium-sized bowl and stir through the remaining oats and the puffed rice.

Melt the coconut oil, almond butter and maple syrup in a small saucepan over low heat then pour over the dry ingredients. Stir gently to combine and, with clean wet hands, press the mixture into the prepared tin. Refrigerate for an hour.

Meanwhile put the chocolate in a heatproof bowl and microwave for 30 seconds at a time, stirring after each time, until melted and smooth. Alternatively, use the double-boiler method: put the chocolate in a heatproof bowl over a saucepan with about 2 inches of simmering water (make sure the water doesn't touch the base of the bowl). Melt the chocolate in the bowl, stirring occasionally until smooth.

Spread over the oat mixture then sprinkle with desiccated coconut. Return to the fridge until set and slice into 16 pieces.

STRAWBERRY CACAO CHIA PUDDING

SERVES 1
PREP TIME 5 minutes

60 g (2¼ oz) strawberries, hulled and halved
2 tablespoons chia seeds
80 ml (2½ fl oz/⅓ cup) almond milk
2 teaspoons honey
1 teaspoon natural vanilla extract
1 tablespoon cocoa powder

Set aside 3 of the halved strawberries, 2 teaspoons of the chia seeds and 1 teaspoon of the honey. Combine the remaining ingredients in a blender and blend until smooth.

Transfer to a glass and top with the remaining chia seeds and halved strawberries, then drizzle over the remaining honey to serve.

RASPBERRY BANANA BREAD

SERVES 12
PREP TIME 12 minutes
COOK TIME 50 minutes

100 g (3½ oz) quinoa flour
60 g (2¼ oz) almond meal
45 g (1⅔ oz/½ cup) desiccated coconut
2 teaspoons baking powder
2 tablespoons chia seeds
¼ teaspoon salt
175 g (6 oz) Greek-style yoghurt
2 tablespoons milk
2 tablespoons honey
3 very ripe bananas, mashed
125 g (4½ oz/1 cup) frozen raspberries

Preheat the oven to 160°C (320°F) and lightly grease a 20 × 10 (8 × 4 inch) loaf (bar) tin.

Combine the quinoa flour, almond meal, coconut, baking powder, chia seeds and salt in a medium-sized bowl.

Mix the yoghurt, milk, honey and banana together, then gradually add this mixture to the dry ingredients.

Gently stir through the raspberries then pour into the prepared tin and bake for 50 minutes, or until a skewer inserted into the centre comes out clean. If you find it's browning too much before it's cooked, cover loosely with foil.

Allow to cool in the tin, then turn onto a wire rack and slice once completely cooled.

HEALTHY BANANA SPLIT

SERVES 2
PREP TIME 10 minutes
COOK TIME 2 minutes

1 teaspoon honey
1 teaspoon cocoa powder
1 teaspoon hot water
1 tablespoon chopped almonds
1 tablespoon shredded coconut
1 banana, halved lengthways
70 g (2½ oz/¼ cup) Greek-style yoghurt
2 fresh cherries

Mix the honey, cocoa and hot water in a small bowl to make a chocolate sauce.

Heat a small non-stick frying pan over medium heat. Add the almonds and coconut, and toss for 1–2 minutes, until golden.

Arrange the banana halves on two plates and spoon on the yoghurt. Drizzle over the chocolate sauce, sprinkle with the almond and coconut mixture and top each portion with a cherry.

Most high-protein foods are also incredibly healthy. Therefore, simply by changing your dietary intake and eating more high-protein snacks, such as the ones on these pages, you'll not only be consuming more whole foods, but you'll also be improving your health at the same time. These snacks also tend to have a much lower energy density than high-fat and high-sugar foods.

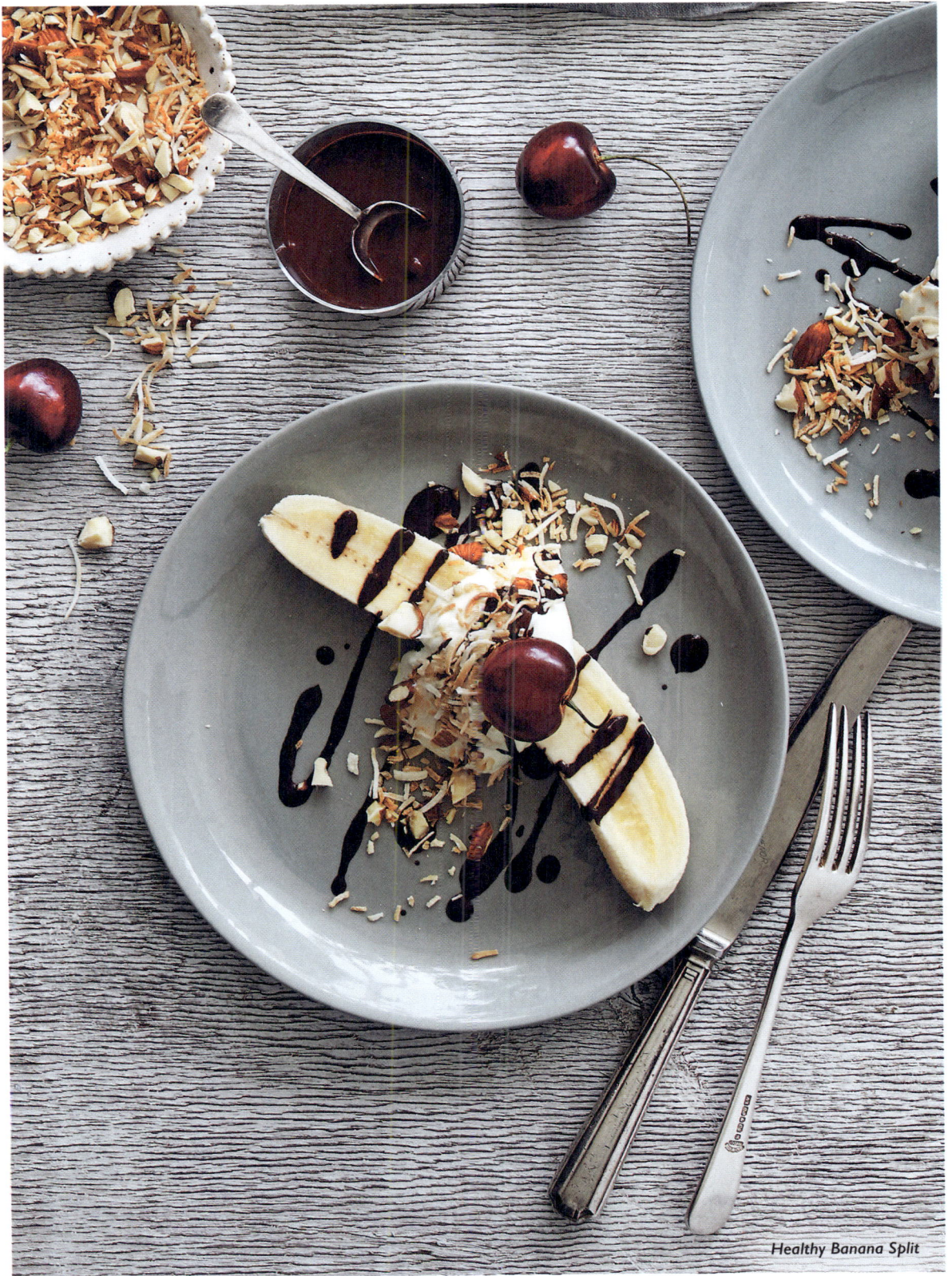

Healthy Banana Split

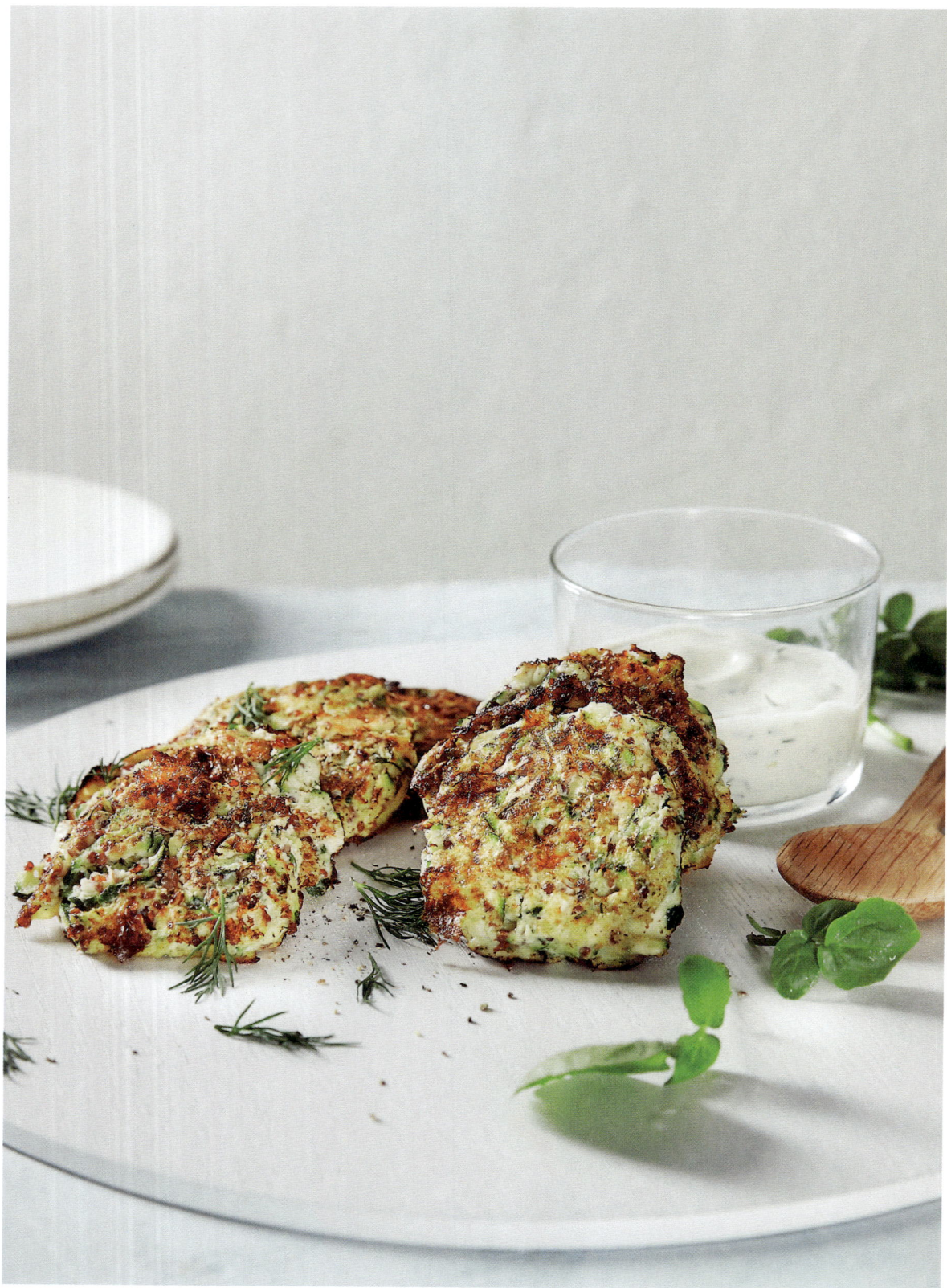

QUINOA ZUCCHINI FRITTERS

SERVES 6 **PREP TIME** 15 minutes **COOK TIME** 20 minutes

50 g (1¾ oz/¼ cup) red quinoa,
  washed
¼ teaspoon salt
2 zucchini (courgettes),
  coarsely grated
135 g (4¾ oz/½ cup) cottage
  cheese
2 large eggs
50 g (1¾ oz/1 cup) baby spinach
  leaves
3 tablespoons finely chopped dill
salt and pepper, to taste
2 tablespoons olive oil

DILL YOGHURT
130 g (4½ oz/½ cup) Greek-
  style yoghurt
1 tablespoon chopped dill
¼ teaspoon salt

Place the quinoa, 125 ml (4 fl oz/½ cup) water and the salt in a saucepan and bring to the boil. Simmer, covered, for 15 minutes, or until cooked, then allow to stand, covered, for 5 minutes.

Place the grated zucchini in a colander and leave for 10 minutes. Squeeze out as much liquid as possible after this time.

Put the cheese and eggs in a food processor and whizz until smooth. Add the spinach and pulse to combine. (Don't purée unless you like green fritters.) Fold through the cooked quinoa, zucchini and 2 tablespoons of dill until well combined, then season with salt and pepper.

Heat the oil in a medium frying pan over medium–high heat. Add heaped tablespoon batches of batter to the pan and cook for about 3 minutes on each side.

Combine all the ingredients for the dill yoghurt in a small bowl and serve with the fritters.

WHOLEGRAIN TOAST WITH RICOTTA AND SPROUTS

SERVES 1
PREP TIME 5 minutes
COOK TIME 3 minutes

1 slice wholegrain (or gluten-free) bread
2 tablespoons ricotta cheese
30 g (1 oz/½ cup) alfalfa sprouts
½ teaspoon black sesame seeds
salt and pepper

Toast the bread, then spread with the ricotta, and top with the alfalfa sprouts and sesame seeds. Season with salt and pepper.

CORN THINS WITH PEANUT BUTTER, BANANA AND COCONUT

SERVES 1
PREP TIME 5 minutes

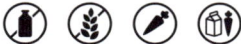

2 teaspoons natural peanut butter
2 Corn Thins
½ banana, sliced
2 teaspoons shredded or desiccated coconut

Spread the peanut butter over the Corn Thins, then top with sliced banana and sprinkle with coconut.

CHEWY RASPBERRY OAT BARS

MAKES 6
PREP TIME 10 minutes
COOK TIME 20 minutes

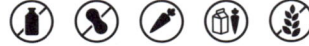

60 g (2¼ oz/¼ cup) unsweetened apple sauce
60 ml (2 fl oz/¼ cup) maple syrup
1 ripe banana, mashed
1 teaspoon natural vanilla extract
160 g (5⅔ oz) rolled (porridge) oats, or quinoa flakes if gluten free
2 tablespoons chia seeds
100 g (3½ oz) raspberries

Preheat the oven to 160°C (320°F). Line a square 20 cm (8 inch) baking tin with baking paper.

Combine the apple sauce, maple syrup, banana and vanilla in a bowl. Add the oats and chia seeds, and mix to combine.

Gently fold through the raspberries and transfer the mixture to the prepared tin. Press down gently with the back of a spoon to even out and smooth the top.

Bake for 20 minutes then cool completely on a wire rack before cutting into 6 bars.

If you are resistance training and trying to build lean muscle and sculpt your body, I recommend three snacks per day. Choose snacks that contain protein and carbohydrates.

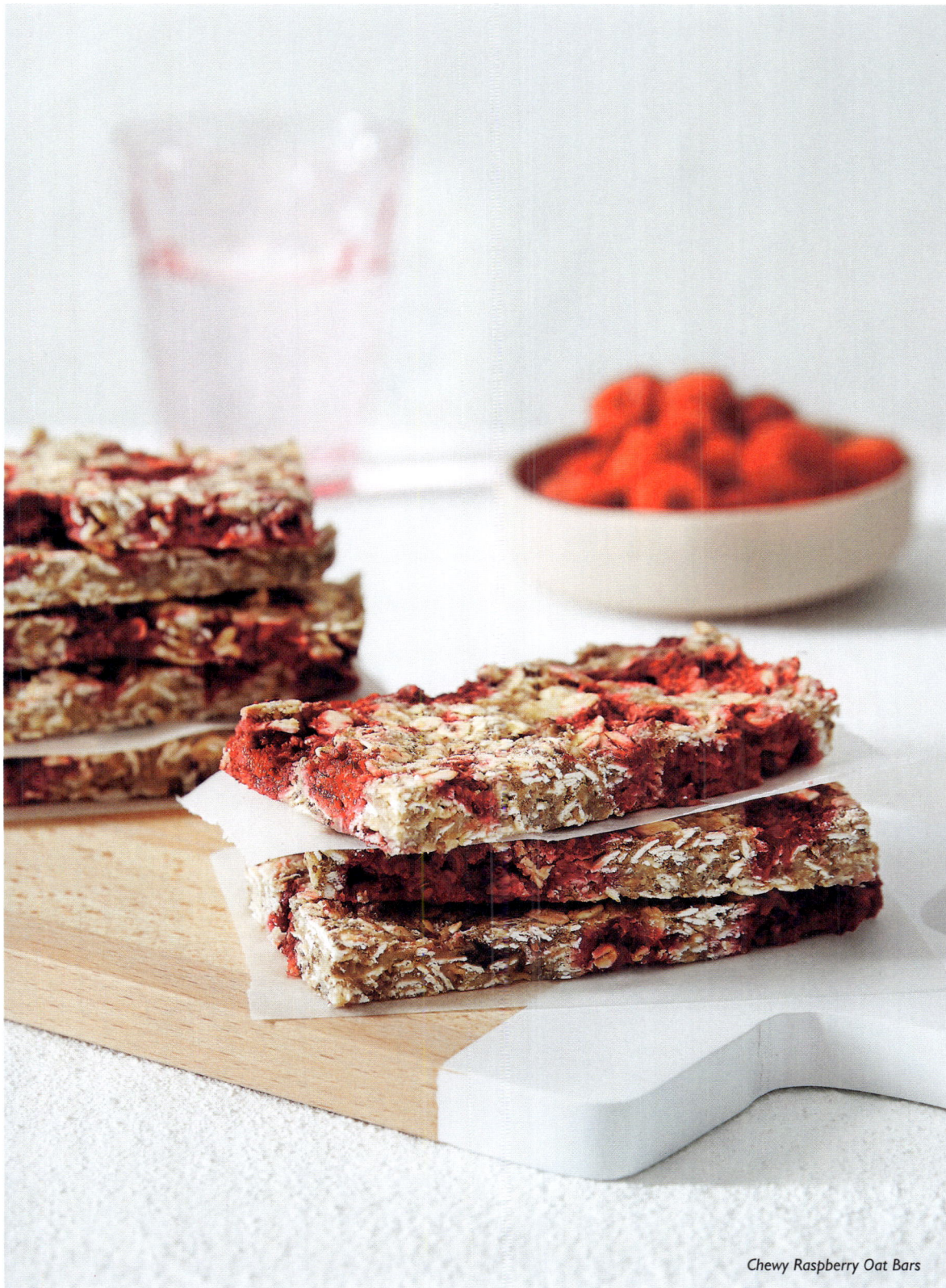

Chewy Raspberry Oat Bars

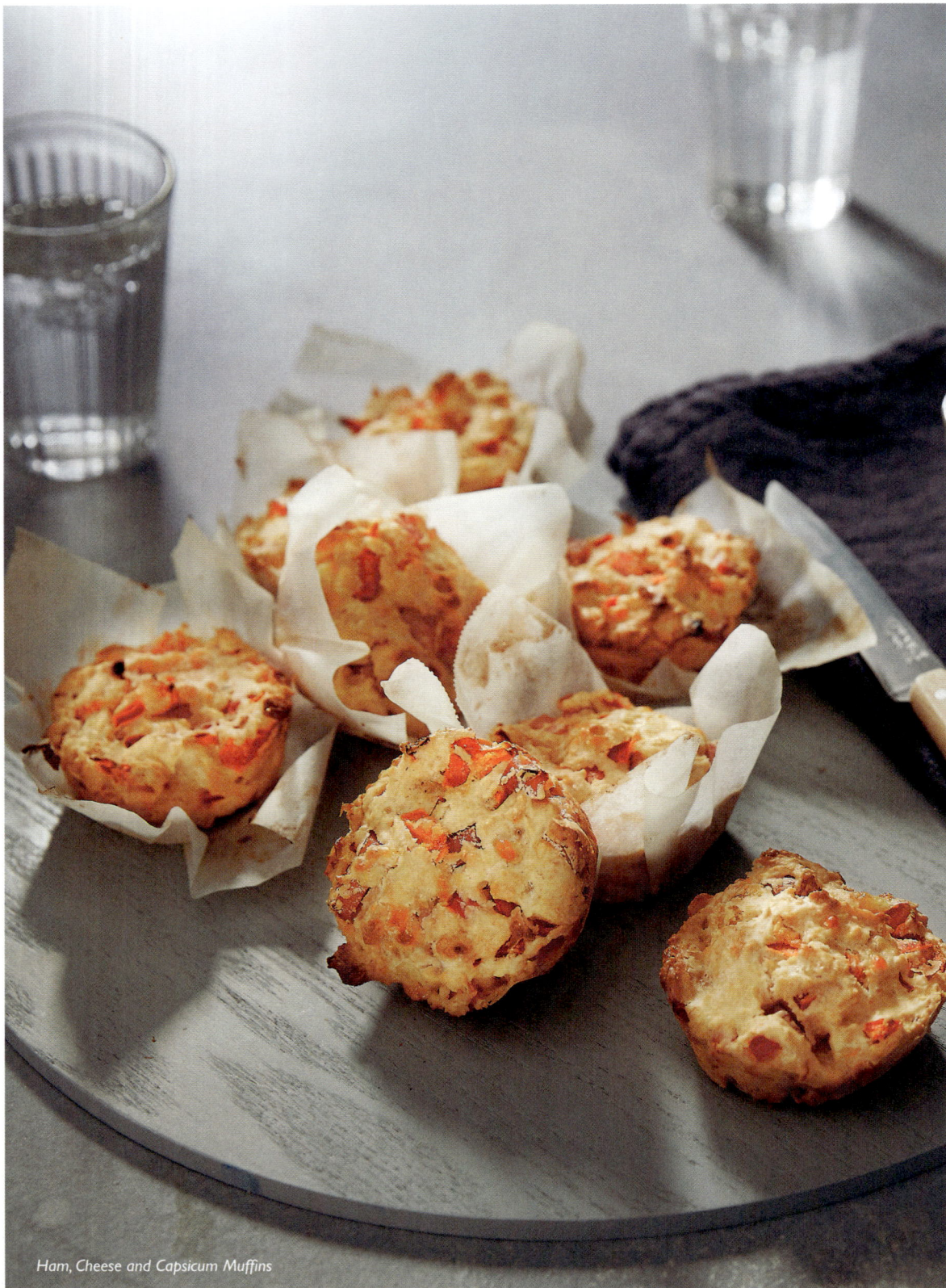

Ham, Cheese and Capsicum Muffins

HAM, CHEESE AND CAPSICUM MUFFINS

MAKES 12
PREP TIME 10 minutes
COOK TIME 25 minutes

100 g (3½ oz/1 cup loosely packed) coarsely grated cheddar cheese
1 small capsicum (pepper), deseeded and diced
1 tomato, diced
200 g (7 oz) ham, diced
300 g (10½ oz/2 cups) wholemeal (whole-wheat) self-raising flour
salt and pepper
1 large egg
250 ml (9 fl oz/1 cup) milk
75 g (2⅔ oz) butter, melted

Preheat the oven to 180°C (350°F) and line a 12-hole standard (60 ml/¼ cup) muffin tin with squares of baking paper.

Set 2 tablespoons of the cheese aside, then mix the remaining cheese with the vegetables, ham and flour in a large mixing bowl. Season with salt and pepper.

Whisk the egg, milk and melted butter together in a small bowl or measuring jug.

Make a small well in the dry mixture and slowly add the wet ingredients. Stir until just combined, and don't overmix! (If the mixture is too dry, add a dash of milk.)

Spoon the mixture into the prepared tin and top with the remaining cheese.

Bake for 20–25 minutes, or until golden brown. Allow to cool in the tin, then either serve warm, or transfer to a wire rack to cool completely

APPLE AND CINNAMON SEEDED LOAF

SERVES 12
PREP TIME 20 minutes
COOK TIME 1 hour 30 minutes

175 g (6 oz/1¾ cups) rolled (porridge) oats
2 teaspoons baking powder
55 g (2 oz/⅓ cup) pepitas (pumpkin seeds)
1 teaspoon ground cinnamon
2 large eggs
200 g (7 oz/¾ cup) Greek-style yoghurt
2 teaspoons natural vanilla extract
60 g (2¼ oz) unsalted butter, melted
90 g (3¼ oz/¼ cup) honey
2 granny smith apples, cored and diced

Preheat the oven to 180°C (350°F) and line a loaf (bar) tin with baking paper.

Place the oats in a food processor, blitz to a rough flour then place in a large mixing bowl with the other dry ingredients and mix well.

Combine the eggs, yoghurt, vanilla, butter and honey in a small bowl.

Slowly add the egg mixture to the dry ingredients and fold through until combined.

Fold through the diced apple then pour the batter into the prepared tin.

Place in the oven to bake for 1½ hours, or until a skewer inserted in the centre comes out clean.

Cool in the tin for a few minutes, then transfer to a wire rack to cool completely. Slice before serving, or store in an airtight container in the fridge for up to 3 days or in the freezer.

TERIYAKI BEEF AND QUINOA SUSHI

SERVES 3 (4 pieces per portion)
PREP TIME 15 minutes
COOK TIME 15 minutes

100 g (3½ oz) tri-coloured quinoa, washed
1 teaspoon rice vinegar
1 teaspoon maple syrup
2 sheets nori
100 g (3½ oz) roast beef, thinly sliced
4 asparagus spears, blanched
1 tablespoon pickled ginger
1 tablespoon teriyaki sauce
tamari, to serve

Combine the washed quinoa with 150 ml (5½ fl oz) water in a small saucepan. Bring to the boil then reduce the heat to low and cover with a lid. Simmer for 15 minutes, or until all the water has been absorbed and the quinoa has puffed up.

Remove the pan from the heat and stir through the vinegar and maple syrup. Spread the quinoa around a baking tray and refrigerate to cool.

Place the nori sheet on a bamboo sushi mat (skip this step if you don't have a mat). Spread an even layer of quinoa over the nori, leaving a 2 cm (¾ inch) area free along the baseline.

Place half of the roast beef, asparagus and ginger in a straight line along the top. Drizzle with half of the teriyaki sauce then roll the sushi into a long, tight cylindrical shape. Repeat the process with the remaining nori sheet.

Slice each roll into six portions and serve with tamari for dipping.

JAFFA ENERGY BITES

SERVES 10
PREP TIME 20 minutes

100 g (3½ oz/1 cup) rolled (porridge) oats (use brown rice or quinoa flakes if gluten-free)
2 tablespoons honey
25 g (1 oz/¼ cup) desiccated coconut
140 g (5 oz/½ cup) natural peanut butter
zest and juice of 1 orange
40 g (1½ oz) dark chocolate (70%)

Pulse the oats, honey, coconut, peanut butter and orange zest and juice in a food processor to combine.

Scoop teaspoons of the mixture into 10 balls and place on a tray.

Meanwhile melt the chocolate in a heatproof bowl and microwave for 30 seconds at a time, stirring after each time, until melted and smooth. Alternatively, use the double-boiler method on page 73.

Drizzle the chocolate over the balls and place in the fridge for 10–15 minutes. Store in an airtight container for up to a week.

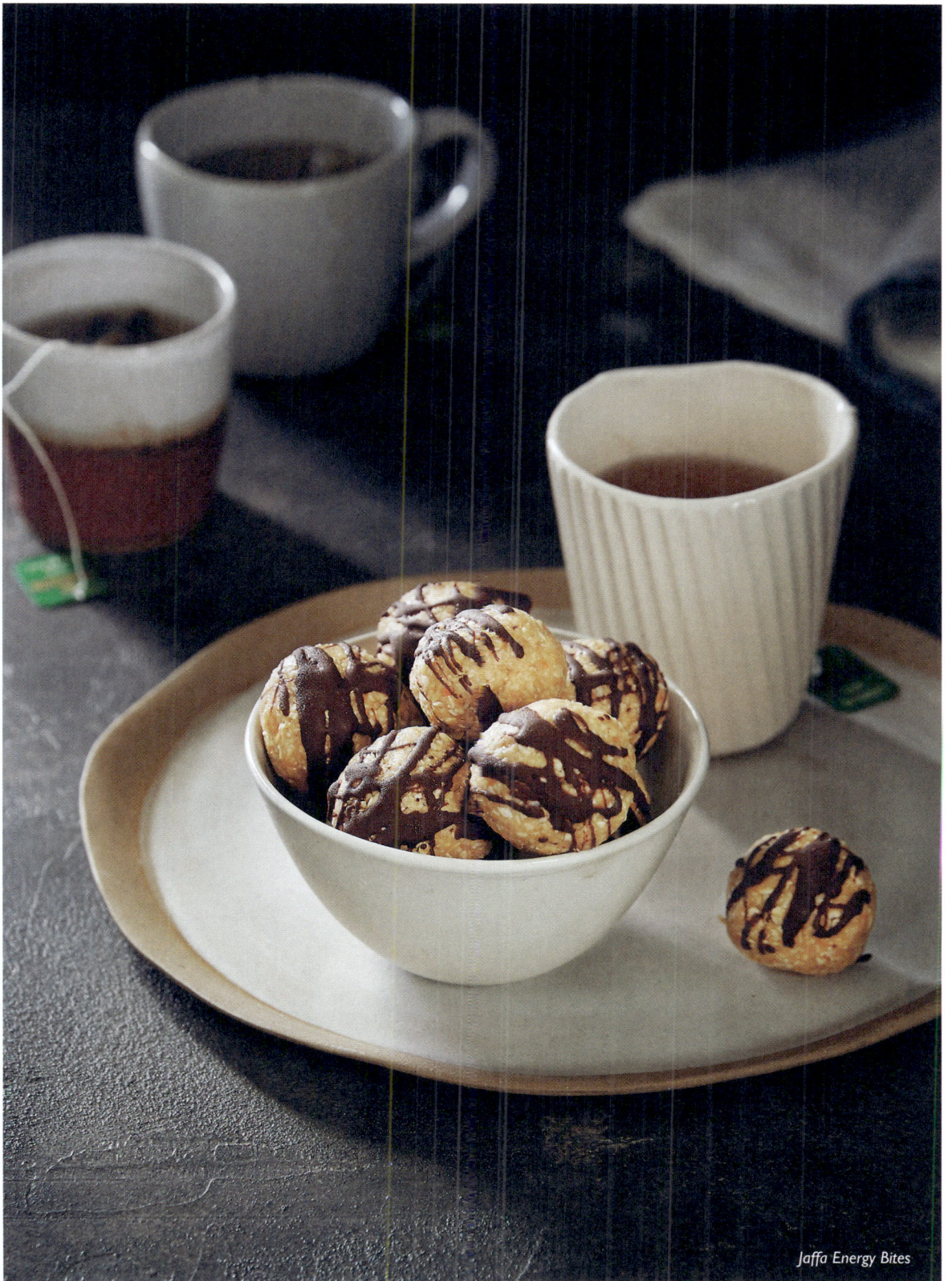

Jaffa Energy Bites

PROTEIN MAKES SKIN GLOW AND
MUSCLES GROW. AMP UP YOUR INTAKE
WITH A PROTEIN-PACKED SNACK!

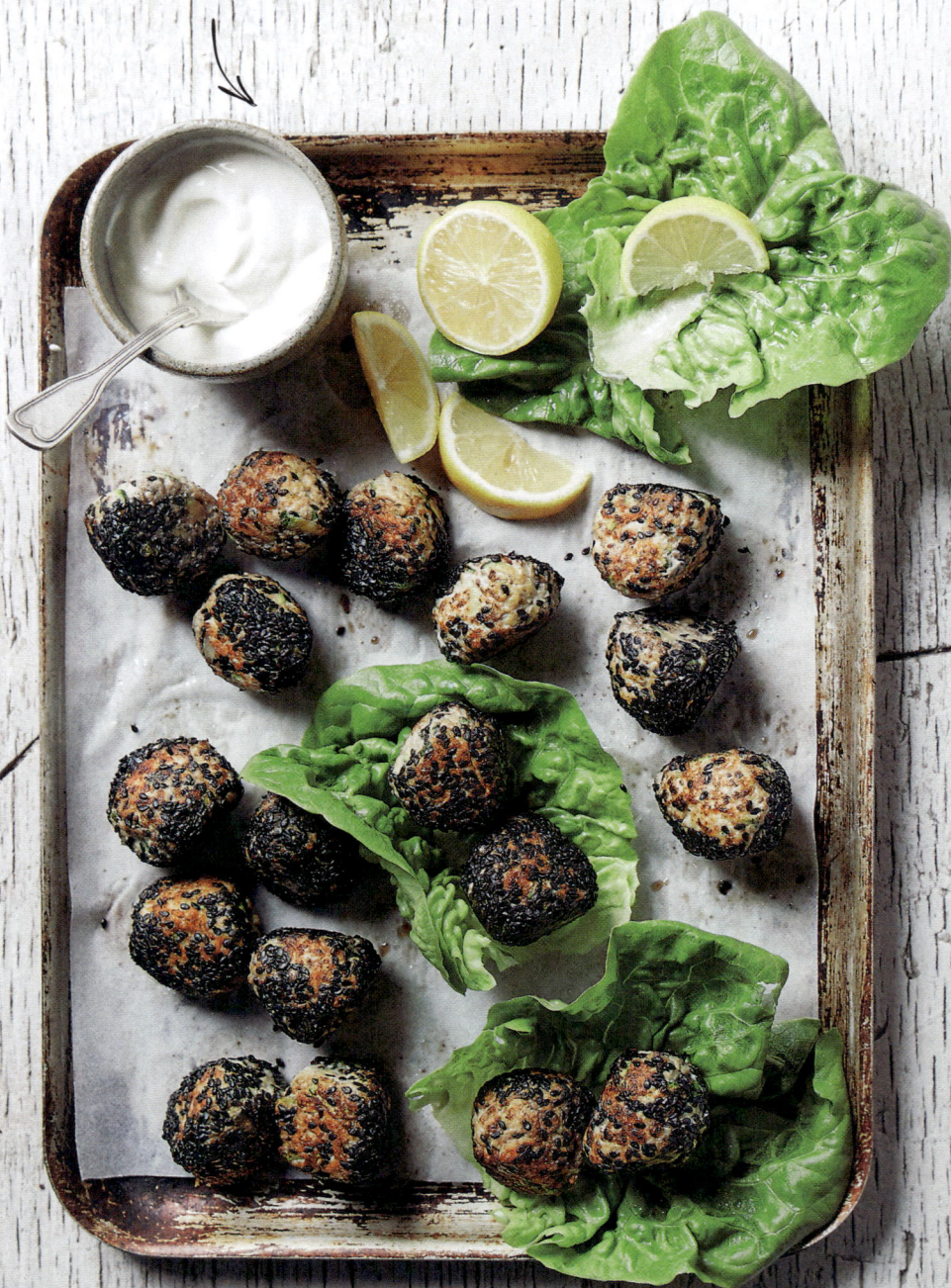

CHICKEN AND CHIA MEATBALLS

MAKES 24 (2–3 per snack) **PREP TIME** 15 minutes **COOK TIME** 15 minutes

20 g (¾ oz) black chia seeds
500 g (1 lb 2 oz) minced (ground) chicken
1 tablespoon minced ginger
½ onion, coarsely grated
100 g (3½ oz) coarsely grated zucchini (courgette)
small handful of coriander (cilantro), coarsely chopped
½ teaspoon salt
pepper, to taste
40 g (1½ oz/¼ cup) sesame seeds
1 tablespoon olive oil
70 g (2½ oz/¼ cup) Greek-style yoghurt
large lettuce leaves, for serving (optional)

Preheat the oven to 180°C (350°F). Line a baking tray with baking paper and set aside.

Combine the chia seeds with 60 ml (2 fl oz/¼ cup) water in a bowl, stir and set aside for about 10 minutes, or until the water is absorbed and the mixture has formed a gel.

In a large bowl combine the chicken, ginger, onion, zucchini, coriander, salt and pepper. Mix to combine then stir through the chia gel. With damp hands, portion the mixture into about 30 g (1 oz/1½ tablespoon) amounts and roll into balls.

Roll the meatballs in the sesame seeds to coat.

Heat a large non-stick frying pan over medium heat. Add the olive oil and cook the meatballs in batches for 5 minutes, or until well browned. Transfer to the prepared baking tray and bake for a further 5 minutes, or until cooked through.

Serve the meatballs with yoghurt and wrap them in a lettuce leaf for extra crunch.

SUPPORT YOUR GOALS

- If your goal is to lose a few kilos, you can enjoy up to two snacks per day. If you're not hungry, don't eat both snacks. Easy!

- If you're working on gaining a little extra muscle and strength, bump up to three snacks per day. Again, if you don't feel you need those three snacks every day, that's okay, too.

- If you're extra active or training for long periods of time (running a marathon? I'm talking to you!), you might need some extra carb-love.

COMFORT FOOD & GOOD-MOOD SNACKS

HOW TO CONTROL EMOTIONAL EATING

We've all eaten when we weren't hungry. I have, of course I have! Everyone experiences moments of zombie snacking, but eating these types of snacks has never kept me on track with my goals.

It's really easy to over-snack with a treat here and there, free snacks in the work kitchen or a little something-something while you're cooking dinner. Over time, this zombie snacking can undo all your hard work—no matter how many times a week you exercise. I'm not the snack police (promise!), but I am going to break down two ways that snacking can sabotage your healthy lifestyle.

1. Emotional snacking

Occasionally, using food to make yourself feel better is okay. But when it becomes habitual, it can affect our health and leave us feeling crappy.

There are many reasons why we emotionally snack (stress, hormones, anxiety, boredom), but food is not the antidote. It's important to find other things that make you feel happy or comforted and draw from these instead.

2. Snacking in the dark

I've been guilty of this one. Whether you're working late or lying in bed thinking about everything, it's easy to head to the fridge and snack on the first thing you see.

Eating well beyond bedtime can lead to poor food choices and bad sleep hygiene, as we tend to reach for sugar snacks late at night and these disrupt our sleep as the body keeps you awake as it works on digesting the food.

Next time you think you need a snack, it's worth doing a quick head check.

1. THE MENTAL CHECK-IN

Ask yourself, *How am I feeling right now?* And be specific with the question by tagging on whatever it is you are doing in that specific moment. *How am I feeling right now (as I stand in the pantry after the kids are in bed)? Am I hungry or am I just super tired?*

2. BODY SCAN

Your body will speak to you if you listen. Are your shoulders tense? Is your jaw tight? Are you clenching your toes? Do you have body aches or a headache? Are your muscles heavy and tired? Do a quick body scan of how you are feeling right now.

3. BREATHE

Nearly everyone I meet isn't breathing correctly. Yep, there's a wrong way to breathe. Shallow chest breaths will make you feel stressed and can increase cravings. Breathing right is the best advice I can give you. Take a full, deep breath into your diaphragm. Focus on the inhale for 5 seconds, and then on the exhale for 5 seconds. This will help de-clutter and de-stress your mind. Focus on expanding your ribcage as you breathe and breathing down to your belly. The more you practise this, the easier the process will become—promise!

No matter your mood, the snacks in this chapter will help you feel great. Some give you stamina and energy by keeping blood glucose levels stable, others provide a brain boost via their positive effect on the gut with fibre and prebiotics. And others are pure comfort; they will put a smile on your face because they taste amazing.

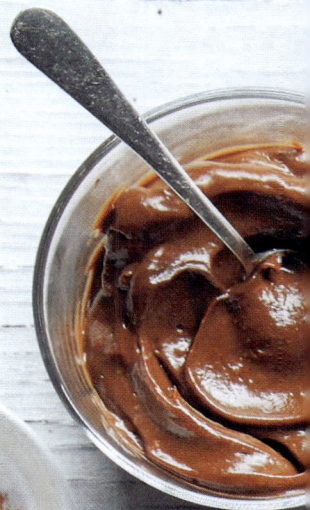

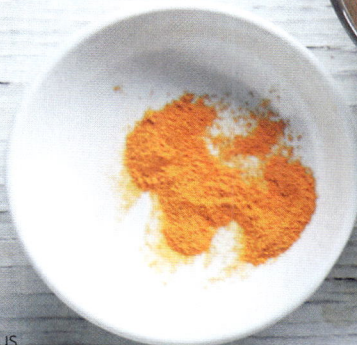

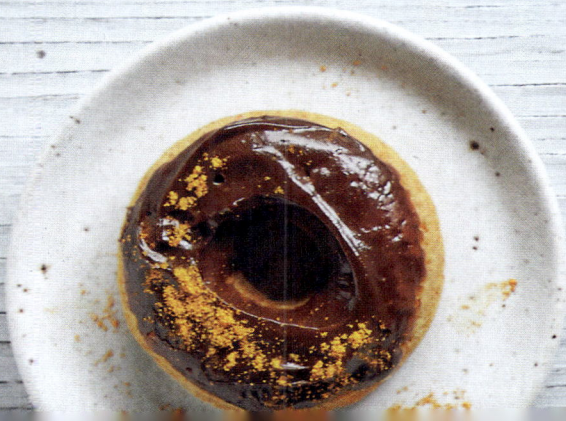

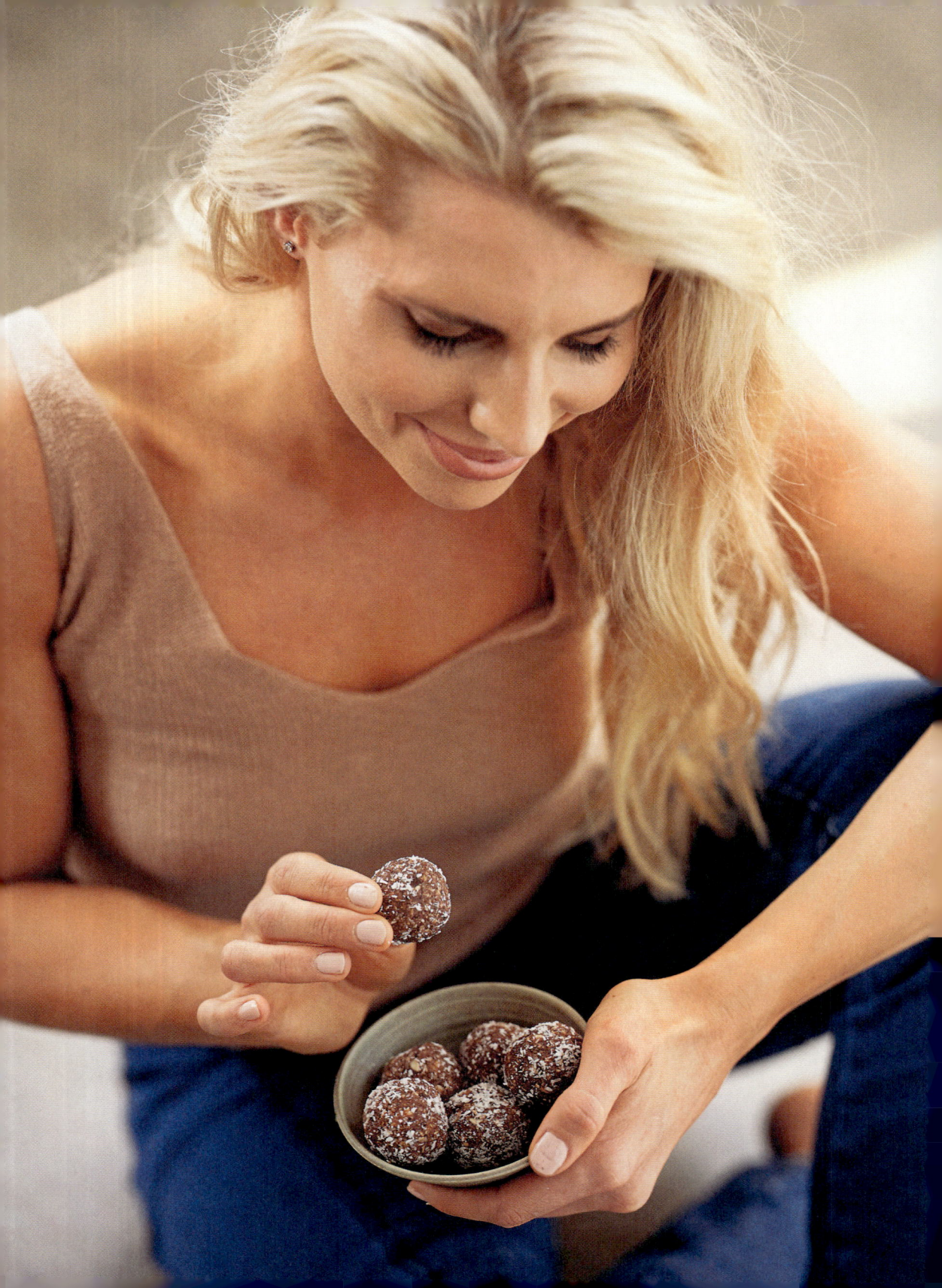

MY MANTRAS FOR MINDFUL SNACKING

Here are six mantras to help you practise mindful snacking (no cross-legged meditation, incense sticks or crystals required—though I do love all those things).

1. SNACK LIKE A SNAIL.

It takes about 20 minutes for your brain to register that you're full. Eating slowly gives your brain time to realise you're satisfied and this prevents you from eating the whole batch of bliss balls.

2. TUNE INTO YOUR TUMMY. LISTEN TO YOUR GUT.

We often listen to our minds or feed our emotions without tuning in to our bellies. If your stomach is rumbling, you've smashed a workout or you're in between meals, you probably are peckish—listen to your body and see if it's your mind or belly talking.

3. SNACK SITTING DOWN.

When we snack on the go, we're more likely to eat mindlessly—most of the time we forget we even ate. Sitting down (even for a minute) allows you to enjoy the physical act of snacking and reap the benefits of a mini mental recharge.

4. EXCESS SUGAR AND SALT ARE NO GOOD FOR YOU.

Potato chips and supermarket muesli bars are not snacks, they are energy zappers. Feed your hunger with wholesome and nutritious homemade snacks to curb sugar cravings and keep you satisfied.

5. MAKE FRIENDS WITH YOUR SNACK. FORM A BOND!

Now, you don't need to get too deep; but do take a moment to consider where each ingredient comes from (the farmer who grew it, the animal it came from, the process involved in growing or harvesting that ingredient) and your involvement in putting the ingredients together—you'll appreciate just how much effort goes into every bite.

6. DON'T STRUGGLE TO JUGGLE YOUR SNACK PLUS A HUNDRED OTHER TASKS.

Sometimes this is impossible—I get it! But if you can, try not to multitask while snacking: put the phone down, don't look at work emails, pause the washing up and just enjoy the single act of snacking.

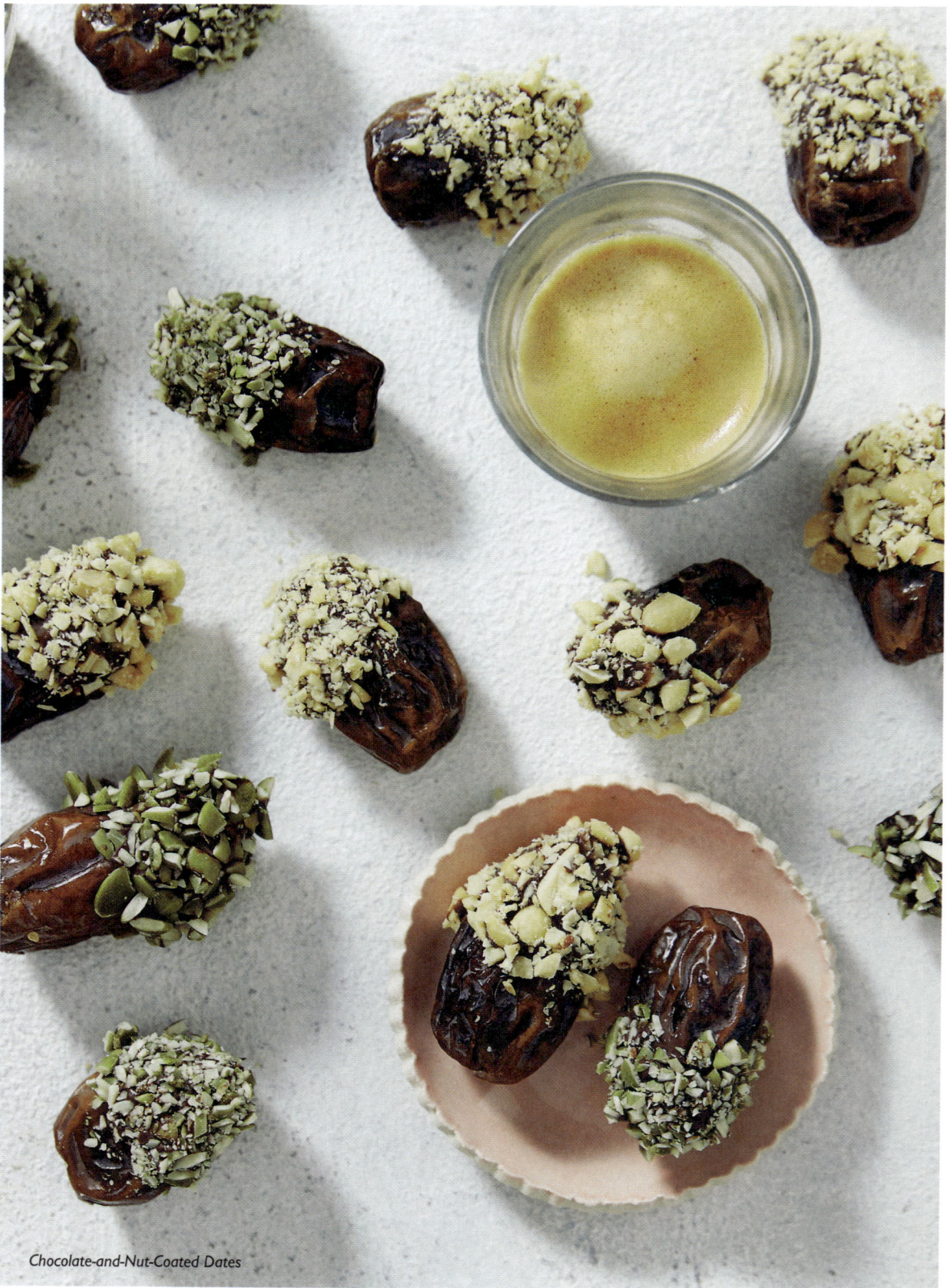

Chocolate-and-Nut-Coated Dates

CHOCOLATE-AND-NUT-COATED DATES

MAKES 16 (4 dates per snack)
PREP TIME 15 minutes
COOK TIME 3 minutes

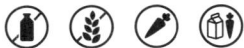

2 tablespoons finely chopped peanuts
2 tablespoons finely chopped pepitas
   (pumpkin seeds)
16 medjool dates, pitted and frozen for
   15 minutes
50 g (1¾ oz) vegan dark chocolate (70%)

Place the peanuts and pepitas in two separate small bowls.

Melt the chocolate in a microwave for 1 minute, and then in 30-second intervals, stirring after each time until fully melted.

Dip half of each date into the melted chocolate and then roll in either the peanuts or pepitas.

CHOCOLATE–BANANA SOFT SERVE

SERVES 2
PREP TIME 5 minutes

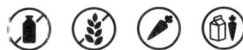

1 large frozen banana
2 tablespoons nut butter of your choice
1 tablespoon cocoa powder

Combine all ingredients in a food processor and blitz until smooth.

MUSHROOM AND CHEDDAR CROSTINI

SERVES 4
PREP TIME 10 minutes
COOK TIME 17 minutes

1 × 70 g wholegrain (or gluten-free) roll,
    sliced into 4 rounds
1 teaspoon olive oil
½ leek (white part only), thinly sliced
2 sprigs thyme, leaves stripped
200 g (7 oz) mushrooms, sliced
1 garlic clove, minced
60 g (2¼ oz) cheddar cheese, grated
salt and pepper

Preheat the oven to 180°C (350°F) and line
a baking tray with baking paper.

Arrange the bread on the tray and bake for
10 minutes, until golden and crisp.

Meanwhile, heat the oil in a non-stick frying
pan over medium heat. Cook the leek and most
of the thyme (reserving a little for serving) for
5 minutes, or until soft. Add the mushrooms and
garlic, season with salt and pepper and cook for
4–5 minutes.

Divide the mushroom mixture between the
crostini and top with cheddar. Sprinkle with the
remaining thyme leaves and some black pepper,
to taste. Return to the oven for 2 minutes, or until
the cheese has melted, and serve. Any remaining
crostini can be stored in an airtight container in
the fridge for 3 days and reheated in the oven at
180°C (350°F) for 5–10 minutes.

GARLICKY PARMESAN TOASTIES

SERVES 2
PREP TIME 5 minutes
COOK TIME 5 minutes

3 tablespoons finely grated parmesan cheese
1 tablespoon finely chopped flat-leaf (Italian)
    parsley
½ teaspoon dried Italian herbs
salt and pepper
1 wholegrain (or gluten-free) long roll, thinly
    sliced (older bread is easier to slice)
1 garlic clove, halved

Preheat the oven grill to medium–high.

Combine the parmesan, parsley and herbs in
a small bowl, and season with salt and pepper.

Grill the slices of bread on one side, then rub the
grilled sides with the cut side of the garlic halves.

Spread the cheese mixture on the uncooked
side of the bread, then grill, cheesy side up, until
melted and golden. Season to taste.

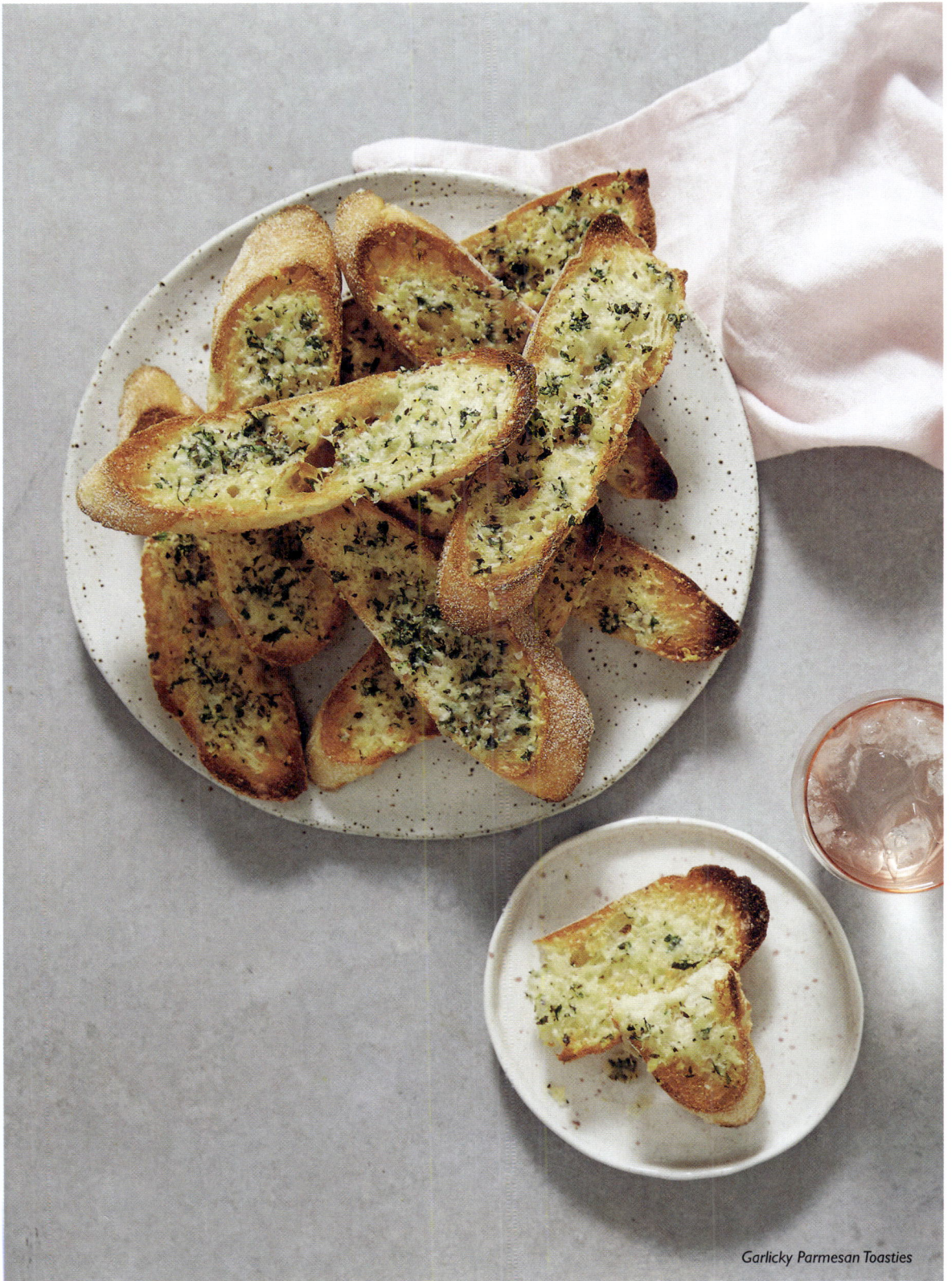

Garlicky Parmesan Toasties

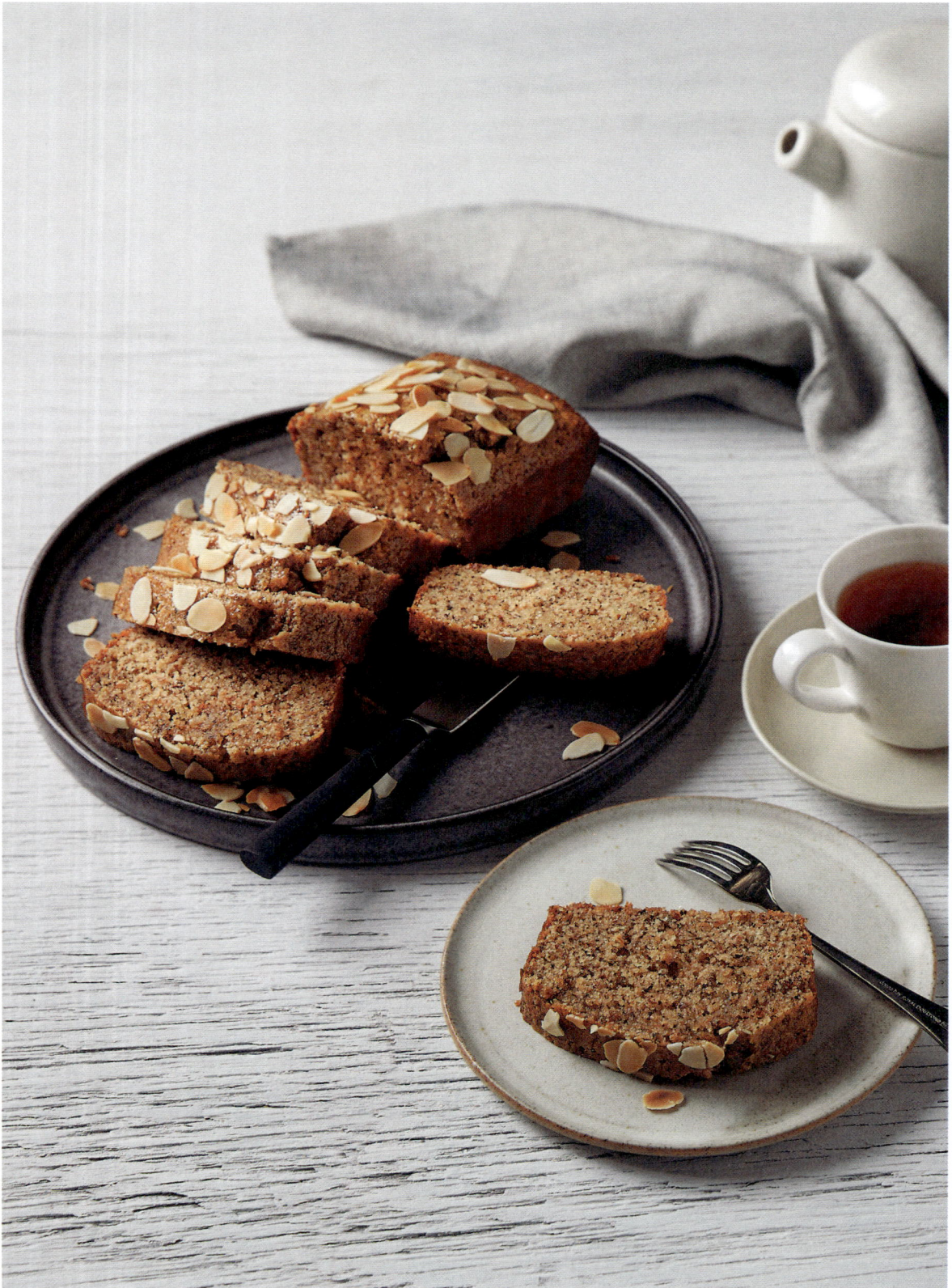

EARL GREY TEA CAKE WITH LEMON COCONUT DRIZZLE

SERVES 14 **PREP TIME** 5 minutes **COOK TIME** 35 minutes

EARL GREY TEA CAKE

135 g (4¾ oz/1 cup) spelt flour

100 g (3½ oz/1 cup) almond meal

1 teaspoon baking powder

½ teaspoon salt

2 teaspoons loose-leaf Earl Grey tea

2 large eggs

80 ml (2½ fl oz/⅓ cup) milk

½ teaspoon natural vanilla extract

80 ml (2½ fl oz/⅓ cup) maple syrup

55 g (2 oz/¼ cup) coconut oil, melted

LEMON COCONUT DRIZZLE

2 tablespoons coconut oil, melted

1 teaspoon lemon juice

1 tablespoon maple syrup

1 tablespoon flaked almonds, to decorate

Preheat the oven to 180°C (350°F) and line a standard loaf (bar) tin with baking paper.

In a large mixing bowl, combine the spelt flour, almond meal, baking powder, salt and tea.

In a separate bowl, whisk the eggs and milk together, then add the vanilla, maple syrup and coconut oil. Whisk together well, then pour a third of the mixture at a time into the dry ingredients, mixing until well combined.

Transfer the mixture to the tin and bake for 35 minutes, or until golden and cooked through.

While the cake is cooling, combine the coconut oil, lemon juice and maple syrup together. Allow the cake to cool, then drizzle the icing all over the top and sprinkle with the flaked almonds. Store in an airtight container for up to 5 days.

RASPBERRY AND RHUBARB OAT SLICE

MAKES ˙6 **PREP TIME** 10 minutes **COOK TIME** 40 minutes

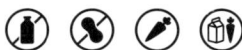

RHUBARB FILLING
300 g (10½ oz) rhubarb,
   trimmed and chopped into
   3 cm (1¼ inch) pieces
155 g (5½ oz/1¼ cups)
   raspberries (fresh or frozen)
3 tablespoons rice malt syrup
1 tablespoon lemon juice
1 tablespoon lemon zest
125 ml (4 fl oz/½ cup) water

CRUMBLE BASE AND TOPPING
200 g (7 oz/2 cups) rolled
   (porridge) oats
2 teaspoons baking powder
1 teaspoon ground cinnamon
95 g (3¼ oz/½ cup) coconut oil,
   melted
180 g (6¼ oz/½ cup) rice malt
   syrup

Preheat the oven to 180°C (350°F). Lightly grease and line a square 23 cm (9 inch) baking tin with baking paper, leaving some paper overhanging at either end to make removing the slice easy.

In a large saucepan over medium heat, combine the rhubarb, raspberries, rice malt syrup, lemon juice and zest and water. Bring to the boil, then turn down the heat to low and simmer for 5–7 minutes. Remove from the heat and set aside.

Place half the oats in a blender and blitz until you've got a floury consistency. Add this oat flour to a large mixing bowl with the remaining dry ingredients. Mix well with a wooden spoon, then add the melted coconut oil and rice malt syrup. Mix all the ingredients together to form the crumble (you can use your hands to do this).

Take three-quarters of the crumble and firmly pack it into the baking tin to form the base of your slice. Bake the base in the oven for 7–10 minutes, or until lightly golden.

Remove from the oven and leave to cool for a few minutes. Once cooled, spoon the rhubarb mixture onto the base and use the back of a spoon to spread it out evenly.

Sprinkle the remaining crumble evenly over the rhubarb then bake in the oven for a further 20 minutes, or until golden brown.

Once cooked, remove from the oven and cool in the tin, then refrigerate for 1 hour or overnight (this helps to set the coconut oil). Slice into 16 squares. These can be kept in an airtight container in the fridge for up to 5 days, or stored in the freezer for up to 3 months.

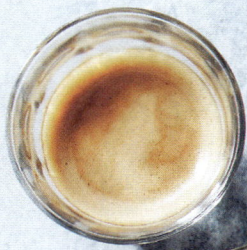

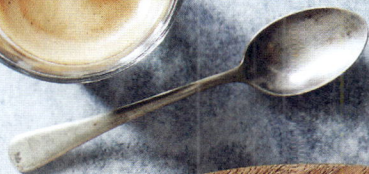

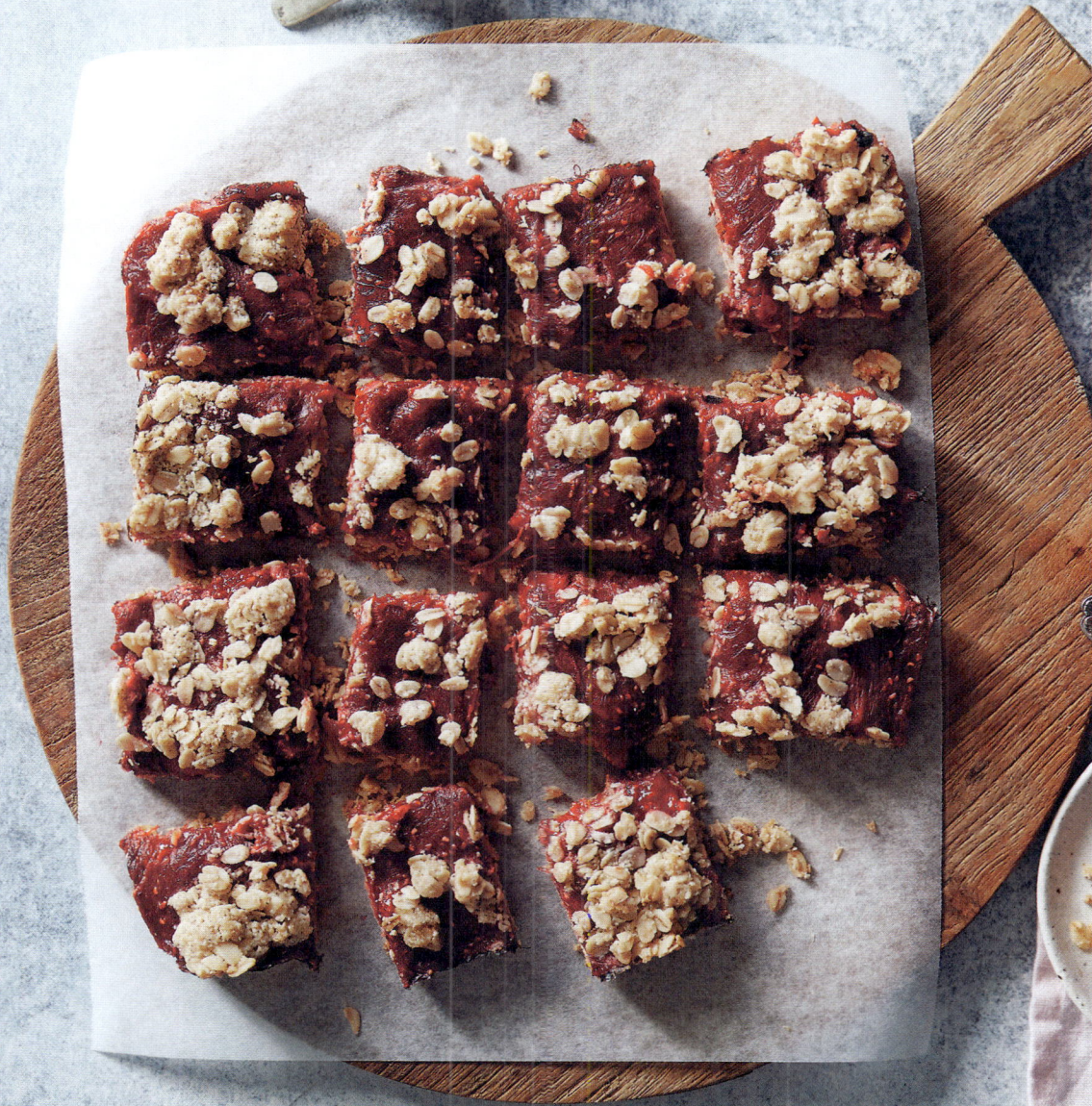

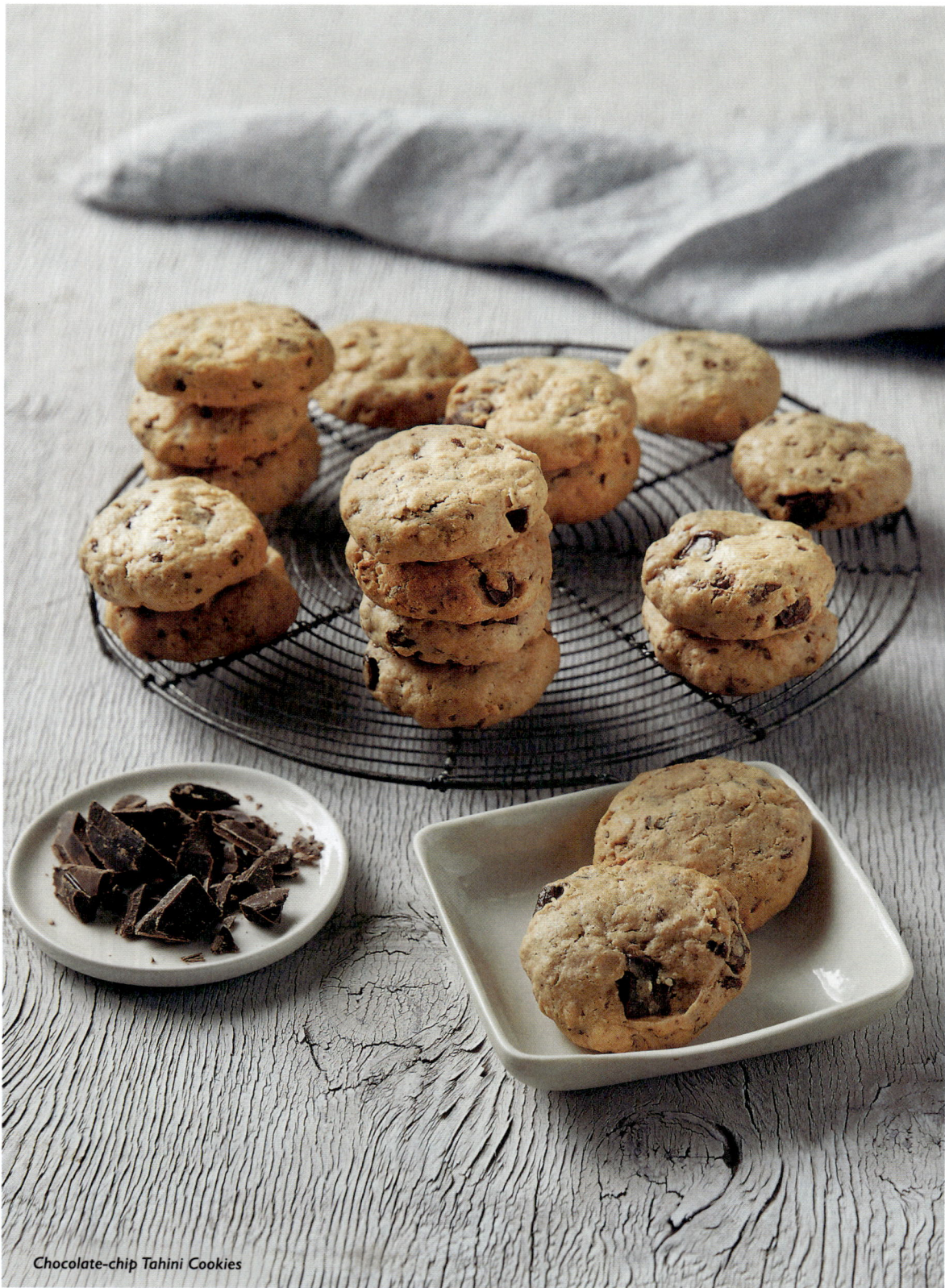

Chocolate-chip Tahini Cookies

CHOCOLATE-CHIP TAHINI COOKIES

MAKES 16
PREP TIME 10 minutes
COOK TIME 15 minutes

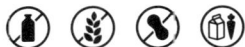

205 g (7¼ oz/¾ cup) tahini
90 g (3¼ oz/¼ cup) rice malt syrup
1 teaspoon vanilla extract
50 g (1¾ oz/½ cup) rolled (porridge) oats (or
   quinoa flakes if gluten-free)
1 egg, whisked
½ teaspoon baking powder
⅛ teaspoon salt
45 g (1⅔ oz/⅓ cup) dark chocolate chips
   (or chopped good-quality dark chocolate)

Preheat the oven to 180°C (350°F). Line a baking tray with baking paper.

Place all of the ingredients except the chocolate in a large mixing bowl and combine well with a fork. Add the chocolate chips and stir through the mixture—it should be nice and sticky, so the cookies will turn out light and airy.

Spoon tablespoon-sized balls of the mixture onto the baking tray and slightly flatten with the back of the spoon. Bake for 10–15 minutes, or until golden.

Cool on the tray for 5 minutes before transferring to a wire rack. Store in an airtight container for up to 5 days.

PISTACHIO, GOJI BERRY AND SWEET POTATO BROWNIES

MAKES 8
PREP TIME 5 minutes
COOK TIME 20 minutes

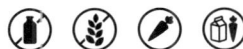

200 g (7 oz) sweet potato, diced
150 g (5½ oz) medjool dates, pitted
40 g (1½ oz) almond meal
2 tablespoons raw cacao powder
pinch salt
1 tablespoon coconut oil, melted
1 tablespoon maple syrup
2 tablespoons goji berries
2 tablespoons pistachio nut kernels
50 g (1¾ oz) vegan dark chocolate (70%)

Preheat the oven to 180°C (350°F) and line a square 20 cm (8 inch) baking tin with baking paper.

Bring a saucepan of water to the boil and steam the sweet potato for 10 minutes, or until softened. Allow to cool, then tip into a food processor and purée with the dates until you have a smooth paste.

Add all of the remaining ingredients except the chocolate to the food processor and blitz a few times to combine.

Spoon the mixture into the prepared tin, smoothing the surface with the back of a spoon, and bake for 20 minutes, or until a toothpick inserted in the centre comes out clean. Cool completely before cutting into eight.

Melt the chocolate in a heatproof bowl and microwave for 30 seconds at a time, stirring after each time, until melted and smooth. Alternatively, use the double-boiler method on page 73.

Drizzle the melted chocolate over the brownies and allow to set for a few minutes. Slice into squares, then store in an airtight container in the fridge for up to 5 days.

CHUNKY CHOCOLATE BLISS BALLS

MAKES 14
PREP TIME 20 minutes

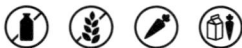

160 g (5⅔ oz) pitted medjool dates
70 g (2½ oz/⅔ cup) rolled (porridge) oats
(use brown rice flakes or quinoa flakes
if gluten free)
3 tablespoons crunchy natural peanut butter
45 g (1⅔ oz) vegan dark chocolate (70%),
coarsely chopped
1 tablespoon chia seeds

FOR ROLLING
20 g (¾ oz) coarsely chopped walnuts

Place the dates in a bowl, cover with boiling water and set aside to soften for 10 minutes. Line a baking tray with baking paper.

Drain the soaked dates then pulse in a food processor to form a ball.

Add the oats, peanut butter, chocolate and chia seeds to the food processor, and pulse in bursts until the mixture is just combined. DO NOT overmix; you want texture.

Roll tablespoons of the mixture into balls, then roll these in the walnuts to coat. Place on the lined tray and freeze for 15 minutes, then store in the fridge in an airtight container, or freeze for up to 3 months.

PEANUT BUTTER OAT BARS

MAKES 12
PREP TIME 20 minutes
COOK TIME 2 minutes

80 g (2¾ oz/½ cup) pitted medjool dates
100 g (3½ oz/1 cup) rolled (porridge) oats (use
brown rice or quinoa flakes if gluten-free)
90 g (3¼ oz/⅓ cup) peanut butter
1 ripe banana
50 g (1¾ oz) butter, melted
30 g (1 oz) dark chocolate (70%)

Line a rectangular baking tin with baking paper.

Place all of the ingredients except the chocolate in a food processor and blitz until the mixture comes together, scraping down the side as you go. The mixture should stick together when pressed with your hands. If the mixture is too dry, add water a teaspoon at a time. If it's too wet, add an extra tablespoon of oats.

Transfer the mixture to the prepared tin and press down gently so it's evenly spread out.

Place in the freezer for at least 1 hour to set. Once set, remove from the freezer.

Roughly chop the chocolate and place in a heatproof bowl. Microwave for 30 seconds at a time, stirring after each time, until melted and smooth. Alternatively, use the double-boiler method on page 73.

Drizzle the chocolate all over the chilled mixture and return to the freezer for a few minutes to set.

Once the chocolate has set, carefully remove from the tin and slice into 12 bars. Store in an airtight container in the fridge for up to 5 days.

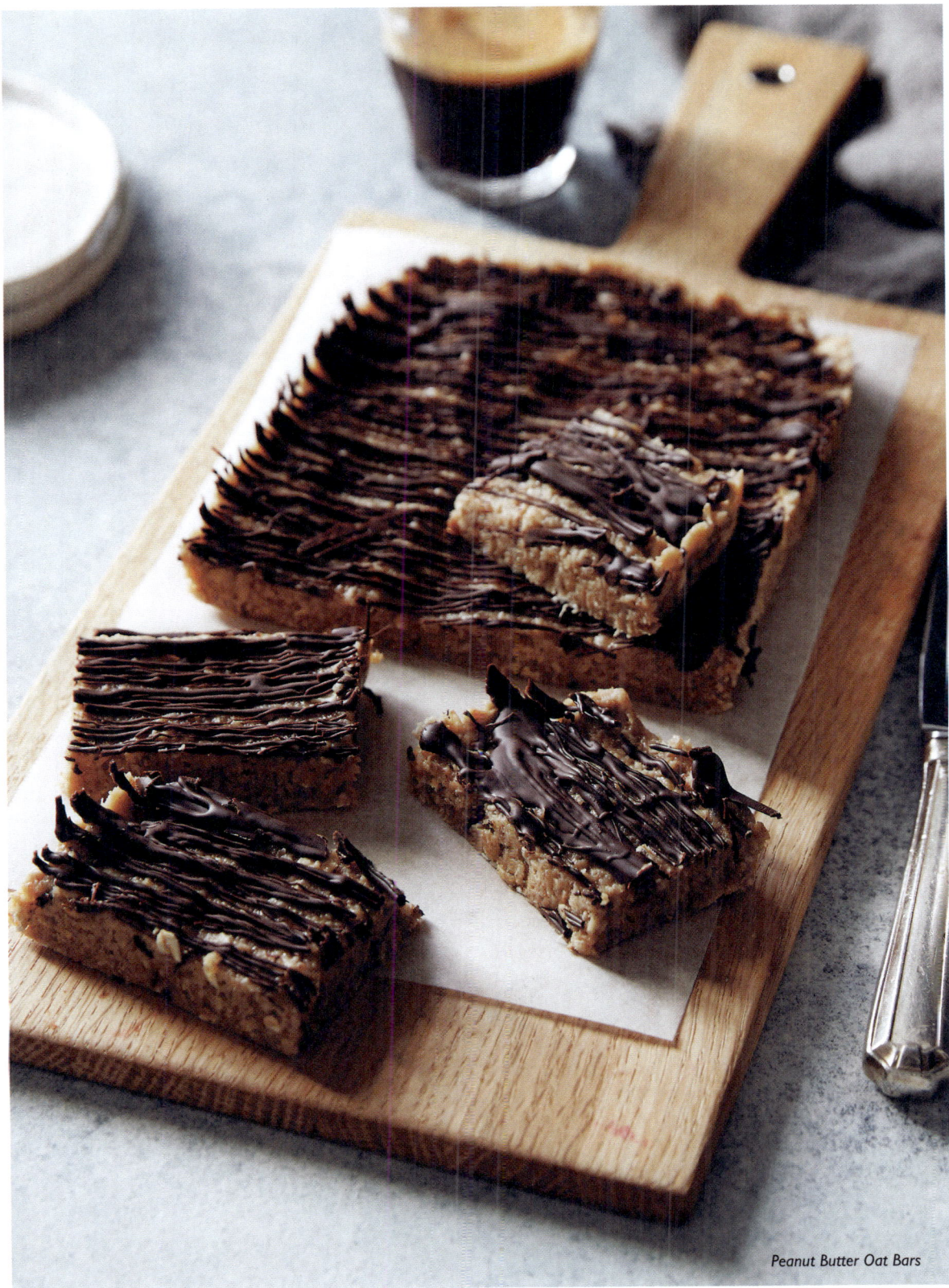

Peanut Butter Oat Bars

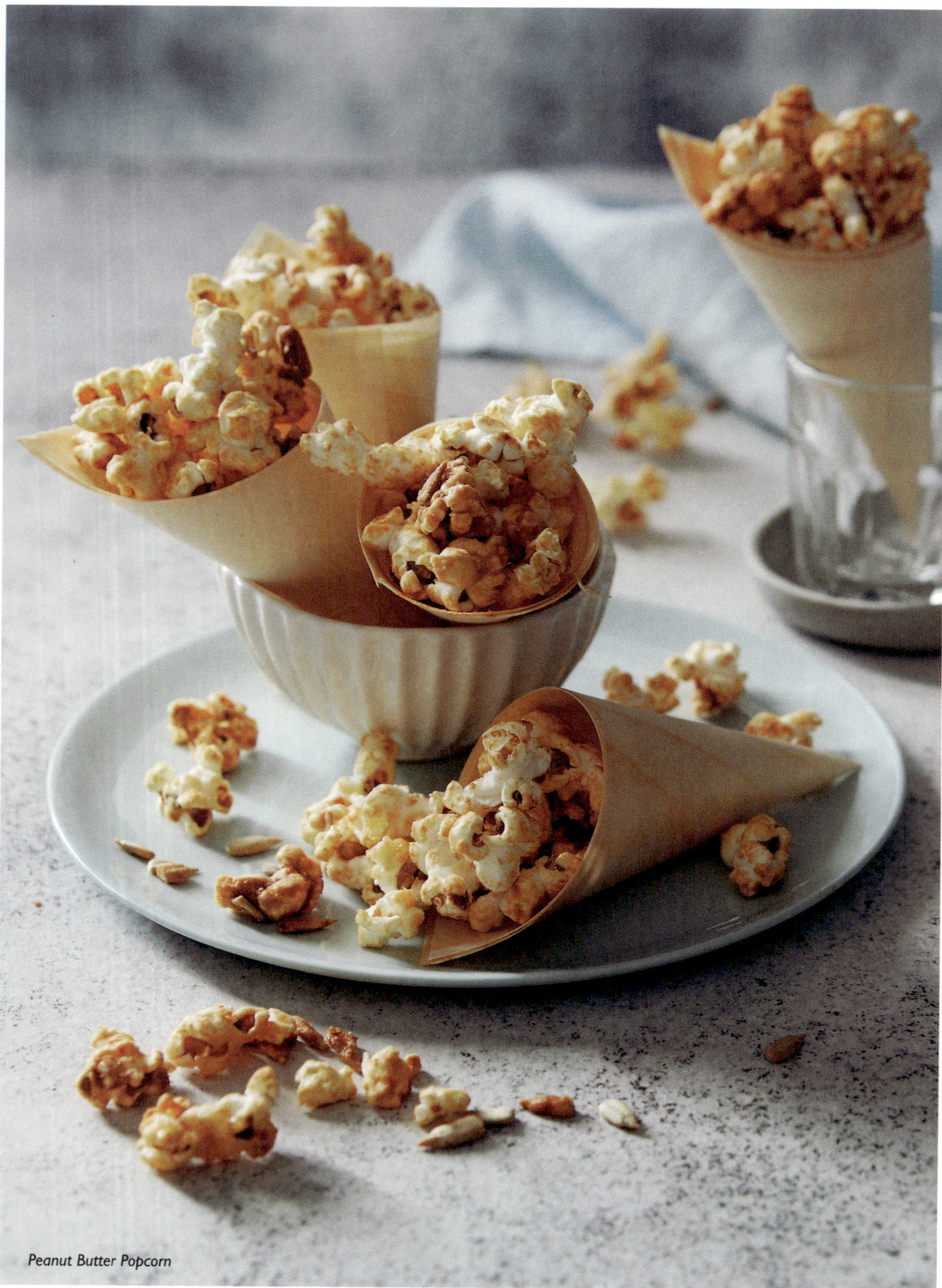

Peanut Butter Popcorn

PEANUT BUTTER POPCORN

SERVES 12
PREP TIME 5 minutes
COOK TIME 15 minutes

1 tablespoon olive oil
115 g (4 oz/½ cup) popping corn
140 g (5 oz/½ cup) natural, crunchy peanut
   butter
90 g (3¼ oz/¼ cup) honey
40 g (1½ oz/¼ cup) sunflower seeds
¼ teaspoon salt

Preheat the oven to 180°C (350°F) and line a baking tray with baking paper.

Heat the oil in a medium saucepan over medium–high heat. Add the popcorn, then cover and cook for a few minutes, shaking constantly to prevent burning until the corn stops popping. (Warning, don't be tempted to take a sneak peek until after the popping stops!)

Combine the rest of the ingredients in a large bowl and mix until well combined, then tip the hot popcorn into the bowl, and fold it through the flavours until well coated.

Transfer to the prepared baking tray and spread out to a thin layer. Bake for 10 minutes, or until golden. Cool slightly before serving.

GRILLED PEACHES WITH VANILLA YOGHURT

SERVES 2
PREP TIME 5 minutes
COOK TIME 10 minutes

2 peaches, halved, stones removed
20 g (¾ oz) walnuts, coarsely chopped
1 vanilla bean, split lengthways
95 g (3¼ oz/⅓ cup) Greek-style yoghurt
1 teaspoon honey

Preheat the oven grill to medium.

Place the peach halves, cut side up, on a roasting tray and grill for 10 minutes, or until beginning to soften.

Meanwhile, add the walnuts to the tray and cook for 2 minutes until slightly roasted.

Scrape the seeds from the vanilla bean and stir these through the yoghurt.

Place two peach halves on each plate, drizzle with honey, scatter over the walnuts and serve with the vanilla yoghurt.

Grazing is the enemy of efficient, effective snacking.

ROASTED BEETROOT CRISPS WITH TZATZIKI

SERVES 4
PREP TIME 10 minutes
COOK TIME 20 minutes

2 large beetroot (beets), thinly sliced
2 teaspoons olive oil
salt and pepper

TZATZIKI
1 Lebanese (short) cucumber, seeds removed,
   grated
260 g (9¼ oz/1 cup) Greek-style yoghurt
1 tablespoon lemon juice
1 garlic clove, crushed
2 mint sprigs, finely chopped

Preheat the oven to 200°C (400°F) and line a baking tray with baking paper.

Place the beetroot slices in a bowl, toss with oil, salt and pepper. Spread around the prepared tray and bake for 20 minutes, or until crisp. Remove from the oven and leave to cool.

Meanwhile, squeeze any liquid out of the grated cucumber before combining with the yoghurt, lemon juice, garlic and mint in a bowl to make the tzatziki. Season to your liking.

Serve the tzatziki with beetroot crisps.

BABA GHANOUSH

SERVES 4
PREP TIME 10 minutes
COOK TIME 45 minutes

2 eggplants (aubergines)
2 garlic cloves, unpeeled
2 wholegrain (or gluten-free) pitta breads
1 teaspoon sesame oil
salt and pepper
1 teaspoon sesame seeds
¼ teaspoon ground cumin
130 g (4½ oz/½ cup) Greek-style yoghurt
2 tablespoons tahini
2 tablespoons lemon juice
¼ teaspoon smoked paprika

Preheat the oven to 220°C (425°F) and line two baking trays with baking paper.

Pierce each eggplant a few times with a fork and transfer to the baking tray with the whole garlic cloves. Place in the oven and roast for 20 minutes. Remove the garlic from the tray and continue to roast the eggplant for another 25 minutes, or until completely soft. Remove from the oven and set aside to cool slightly.

Meanwhile, cut the pitta breads into triangles and spread these out on the other baking tray. Brush with the sesame oil, season with salt, and sprinkle with sesame seeds and the cumin. Bake for 8–10 minutes, or until lightly golden and crisp. Cool completely.

Gently slice each eggplant open and scoop the flesh out of the skin. Place in a blender or food processor. Squeeze the roasted garlic out of its skin and add to the food processor with the yoghurt, tahini and lemon juice. Blend until smooth. Taste and adjust seasonings, if needed.

Transfer to a serving bowl, sprinkle over some paprika and serve with pitta crisps. Any remaining dip can be kept covered in the fridge for up to 3 days, and leftover pitta crisps can be stored in an airtight container for up to 3 days.

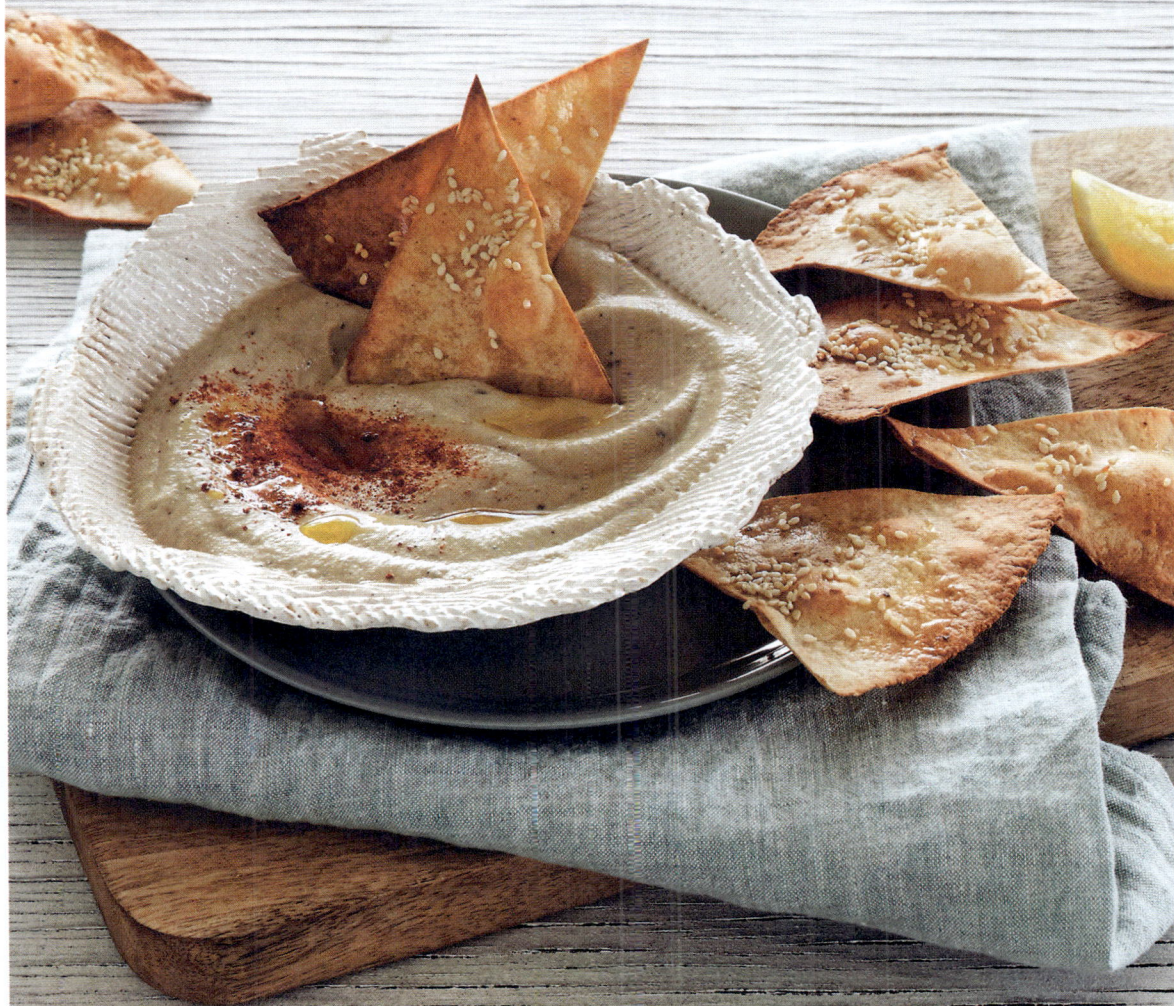

Baba Ghanoush

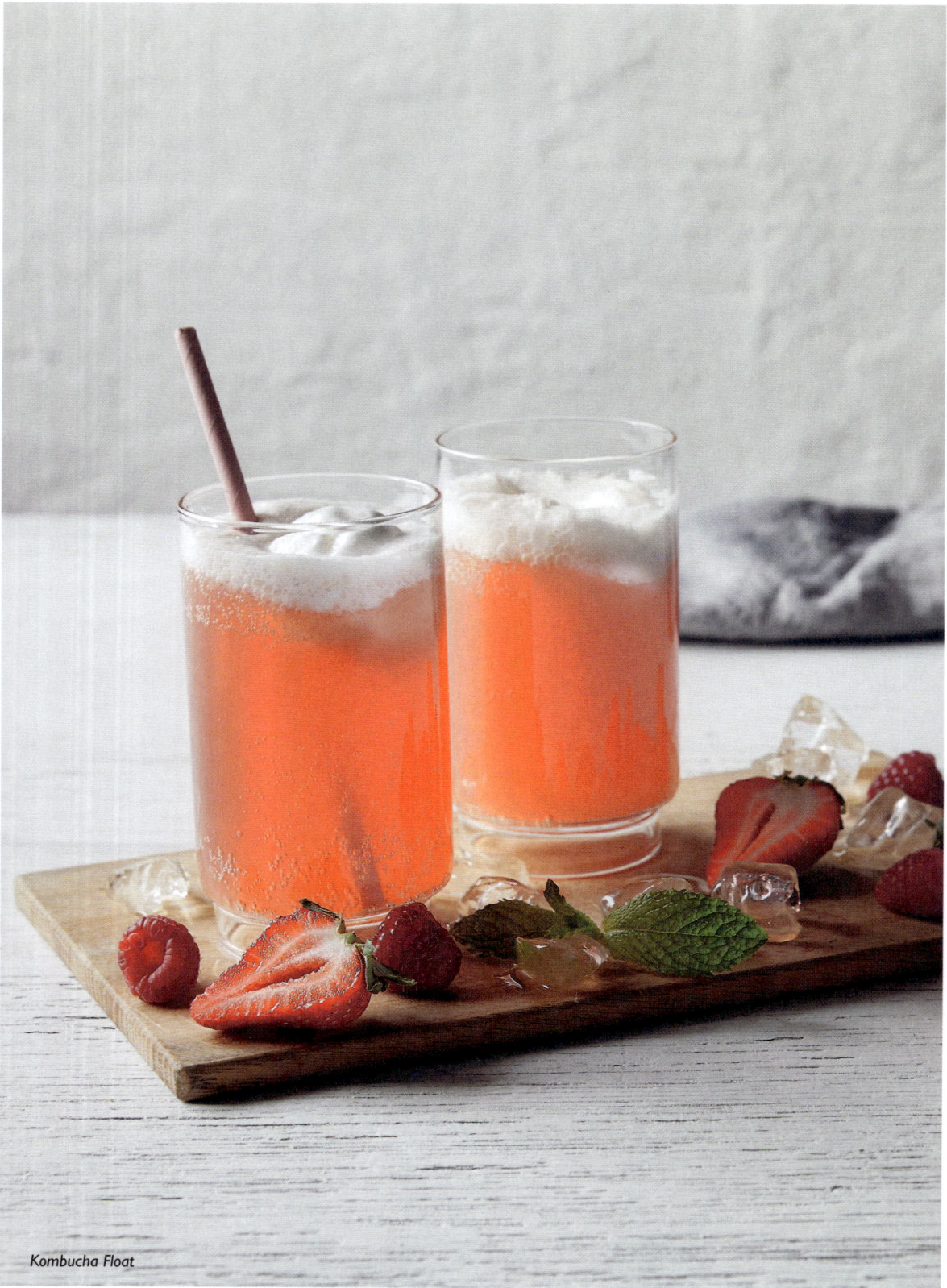

Kombucha Float

KOMBUCHA FLOAT

SERVES 1
PREP TIME 5 minutes

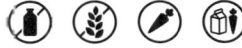

300 ml (10½ fl oz) kombucha (I like a berry-
    flavoured kombucha for this)
1 scoop (60 g/2¼ oz) vanilla or non-dairy
    coconut ice cream
1 mint sprig, leaves picked

Pour the kombucha into a large glass and top with
the ice cream and mint leaves. Serve immediately.

BANANA–NUT SOFT SERVE

SERVES 2
PREP TIME 5 minutes

1 small banana, sliced and frozen
2 tablespoons nut butter of your choice

Combine the ingredients in a small food
processor and blitz until smooth.

SOS, NO-COOK & PORTABLE SNACKS

LIFE-SAVERS

These portable, life-saving snacks will lift you out of your funk, clear out the fog and carry you through to your next meal.

Sometimes, you need a snack, STAT!

Imagine being told you're not snacking enough? (Sounds like a dream to me.) If you're overhauling your lifestyle or simply trying to reduce your daily energy intake, you could be cutting out too much food. And, just like overeating, undereating also has a negative impact on our physical and mental health.

All of us have those days when we're rushed off our feet; and when you're chasing a deadline or taking care of kids or other important stuff, it's easy to miss a meal and keep going until you suddenly realise you're running on empty. Nourishing your body with fresh fruit and veg, healthy fats, lean protein, wholegrains and processed-free snacks is the best way you can support yourself. It helps you to feel energised, focused and satisfied. So if you're feeling a little 'blergh', you may need to up your snack game. And if you're a new mum, I've got some great suggestions for you on page 117.

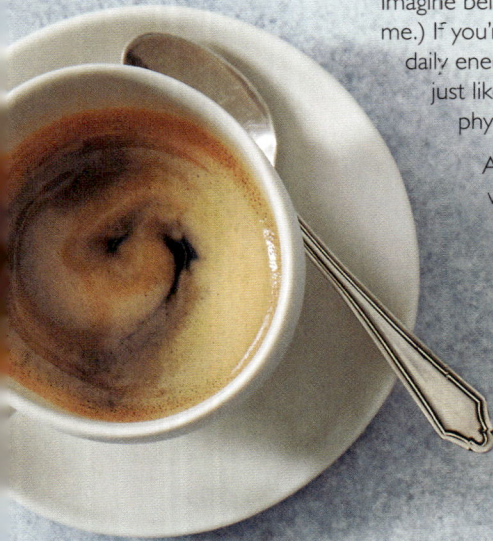

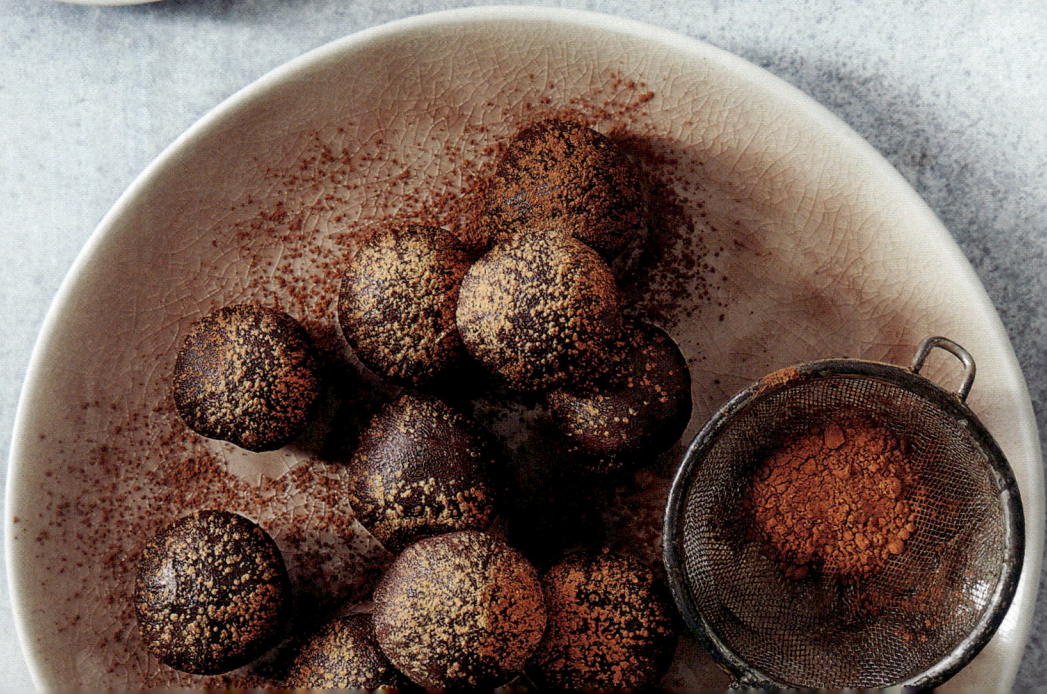

6 SIGNS YOU NEED TO EAT

1. BRAIN FOG

Have you ever looked for your phone only to realise it's in your pocket? Classic brain fog, and a sign that your energy levels are low. You need a snack!

2. INCREASED EXERCISE

If you're training frequently, you may need to increase your protein intake to give your body the building blocks it needs to build new lean muscle tissue. Well, guess what? I've dedicated a whole chapter to post-workout snacks! Goals! Go have a protein rich snack!

3. IRRITABLE AND MOODY

Road rage? Easily irritated? Could burst into tears any second? When your blood sugar drops, this can affect your mood. You may need a tiny bite for a slow and sustained release of insulin, which will bring on a rise in one of your mood's biggest players: serotonin. You need a snack!

4. DIZZINESS

Feel faint if you stand up too quickly? When you don't eat enough, your blood sugar can drop making you feel dizzy (and maybe queasy, too). Dizziness can also mean you're dehydrated, so up your water intake, and you need a snack!

5. ALWAYS HUNGRY

Hello! Ravenous between meals? Perhaps you're not timing your food well throughout the day and need to work in more little snacks. But upping your snacks isn't always about quantity; the quality of what you eat is important. Ditch sugary and salty snacks. You need a protein-based snack!

6. ZERO ENERGY

Pressing snooze, drinking endless cups of coffee and lacking the motivation or get up and go to exercise? Your tank is empty. You're not getting the right nutrients from wholesome fresh food and your body is depleted. You need a snack!

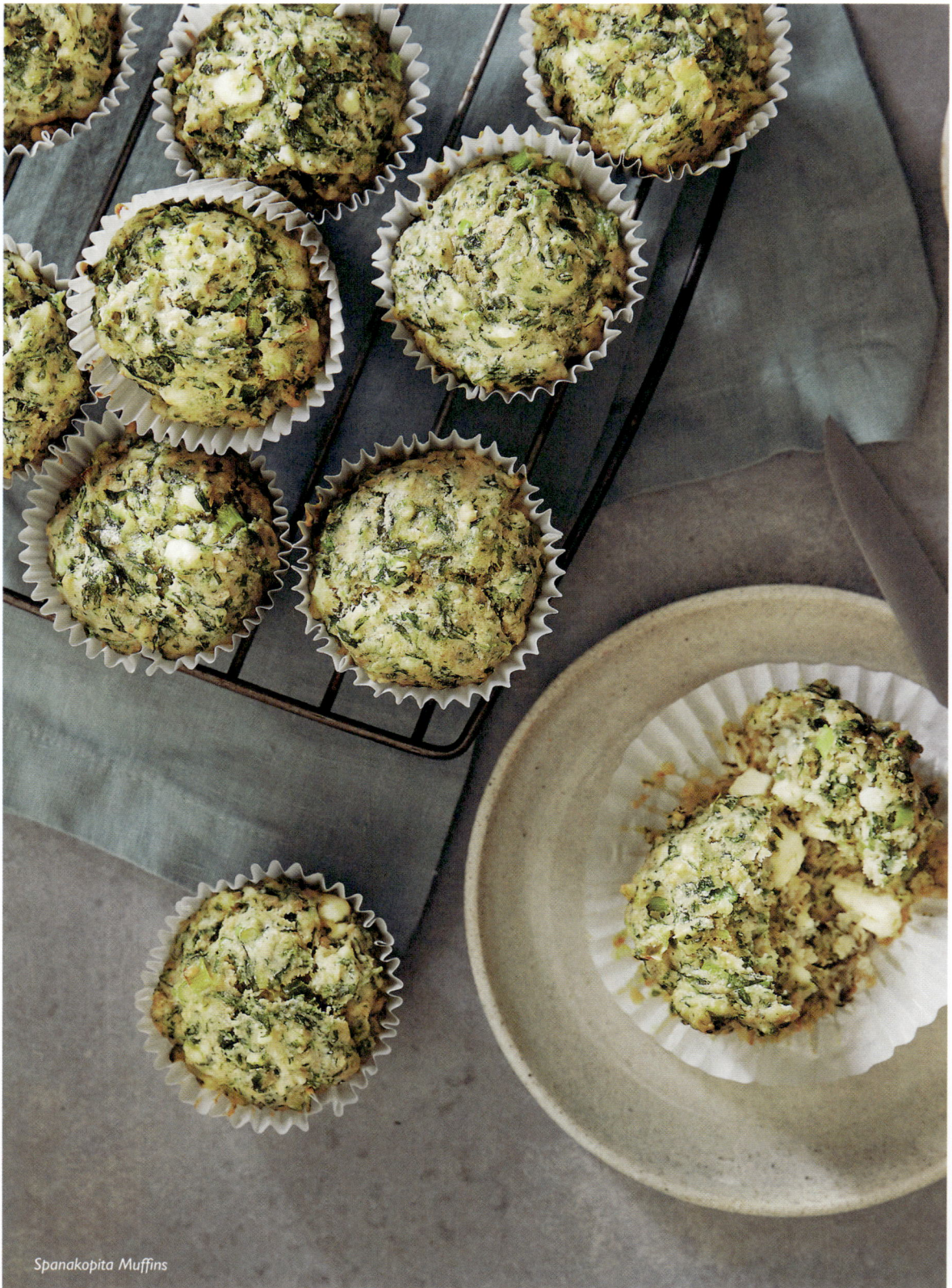

Spanakopita Muffins

SPANAKOPITA MUFFINS

MAKES 12
PREP TIME 10 minutes
COOK TIME 25 minutes

150 ml (5 fl oz) olive oil
120 g (4¼ oz/1 cup) finely chopped spring onions
   (scallions)
2 teaspoons dried oregano
250 g (9 oz) frozen spinach, defrosted and excess
   water squeezed out
300 g (10½ oz/2 cups) wholemeal (whole-wheat)
   flour (or gluten-free if needed)
200 g (7 oz) feta cheese, crumbled
185 ml (6 fl oz/¾ cup) milk
3 eggs, whisked
black pepper

Preheat the oven to 200°C (400°F) and line a
12-hole standard (60 ml/¼ cup) muffin tin with
paper cases.

Heat 60 ml (2 fl oz/¼ cup) of oil in a saucepan
and sauté the spring onions, oregano and spinach
for 2 minutes. Stir through the remaining oil.

Combine the spinach mixture and flour in a large
bowl. Stir through the feta, milk and eggs until just
combined, then sprinkle with pepper.

Spoon the mixture into the paper cases and
bake for 20–25 minutes, or until golden and a
toothpick inserted in one of the muffins comes
out clean.

Serve warm. Any remaining muffins can be stored
in an airtight container in the fridge for up to
3 days or frozen for up to 3 months.

MATCHA, CASHEW AND PISTACHIO BALLS

MAKES 8
PREP TIME 5 minutes

3 medjool dates, pitted
80 g (2¾ oz/½ cup) raw cashew nuts
45 g (1⅔ oz/½ cup) desiccated coconut
20 g (¾ oz) pistachio kernels
2 tablespoons rice malt syrup
¼ teaspoon matcha powder
¼ teaspoon ground cinnamon
pinch of salt

Place all the ingredients in a food processor and
blend until a coarse mixture forms.

Add 2–4 teaspoons of water and continue to
blend until the mixture is a sticky consistency.

Roll into eight tablespoon-sized balls and place
on a plate in the freezer for 2 hours. Store in an
airtight container in the fridge or freezer.

SALTED EDAMAME BEANS

SERVES 2
PREP TIME 5 minutes
COOK TIME 5 minutes

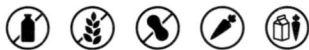

300 g (10½ oz) edamame (soya beans), podded
   (thawed if frozen)
1¼ tablespoons salt

Bring 1.5 litres (52 fl oz/6 cups) water to the boil
in a very large saucepan with 1 tablespoon of salt.
Add the beans and simmer for 5 minutes.

Drain, and sprinkle with the remaining salt to
serve warm or chilled.

RYE CRISPBREADS WITH AVOCADO, RICOTTA AND TOMATO

SERVES 1
PREP TIME 5 minutes

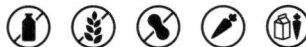

⅛ avocado, mashed
2 rye crispbreads
1 tablespoon ricotta cheese
6 cherry tomatoes, halved
10 g (¼ oz) rocket leaves

Spread the mashed avocado on the crispbreads.
Top with the ricotta, cherry tomatoes and rocket.

MISO SOUP WITH TOFU

SERVES 1
PREP TIME 5 minutes

2 teaspoons white miso paste
50 g (1¾ oz) silken tofu, diced into
   1 cm (½ inch) pieces
1 spring onion (scallion), green part only,
   thinly sliced
1 teaspoon mirin
250 ml (9 fl oz/1 cup) boiling water

Gently combine all of the ingredients in a bowl
and enjoy.

PEACH AND PISTACHIO SNACK CUP

SERVES 2
PREP TIME 10 minutes

260 g (9¼ oz/1 cup) plain yoghurt
½ yellow peach, stone removed, flesh sliced
1 teaspoon maple syrup
1 tablespoon pistachio nut kernels, coarsely
   chopped
50 g (1¾ oz) fresh or frozen cherries

Divide the yoghurt between two small bowls and top with peach slices.

Drizzle over the maple syrup and top with pistachios and cherries to serve.

PEACH AND RICOTTA TOAST WITH BASIL

SERVES 2
PREP TIME 5 minutes
COOK TIME 5 minutes

30 g (1 oz) ricotta cheese
2 slices wholemeal (whole-wheat) sourdough
   bread (or gluten-free bread), toasted
½ yellow peach, thinly sliced
20 g (¾ oz) walnuts, chopped
2 basil sprigs, leaves picked
½ teaspoon chia seeds

Spread the ricotta onto the slices of toasted bread and top each with peach slices.

Garnish with walnuts, basil leaves and chia seeds, then serve.

10 easy, nourishing snack ideas for new mums

Mums all around the world, I salute you! I've always looked up to my mum, but it wasn't until I became a mother myself that my respect for mothers, and anyone who looks after children, took on a whole new meaning. If there's ever an occasion for SOS snacking, new parenthood is it. We're not thinking 'nutritional value' when we're wrecked and sleep-deprived looking after bubs. One of the best ways to look after your baby is to look after yourself. The snacks in this chapter are quick and easy go-tos, as are any of the recipes on the list below. These are some of my favourite nutrient-dense snacks to help keep your energy high, hormones balanced and to have you sleeping (when you can!) like a baby.

Banana and Chia Snack Smoothie page 53
Mini Mushroom Frittatas page 64
Strawberry Cacao Chia Pudding page 73
Wholegrain Toast with Ricotta and Sprouts page 78
Spanakopita Muffins page 115
Smoked Salmon Roulade page 126
Peanut Butter Banana with Toasted Coconut page 153
Cheesy Broccoli Quinoa Bites page 168

HONEY AND SESAME ROASTED CHICKPEAS

SERVES 2
PREP TIME 10 minutes
COOK TIME 30 minutes

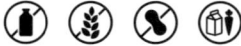

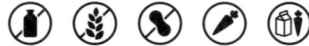

400 g (14 oz) tinned chickpeas, drained
   and rinsed
1 teaspoon honey
1 teaspoon sesame oil
2 teaspoons sesame seeds

Preheat the oven to 210°C (410°F) and line a baking tray with baking paper.

Pat the chickpeas dry with paper towel.

Combine the honey and oil in a large mixing bowl, then add the chickpeas and stir to coat completely.

Spread the chickpeas onto the prepared baking tray, sprinkle with the sesame seeds and bake for 20–30 minutes. The chickpeas can be served straight from the oven, or kept for up to 7 days in an airtight container.

HUMMUS WITH TOASTED PITTA BREAD

SERVES 2
PREP TIME 5 minutes
COOK TIME 3 minutes

1 wholemeal (whole-wheat) pitta
   bread (or gluten-free bread), cut into triangles
75 g (2⅔ oz/⅓ cup) hummus
1 flat-leaf (Italian) parsley sprig, chopped
¼ teaspoon ground cumin
1 teaspoon olive oil

Preheat the oven grill to medium–high, and line a baking tray with baking paper.

Place the pitta triangles onto the tray and grill for 1–2 minutes, then remove from the oven, turn over and cook for another 1–2 minutes, until toasted.

Place the hummus in a small bowl, and top with the parsley, cumin and a drizzle of oil. Serve with the pitta bread.

CRISPBREADS WITH CREAM CHEESE AND RADISH

SERVES 1
PREP TIME 5 minutes

2 tablespoons cream cheese
2 rye crispbreads (round or rectangle)
1 radish, thinly sliced
1 tablespoon micro herbs (optional)
salt and pepper

Spread the cream cheese over the crispbreads, top with radish slices and micro herbs, if using, then season to your liking and serve.

CORN THINS WITH RICOTTA, BASIL AND HONEY

SERVES 1
PREP TIME 5 minutes

2 Corn Thins
2 tablespoons ricotta cheese
¼ lemon, zest thinly sliced
1 basil sprig, leaves picked
1 teaspoon honey

Spread the ricotta over the Corn Thins then top with the lemon zest, basil leaves and a drizzle of honey.

Never be hangry again!

My SOS snacks will rescue you like a lifeguard at Bondi Beach. Stash them in your handbag, your desk drawer or in your glovebox.

CUCUMBER ROLLS WITH CREAM CHEESE

SERVES 2
PREP TIME 5 minutes

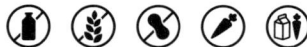

4 tablespoons cream cheese
1 teaspoon lemon juice
1/8 teaspoon chilli flakes
1 garlic clove, crushed
small handful of finely chopped flat-leaf (Italian)
  parsley
salt and pepper
1 telegraph (long) cucumber
1/2 carrot, coarsely grated

Combine the cream cheese, lemon juice, chilli, garlic and parsley in a small bowl and season with salt and pepper. Place in the fridge to chill for 5 minutes.

Using a mandoline or vegetable peeler, slice the cucumber lengthways to make long, thin cucumber ribbons.

Add a tablespoon of the cream cheese mixture to one end of each of the cucumber ribbons and top with grated carrot. Roll up each cucumber ribbon, starting from the end where the cream cheese and carrot is, and serve.

RICE CAKES WITH AVOCADO, TOMATO AND PEPITAS

SERVES 1
PREP TIME 5 minutes

1/4 avocado, mashed
2 rice cakes
1 tomato, sliced
20 g (3/4 oz) rocket
1 teaspoon pepitas (pumpkin seeds), toasted
salt and pepper
juice of 1/4 lemon (optional)

Spread the avocado over the rice cakes, then top with tomato slices, rocket and pepitas.

Season with salt and pepper and squeeze over the lemon juice, if using.

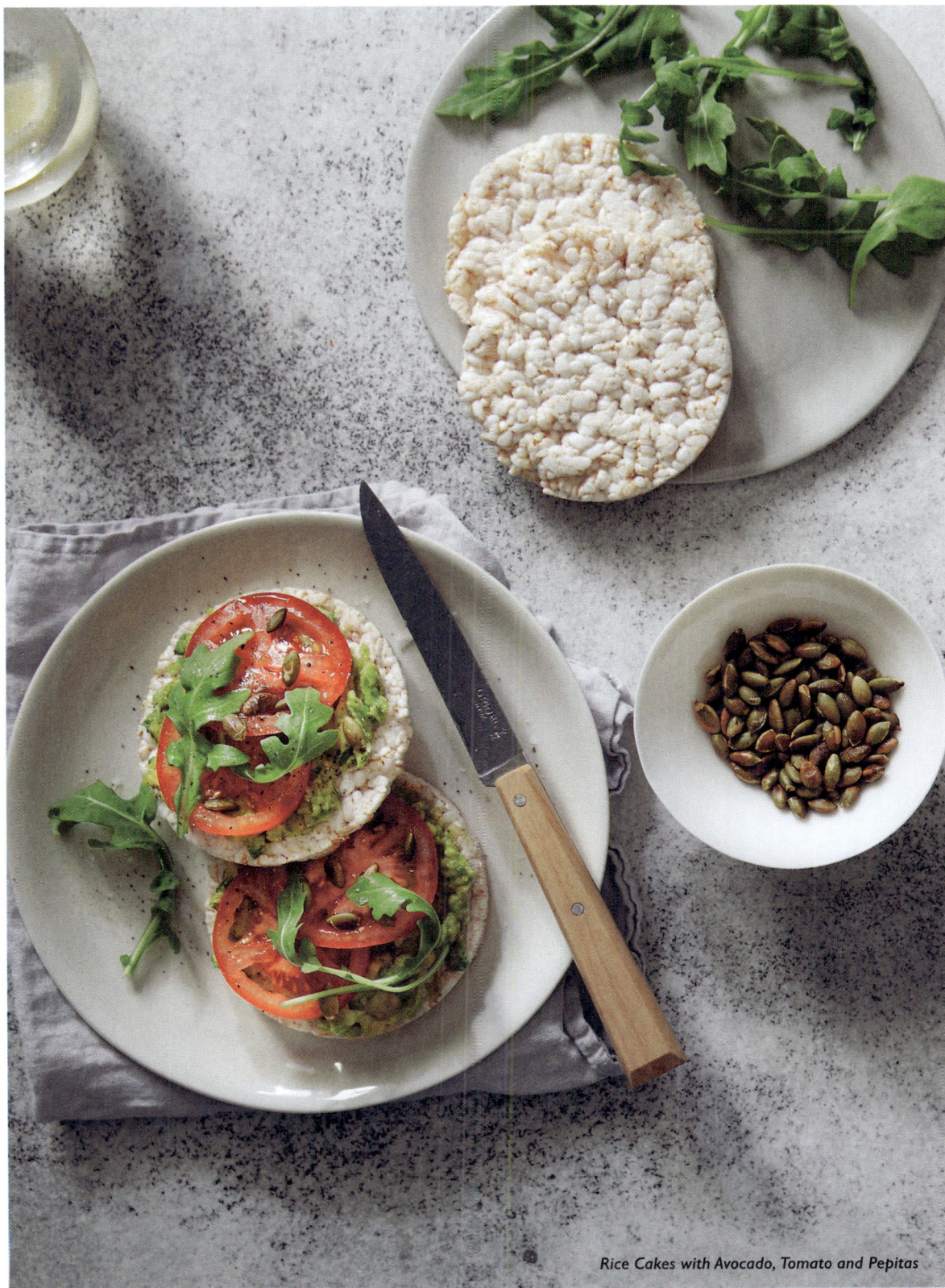

Rice Cakes with Avocado, Tomato and Pepitas

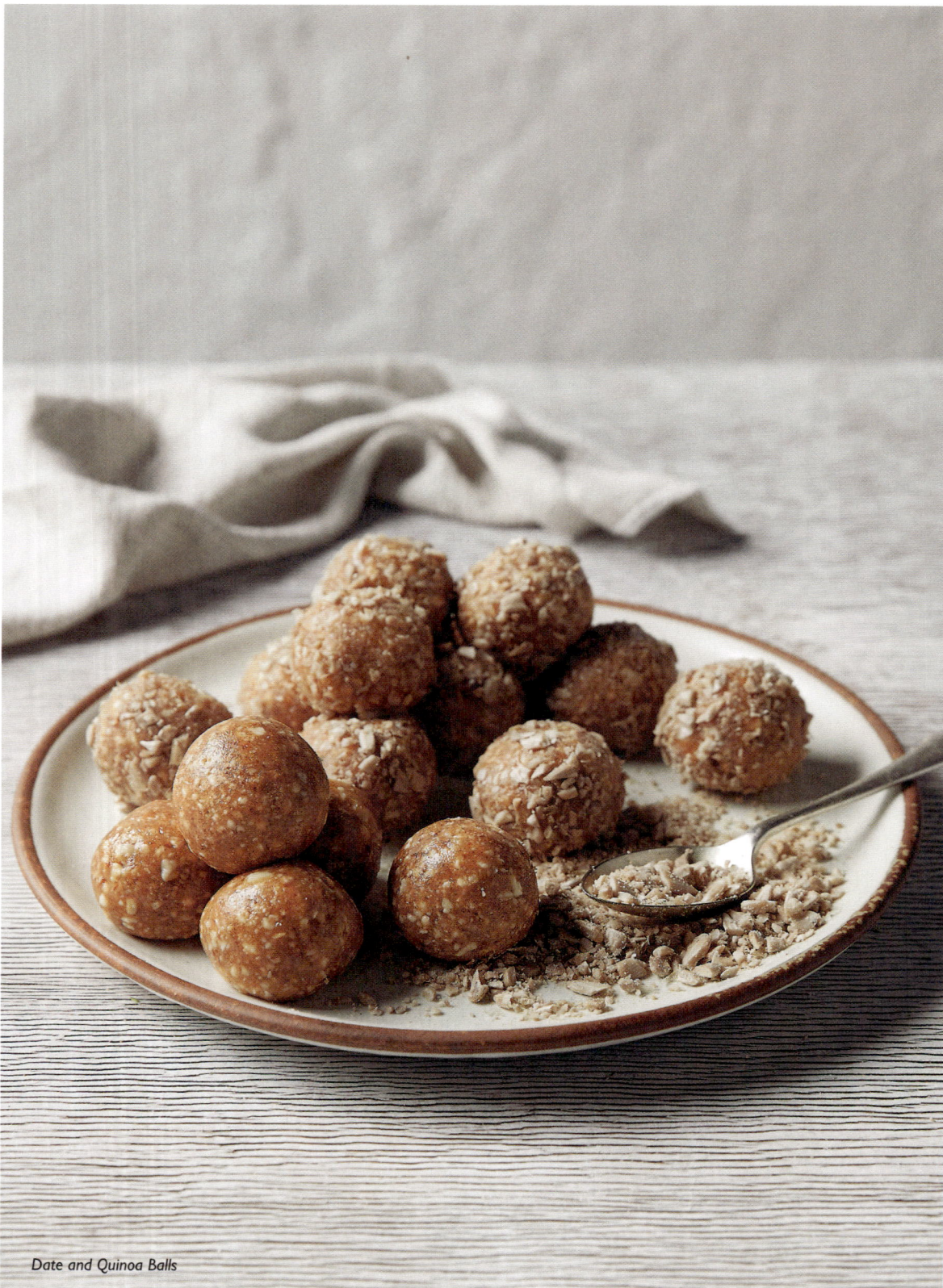

Date and Quinoa Balls

DATE AND QUINOA BALLS

MAKES 18
PREP TIME 15 minutes

40 g (1½ oz/¼ cup) sunflower seeds, for rolling
80 g (2¾ oz/½ cup) pitted medjool dates, chopped
50 g (1¾ oz/½ cup) flaked almonds
30 g (1 oz/½ cup) puffed quinoa (or puffed rice)
80 g (2¾ oz/½ cup) unsalted, roasted cashew nuts
90 g (3¼ oz/¼ cup) honey
65 g (2⅓ oz/¼ cup) tahini

Pulse the sunflower seeds to a fine crumb in a food processor. Put in a bowl and set aside.

Pulse the dates and almonds in the food processor until a fine crumb forms.

Add the puffed quinoa and cashews and, with the motor running, add the honey and tahini and blend until combined and sticky.

With slightly wet hands, roll into tablespoon-sized balls, then roll them in the sunflower seeds until completely coated, and refrigerate for at least 1 hour.

Enjoy with a cup of tea and store in an airtight container in the fridge for up to a week.

HONEY AND ALMOND BLISS BALLS

MAKES 15
PREP TIME 20 minutes
COOK TIME 5 minutes

70 g (2½ oz/⅔ cup) flaked almonds
150 g (5½ oz/1½ cups) almond meal
100 g (3½ oz/⅓ cup) almond butter
90 g (3¼ oz/¼ cup) honey
50 g (1¾ oz) vanilla vegan protein powder
½ teaspoon natural vanilla extract

Preheat the oven to 180°C (350°F).

Place the flaked almonds on a baking tray and bake for 3–4 minutes, or until lightly golden. Cool completely then transfer to a food processor. Pulse the almonds until chopped but not fine. Transfer to a bowl.

Place the almond meal, almond butter, honey, protein powder and vanilla in the food processor and mix well until combined and the mixture holds together when pressed.

Using wet hands, roll tablespoons of the mixture into balls, then roll in the almonds to coat.

Store in an airtight container at room temperature for up to 5 days, or freeze for up to 3 months.

CARROT, DATE AND OAT RAW ENERGY BARS

MAKES 16
PREP TIME 15 minutes

160 g (5⅔ oz/1 cup) almonds
2 tablespoons sunflower seeds
200 g (7 oz) pitted medjool dates
150 g (5½ oz/1½ cups) rolled (porridge) oats
2 teaspoons natural vanilla extract
90 g (3¼ oz/¼ cup) honey
3 tablespoons peanut butter
½ carrot, grated

Line a square 20 cm (8 inch) baking tin with baking paper.

Add the almonds and seeds to a food processor or blender, and blitz until finely chopped.

Add the dates and oats to the food processor and blitz again until combined.

Add all of the remaining ingredients and blitz to combine.

Transfer the mixture to the tin, then smooth and press down with a spatula. Put in the fridge for 2 hours to set, then cut into 16 bars. Store in an airtight container in the fridge for up to 3 days.

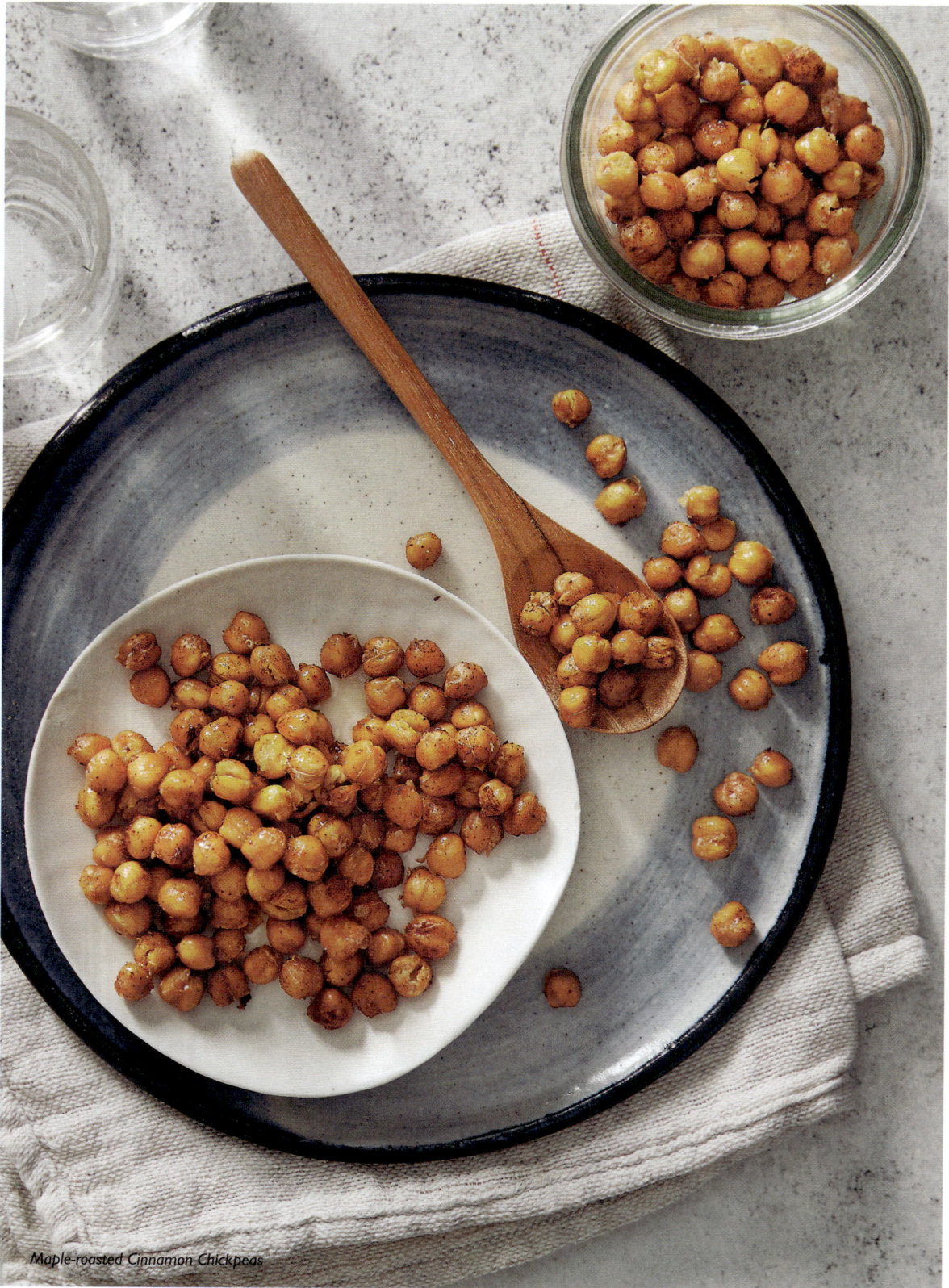

Maple-roasted Cinnamon Chickpeas

MAPLE-ROASTED CINNAMON CHICKPEAS

SERVES 4
PREP TIME 5 minutes
COOK TIME 30 minutes

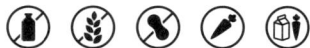

400 g (14 oz) tinned chickpeas,
    drained and rinsed
2 teaspoons olive oil
1 teaspoon maple syrup
¾ teaspoon ground cinnamon
¼ teaspoon salt

Preheat the oven to 200°C (400°F) and line a baking tray with baking paper.

Pat the chickpeas dry with paper towel, then place on the prepared tray and roast for 10 minutes.

Combine the oil, maple syrup, cinnamon and salt in a small bowl. Remove the chickpeas from the oven, drizzle the syrup mixture over them and move the chickpeas around the tray until well coated.

Return the tray to the oven and continue to roast for a further 20–25 minutes, or until golden and crisp.

The chickpeas can be served straight from the oven or kept for up to 7 days in an airtight container.

CHOCOLATE TRAIL MIX

SERVES 2
PREP TIME 5 minutes
COOK TIME 15 minutes

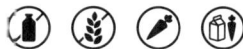

1 teaspoon sesame seeds
1 tablespoon pepitas (pumpkin seeds)
1 teaspoon raw cacao powder or cocoa powder
1 tablespoon flaked almonds
15 g (½ oz/½ cup) puffed brown rice
1 tablespoon maple syrup

Preheat the oven to 160°C (320°F) and line a baking tray with baking paper.

Place all the ingredients in a medium mixing bowl, and stir gently until combined.

Spread the trail mix around the prepared tray and bake for 7 minutes. Remove from the oven, stir and then return to the oven for a further 5 minutes, or until crisp and golden.

Store in an airtight container for up to 7 days.

KIMCHI

SERVES 8
PREP TIME 1 hour 15 minutes

½ wombok (Chinese cabbage), cut into 5 cm
  (2 inch) slices
40 g (1½ oz/⅓ cup) salt
6 garlic cloves
2 cm (¾ inch) piece fresh ginger
4 long red chillies, coarsely chopped
2 tablespoons fish sauce
4 spring onions (scallions), sliced into 5 cm
  (2 inch) lengths

Place the cabbage in a large bowl and sprinkle
with the salt. Add 250 ml (9 fl oz/1 cup) water
and mix well. Cover and set aside for 1 hour.

Transfer the soaked cabbage to a colander and
rinse it under cold water three times. Drain well,
then transfer to a clean glass or ceramic bowl.

Using a mortar and pestle or a food processor,
pound the garlic, ginger and chillies to a paste. Stir
this mixture through the cabbage, along with the
fish sauce and spring onions, mixing well.

Seal in a large glass jar, leaving a gap at the top.
Leave at room temperature to ferment for 3 days,
then store in the fridge for up to 3 months.

SMOKED SALMON ROULADE

SERVES 2
PREP TIME 5 minutes

75 g (2⅔ oz/¼ cup) cottage cheese
½–1 teaspoon horseradish cream (depending
  on your liking)
finely grated zest of ¼ lemon, plus extra for
  garnish
1 teaspoon finely chopped dill, plus extra for
  garnish
1 zucchini (courgette), cut into long ribbons
  (see method for cucumber ribbons on page
  120)
4 slices smoked salmon, cut into long strips
  3 cm (1¼ inch) wide

Place the cottage cheese, horseradish cream,
lemon zest and dill in a small bowl and mix to
combine.

Place the zucchini on a board, lay the salmon on
top and spread the cottage cheese mixture onto
the salmon.

Roll the zucchini and salmon together to form
a roll, and repeat with the other slices of salmon
and zucchini until all ingredients have been used.

Garnish with the extra lemon zest and dill.

It's no-cook time

(AKA you're feeling lazy and don't want to spend time in the kitchen.)

Oven, stove and microwave be gone! If you want something easy and no fuss,
these delicious snacks require minimal effort yet boast maximum flavour.

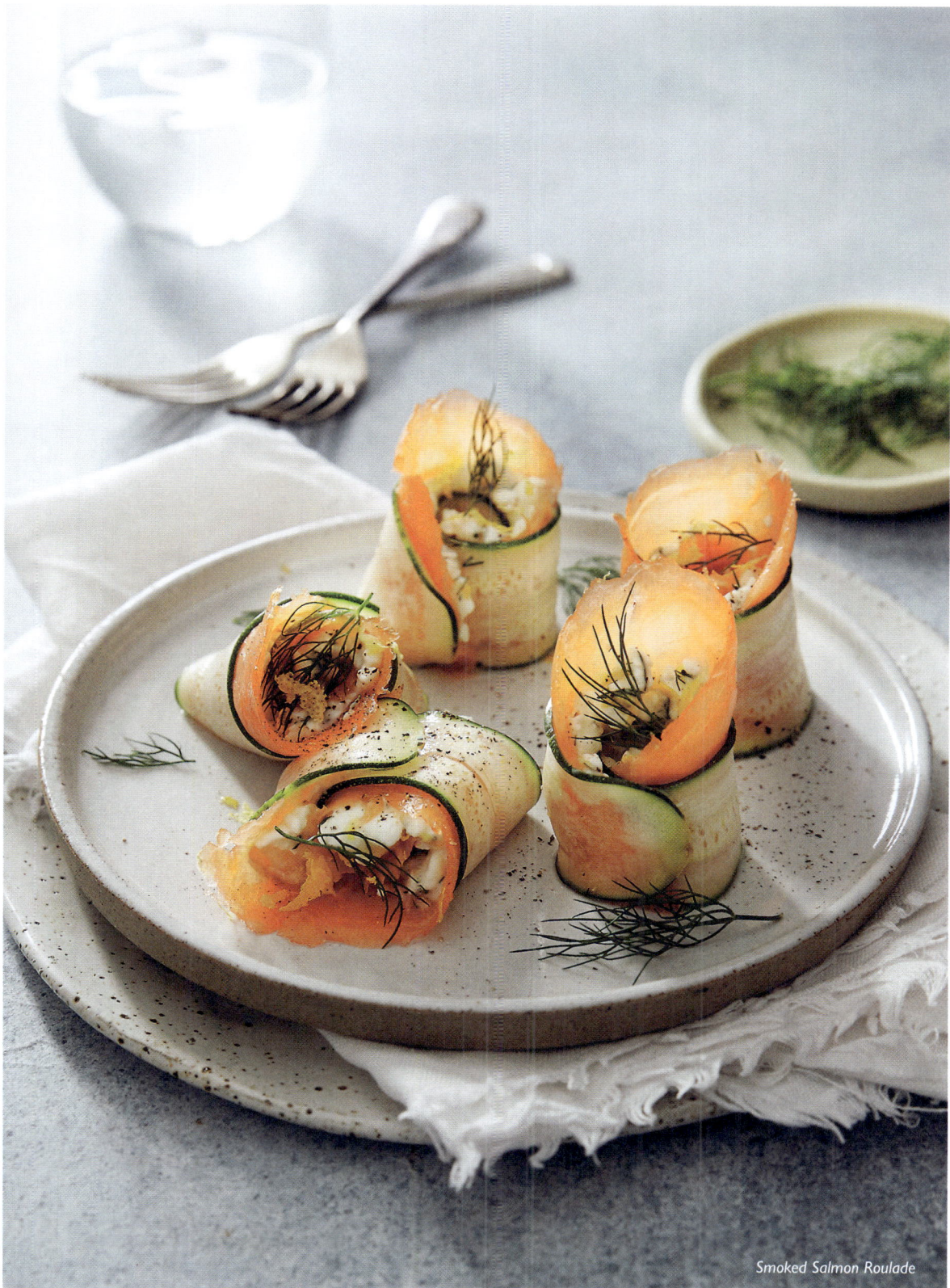

Smoked Salmon Roulade

LAMINGTON WITH RASPBERRY CHIA JAM

MAKES 16
PREP TIME 35 minutes

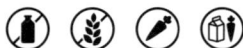

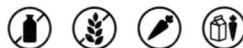

BASE
150 g (5½ oz/1½ cups) almond meal
120 g (4¼ oz/1 cup) coconut flour
65 g (2⅓ oz/¾ cup) desiccated coconut
180 g (6¼ oz/½ cup) rice malt syrup
3 tablespoons coconut oil, melted
1 teaspoon natural vanilla extract

RASPBERRY JAM
125 g (4½ oz/1 cup) frozen raspberries
2 tablespoons chia seeds

TOPPING
1 tablespoon coconut oil, melted
1 tablespoon raw cacao powder
1½ tablespoons desiccated coconut

Line a 20 cm (8 inch) square cake tin with baking paper, leaving some paper overhanging at either end to make removing the slice easy. Lightly grease the areas of the tin on the sides not covered by the baking paper.

Blend all of the base ingredients together in a blender. (The mixture needs to be very firm to hold its shape in the tin, but if it's too firm add ½–1 tablespoon water.)

Press half the mixture into the prepared tin and place in the freezer for 20 minutes.

Blend the raspberries and chia seeds together in a blender until smooth, then pour this mixture over the chilled base and spread evenly.

Gently top with the remaining base mixture and press gently to spread around. Return to the freezer for 10 minutes.

Combine the coconut oil and cacao and spread all over the cake. Sprinkle with the coconut and chill for another 5 minutes before serving.

Cut into 16 slices and store in an airtight container in the fridge for up to 5 days, or freeze for up to 3 months.

RAW CHERRY COCONUT SLICE

MAKES 16
PREP TIME 5 minutes

BASE
65 g (2⅓ oz/1 cup) shredded coconut
160 g (5⅔ oz/1 cup) almonds
150 g (5½ oz/1 cup) frozen, pitted cherries
90 g (3¼ oz/¼ cup) rice malt syrup
2 tablespoons coconut oil
⅛ teaspoon salt

TOPPING
80 g (2¾ oz/⅓ cup) coconut oil, melted
30 g (1 oz/¼ cup) raw cacao powder
90 g (3¼ oz/¼ cup) rice malt syrup

Line a square 20 cm (8 inch) baking tin with baking paper, leaving some paper overhanging at either end to make removing the slice easy. Lightly grease the areas of the tin on the sides not covered by the baking paper.

Put the shredded coconut and almonds into a food processor and blitz to a coarse flour.

Add the cherries, rice malt syrup, coconut oil and salt to the food processor, and pulse again until a sticky mixture is formed. Place this mixture into the prepared tin, and press down firmly until the base is level and compact.

Combine the topping ingredients with a fork in a small bowl until smooth. Pour this mixture all over the slice, and place in the freezer for 2–3 hours. Slice into 16 squares and store in an airtight container in the fridge for up to 5 days, or freeze for up to 3 months.

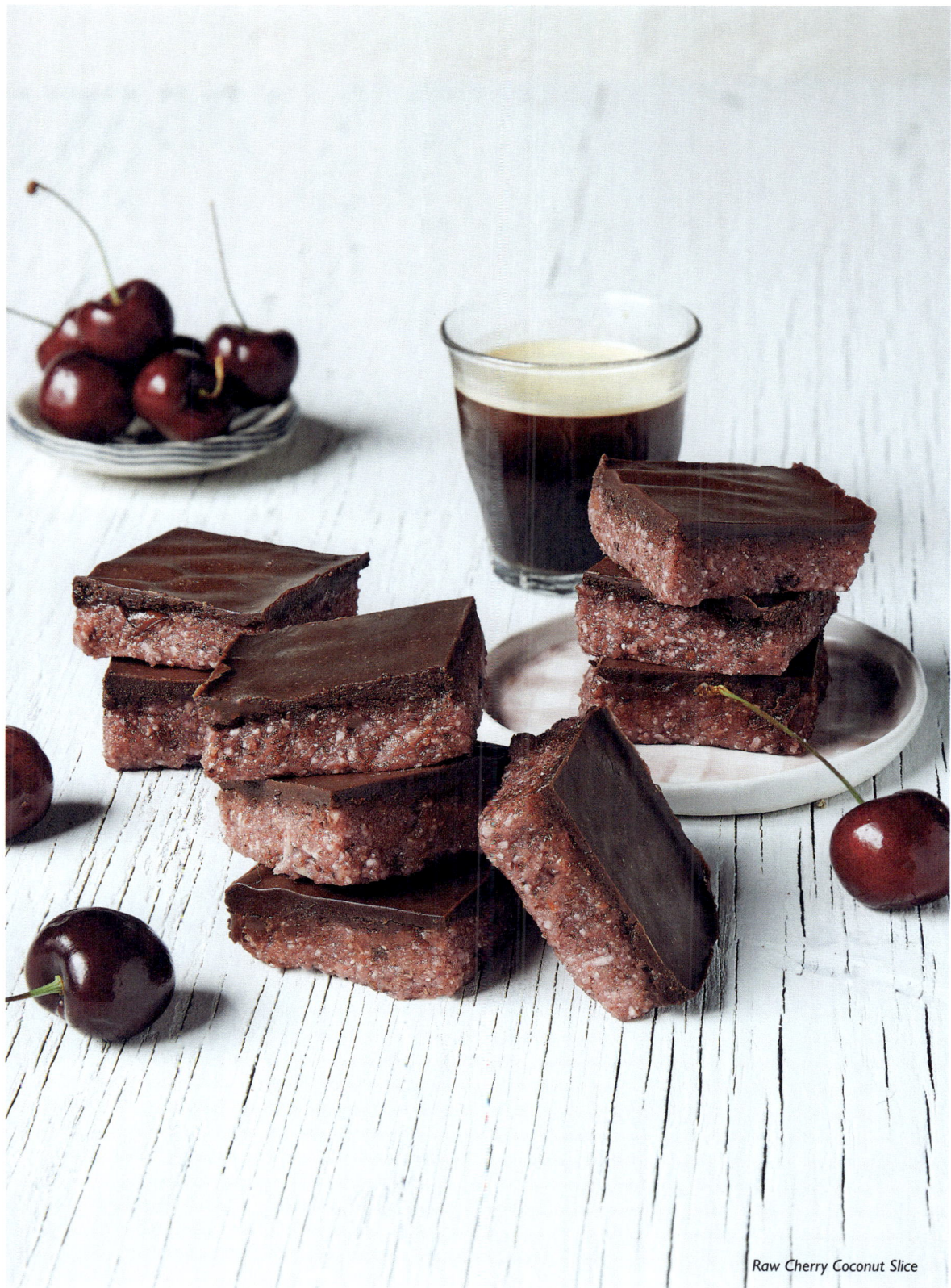

Raw Cherry Coconut Slice

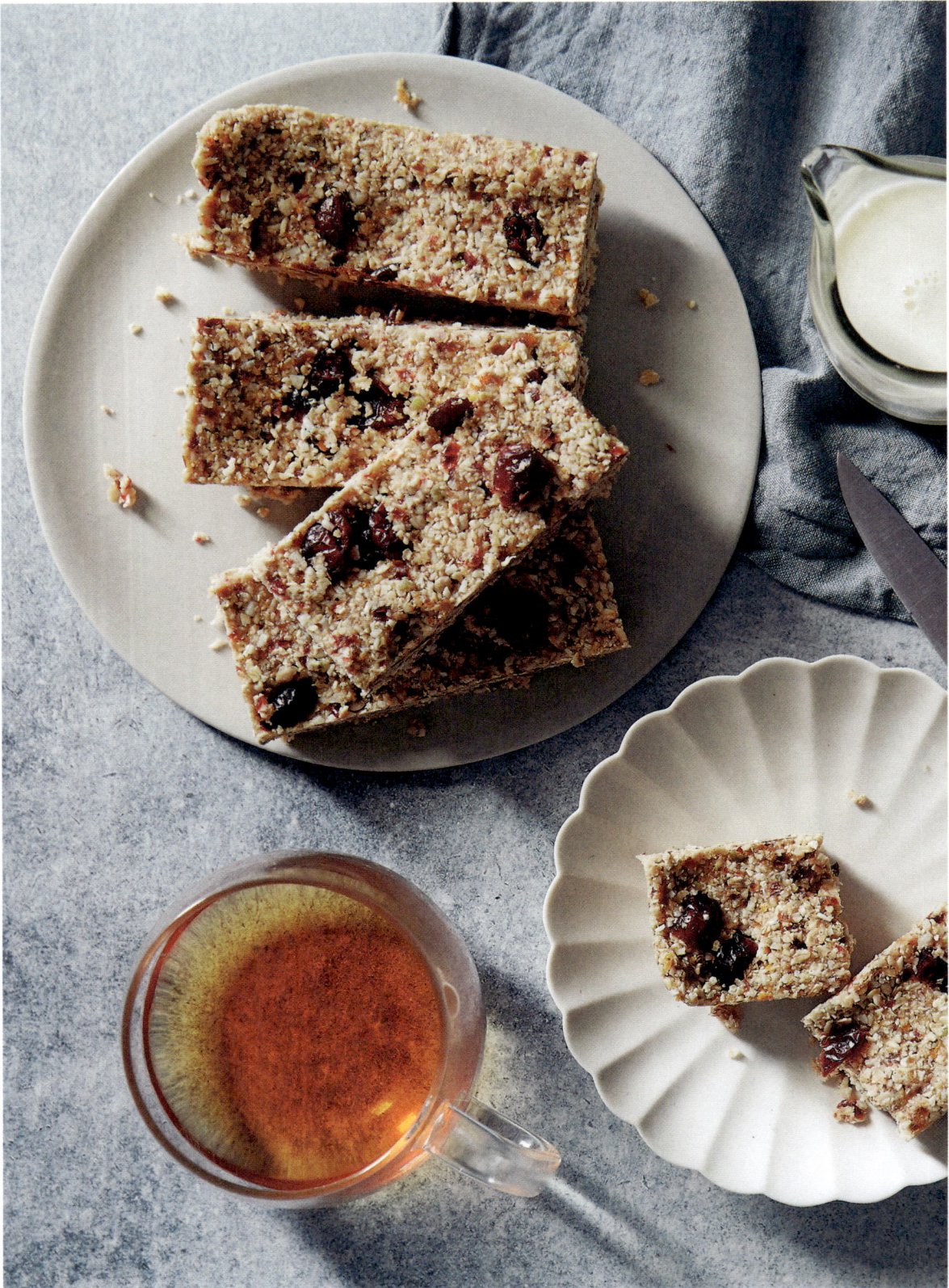

EASY CRANBERRY NO-BAKE BARS

MAKES 20 **PREP TIME** 20 minutes

350 g (12 oz) pitted medjool dates
juice and finely grated zest of
   1 orange
1 tablespoon honey
½ teaspoon ground cinnamon
1 tablespoon protein powder
110 g (3¾ oz) pepitas (pumpkin
   seeds)
40 g (1½ oz) sunflower seeds
250 g (9 oz/2½ cups) rolled
   (porridge) oats
90 g (3¼ oz/1⅓ cups) shredded
   coconut
80 g (2¾ oz) dried cranberries

Line the base and sides of a 30 × 20 cm (12 × 8 inch) baking dish with baking paper, leaving some paper overhanging at either end to make removal easy.

Put the dates, orange juice and zest, honey, cinnamon and protein powder in a food processor and pulse to combine.

Add the pepitas, sunflower seeds, half the oats and 55 g (2 oz/¾ cup) of the coconut to the processor and whizz until the mixture is finely chopped and starts to come together.

Transfer the mixture to a bowl and add the cranberries and remaining oats. Stir until well combined. If the mixture is a little dry, you can add 1 tablespoon water at a time until the desired consistency is reached.

Press the mixture into the prepared dish and sprinkle with the extra coconut. Refrigerate for at least 6 hours, or overnight until firm. Remove the slice from the dish (use the overhanging baking paper to help you do this) and cut into 20 bars. Store in an airtight container in the fridge for up to 5 days, or store in the freezer for up to 3 months.

LEMONY PEA PESTO ON WHOLEMEAL SOURDOUGH TOAST

SERVES 2
PREP TIME 5 minutes
COOK TIME 3 minutes

2 slices wholemeal sourdough bread, toasted

PESTO
75 g (2⅔ oz/½ cup) frozen peas, thawed
1 tablespoon finely grated parmesan cheese
2 teaspoons olive oil
1 mint sprig, leaves picked
small handful of basil leaves, plus a few to serve
½ garlic clove, minced
finely grated zest and juice of ½ lemon
salt and pepper

Blitz all of the pesto ingredients in a food processor until they form a paste. Taste and adjust the seasoning, if needed.

Spread on the toast and top with some basil leaves to serve.

FETA, TOMATO AND BASIL BRUSCHETTA

SERVES 2
PREP TIME 5 minutes
COOK TIME 5 minutes

2 slices sourdough (or gluten-free) bread, toasted
150 g (5½ oz) cherry tomatoes, quartered
30 g (1 oz) feta cheese, diced
2 basil sprigs, leaves picked
extra virgin olive oil
salt and pepper

Top the toast with the tomato, feta, basil, and a drizzle of extra virgin olive oil, then season to serve.

LEMON AND ARTICHOKE DIP

SERVES 8
PREP TIME 5 minutes

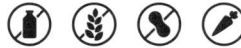

400 g (14 oz) tinned cannellini beans, drained and rinsed
400 g (14 oz) jar artichoke hearts in brine, drained
2 garlic cloves, crushed
finely grated zest and juice of 1 lemon
2 tablespoons horseradish cream
¼ teaspoon lemon pepper
1 thyme sprig, leaves stripped

TO SERVE
¼ teaspoon smoked paprika
1 celery stalk, cut into batons
1 carrot, cut into batons
1 red capsicum (pepper), cut into batons

Combine all of the dip ingredients in a food processor, and pulse until almost smooth (it's nice to leave a little chunkiness for texture).

Refrigerate for 30 minutes, then sprinkle over the smoked paprika before serving with the vegetable crudités.

BALSAMIC STRAWBERRY BRUSCHETTA

SERVES 1
PREP TIME 10 minutes

1 slice of wholegrain (or gluten-free) bread
1 tablespoon fresh ricotta cheese
6 strawberries, hulled and quartered, and soaked in 1 tablespoon balsamic vinegar for 10 minutes
a few small basil leaves, to serve

Toast the bread and spread with ricotta. Strain the strawberries, then arrange on top of the ricotta, and top with torn basil leaves to serve.

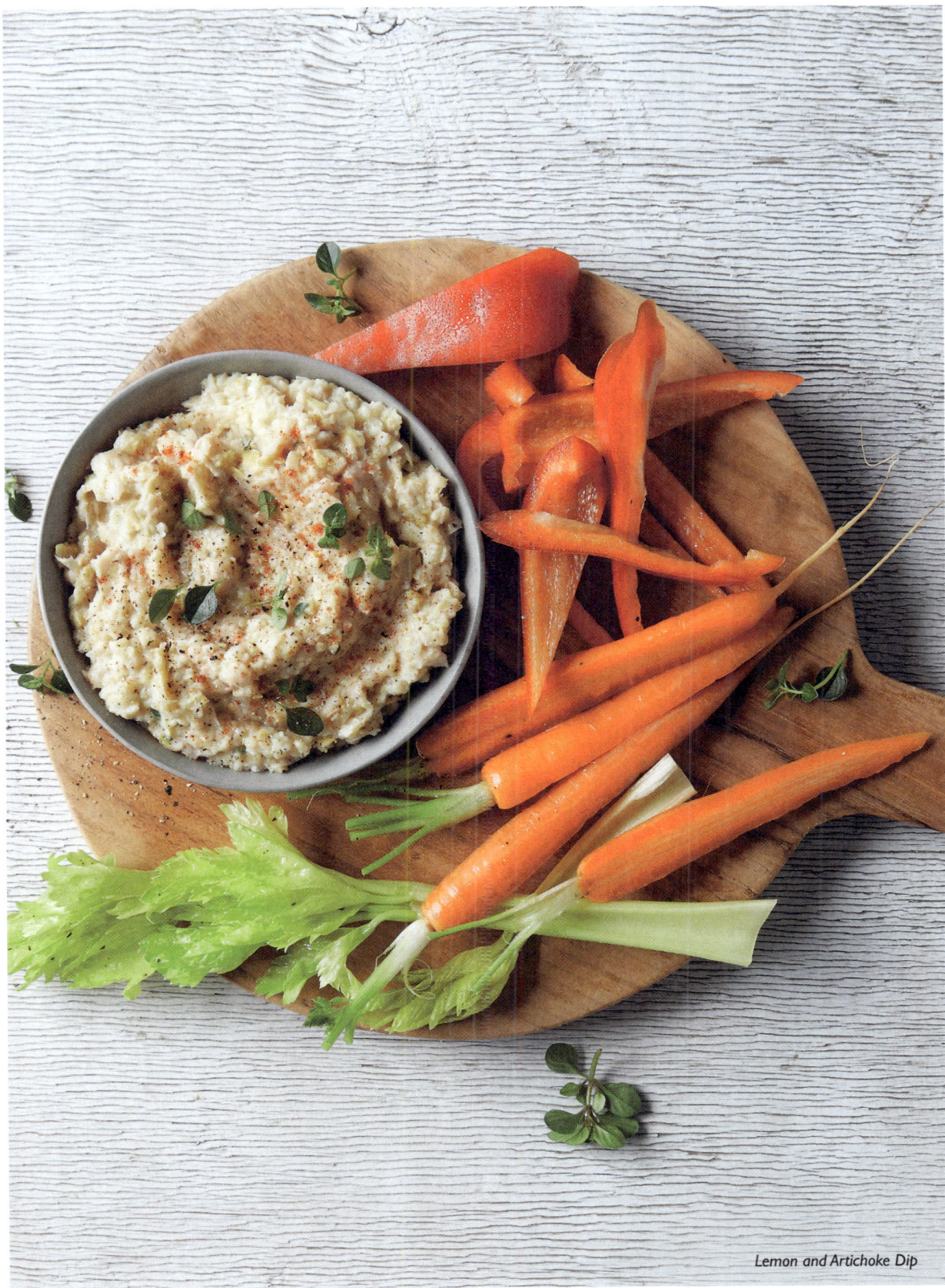

Lemon and Artichoke Dip

BRUNCH SNACK BOX

SERVES 1
PREP TIME 5 minutes

70 g (2½ oz/¼ cup) Greek-style yoghurt
1 tablespoon toasted muesli or granola
   (gluten free if required)
½ apple, cut into wedges
2 walnuts

Top the yoghurt with the muesli and serve with the apple wedges and walnuts.

NIGHTCAP SNACK BOX

SERVES 1
PREP TIME 5 minutes
COOK TIME 3 minutes

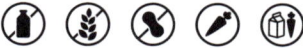

1 chai tea bag
125 ml (4 fl oz/½ cup) boiling water
60 ml (2 fl oz/¼ cup) soy milk (or milk of choice)
2 medjool dates, pitted
10 g (¼ oz) square vegan dark chocolate (70%)
3 strawberries, to serve

Steep the tea bag in a latte glass, cup or mug with the boiling water for a few minutes. Add the milk, stir and remove the tea bag.

Serve with dates, chocolate and strawberries.

LET'S GO MEXICO SNACK BOX

SERVES 1
PREP TIME 5 minutes

50 g (1¾ oz/⅓ cup) chopped capsicum (pepper)
50 g (1¾ oz/¼ cup) chopped tomatoes
1 coriander (cilantro) sprig, finely chopped
salt and pepper
15 g (½ oz) plain baked corn chips
20 g (¾ oz) cheddar cheese, sliced
30 g (1 oz) pineapple, sliced

Combine the capsicum, tomato and coriander, and season to taste with salt and pepper.

Serve with the remaining ingredients.

WHEN YOU CAN'T DECIDE WHAT TO EAT, WHY NOT PACK IT ALL?
Designed to give you options, my snack boxes are colourful, fresh and nutritious.

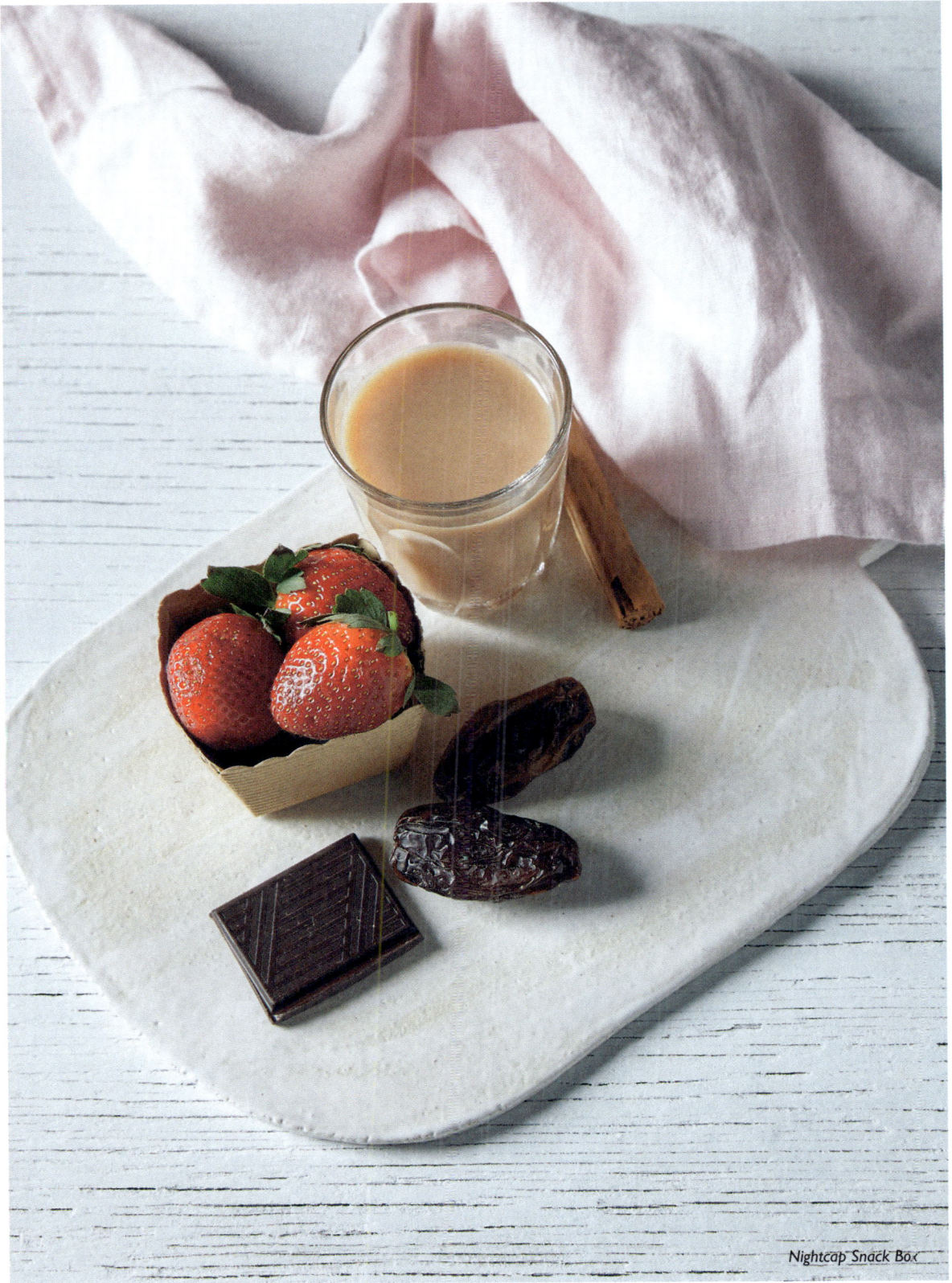

Nightcap Snack Box

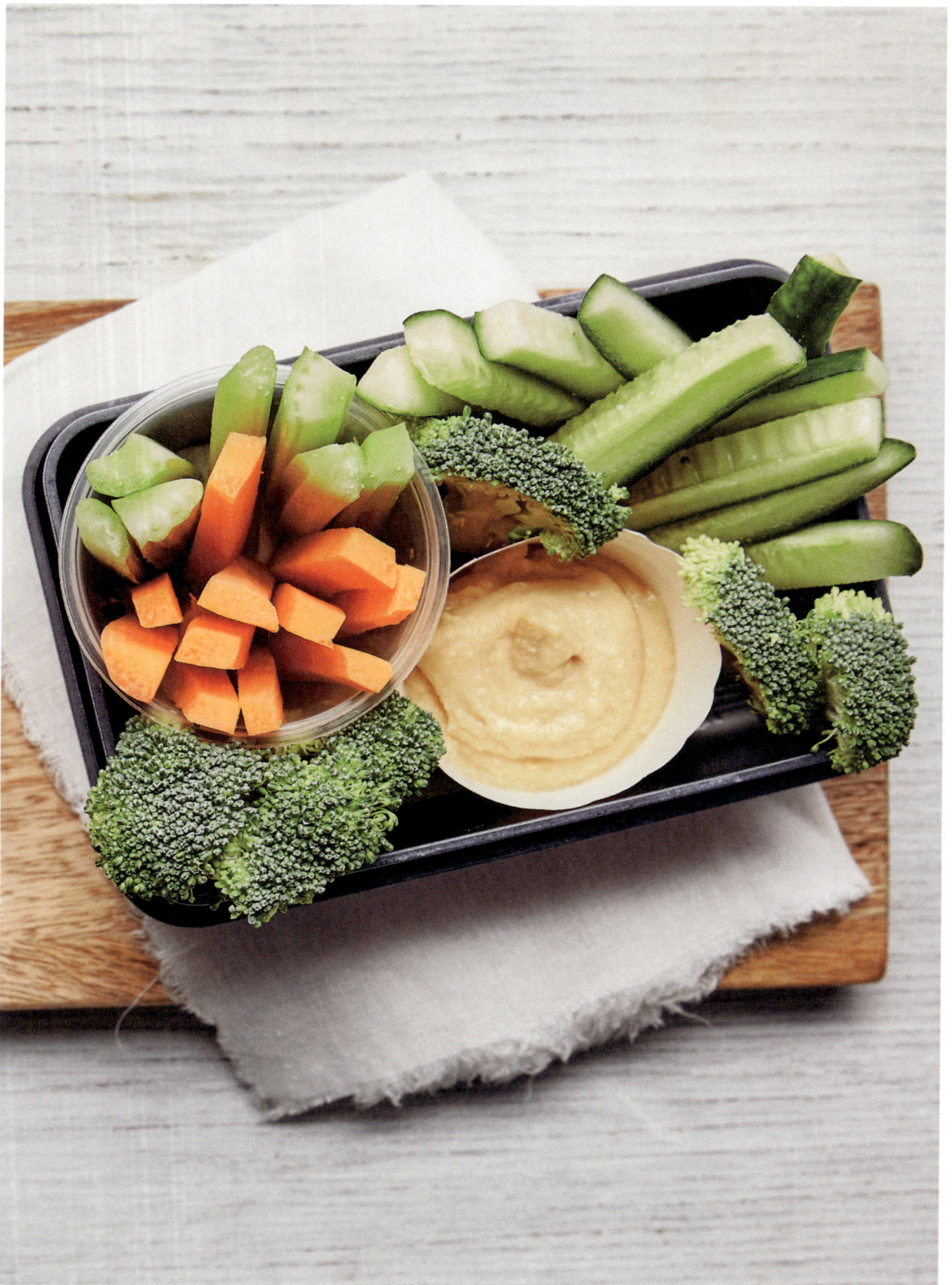

STICKS AND DIP SNACK BOX

SERVES 1
PREP TIME 5 minutes

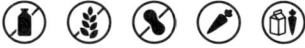

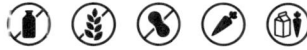

1 carrot, cut into batons
1 Lebanese (short) cucumber, halved and cut
    into batons
30 g (1 oz) broccoli, broken into small florets
1 celery stalk, cut into sticks
2 tablespoons hummus

Prepare the vegetables and serve with the hummus.

MEZZE SNACK BOX

SERVES 1
PREP TIME 5 minutes

8 grapes
4 Sicilian olives
8 cherry tomatoes
1½ tablespoons hummus
¼ red capsicum (pepper), deseeded and thinly
    sliced

Assemble all of the ingredients in a snack box and enjoy!

NOT
ALL HEROES
WEAR CAPES.

CHAPTER 6

KID-FRIENDLY SNACKS

Even the fussiest of eaters can't resist these snacks. Get inspired with my lunchbox and after-school snack ideas (these won't ruin their appetites, promise). There are also nut-free recipes.

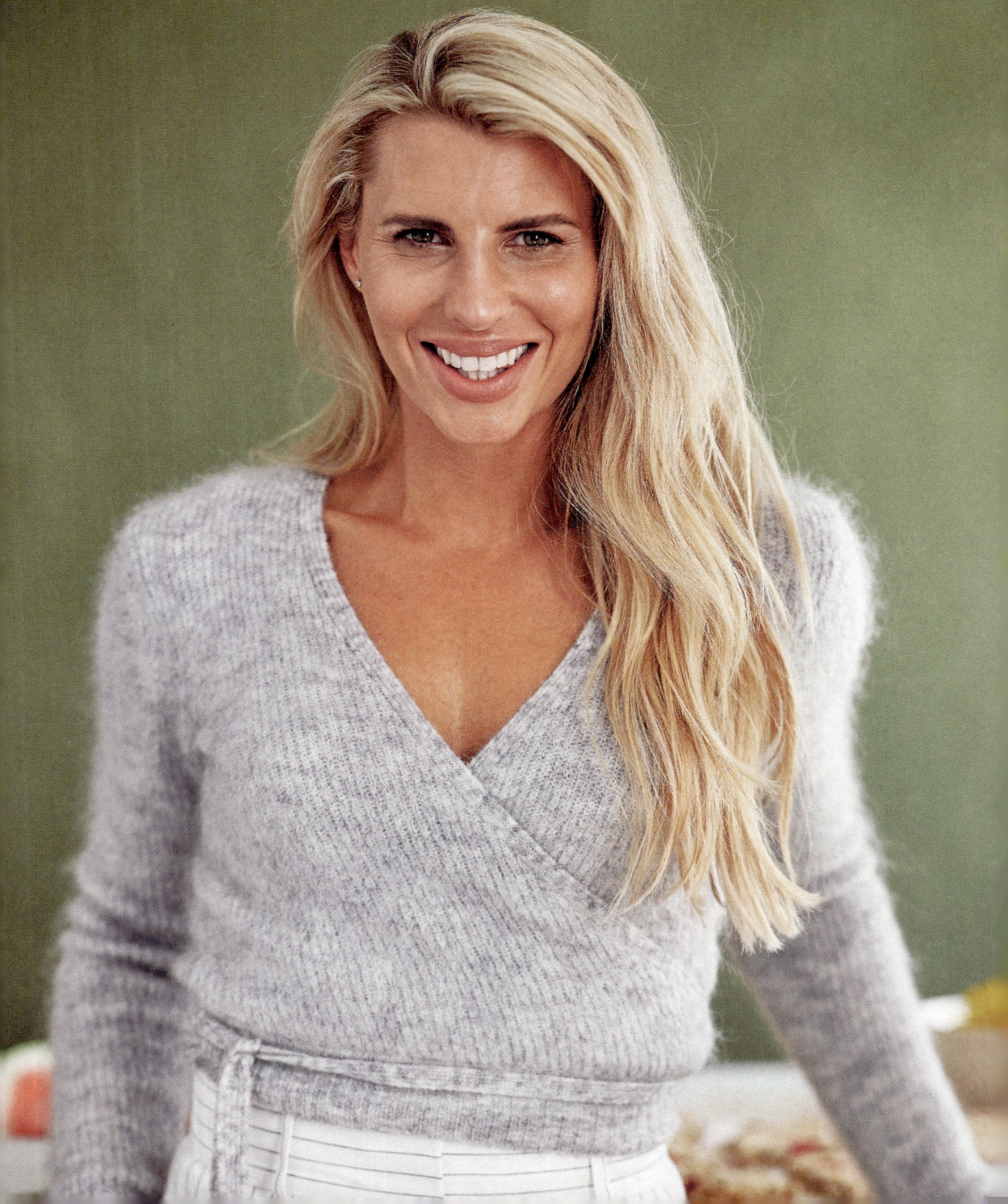

Kid-friendly ways to set healthy snack habits for life

Good eating habits start at home. As a parent, I think we have a huge responsibility to set good examples for our kids; how we snack—the frequency, quantity and quality of our snacks—is how *they'll* decipher what's good and what's not. Instilling these good habits early on will help them grow into strong, healthy beings.

Now, I understand not everything always goes to plan. One day you have a little angel who can't get enough vegetables, the next you have a screaming child who will only eat cheese sandwiches. Here are some ways to implement good snacking and eating habits:

1. BE A ROLE MODEL

A child's observation is a powerful tool, so it's important we practise what we preach (most of the time!). If they see you eating a bag of chips before dinner, they won't understand why they can't. If they see you snacking after lunch or right up until bedtime, they'll assume that's normal eating behaviour. Children will mirror you, so let them see you snacking on healthy foods and eat only when you're hungry at spaced intervals around your main meals.

2. AVOID SNACKING JUST BEFORE MAIN MEALS

Preparing meals takes time (and sometimes a lot of energy). Don't let your efforts go to waste by allowing your kids to snack just before mealtimes. It's hard to teach kids patience when feeding them can be one of the most impatient times of the day, but learning to wait is really important for them to regulate their appetite. Food prepping together can also be fun! Remember, children love to help. So, whether they're setting the table or washing some veggies, they'll learn new skills and forget about wanting a snack.

3. BUMS ON SEATS

I can't stress the importance of sitting down and eating mindfully. Treat a snack like a mini meal, limit distractions, enjoy each mouthful and chew properly. Eating slowly ensures better digestion and greater satisfaction.

4. TEACH THEM HOW TO LISTEN TO THEIR TUMMIES

Kids (like adults) can mistake boredom for hunger, so help them understand the difference. Ask them if they've got hunger pains, and if they don't, steer them towards an activity.

It's also okay to feel a little peckish at times but it's super important to give them healthy snacks that keep their tummies full for longer. Treats are fun too, but treats are not 'all-the-time' snacks.

5. TRY NOT TO USE SNACKS AS REWARDS

It's hard to not give in sometimes, I get it. Kids are cute, but they are persistent. If we constantly reward them with treats, they'll associate happiness with unhealthy foods. It can take more than 10 tries to get a kid on board with a new snack. Tedious? Yes. Worth it? For sure! Try asking them why they don't like eating a certain food. Sometimes cooking or serving it in a more exciting way can be enough to change their mind.

6. HELP KIDS RESPECT SNACKS

In the same way you've taught them to respect their friends, family and toys, teach them to also respect snacks—and food in general. Encourage them not to be wasteful, to listen to their tummy and feelings, to not fear bruised fruit and veggies, and to enjoy the preparation and eating of food.

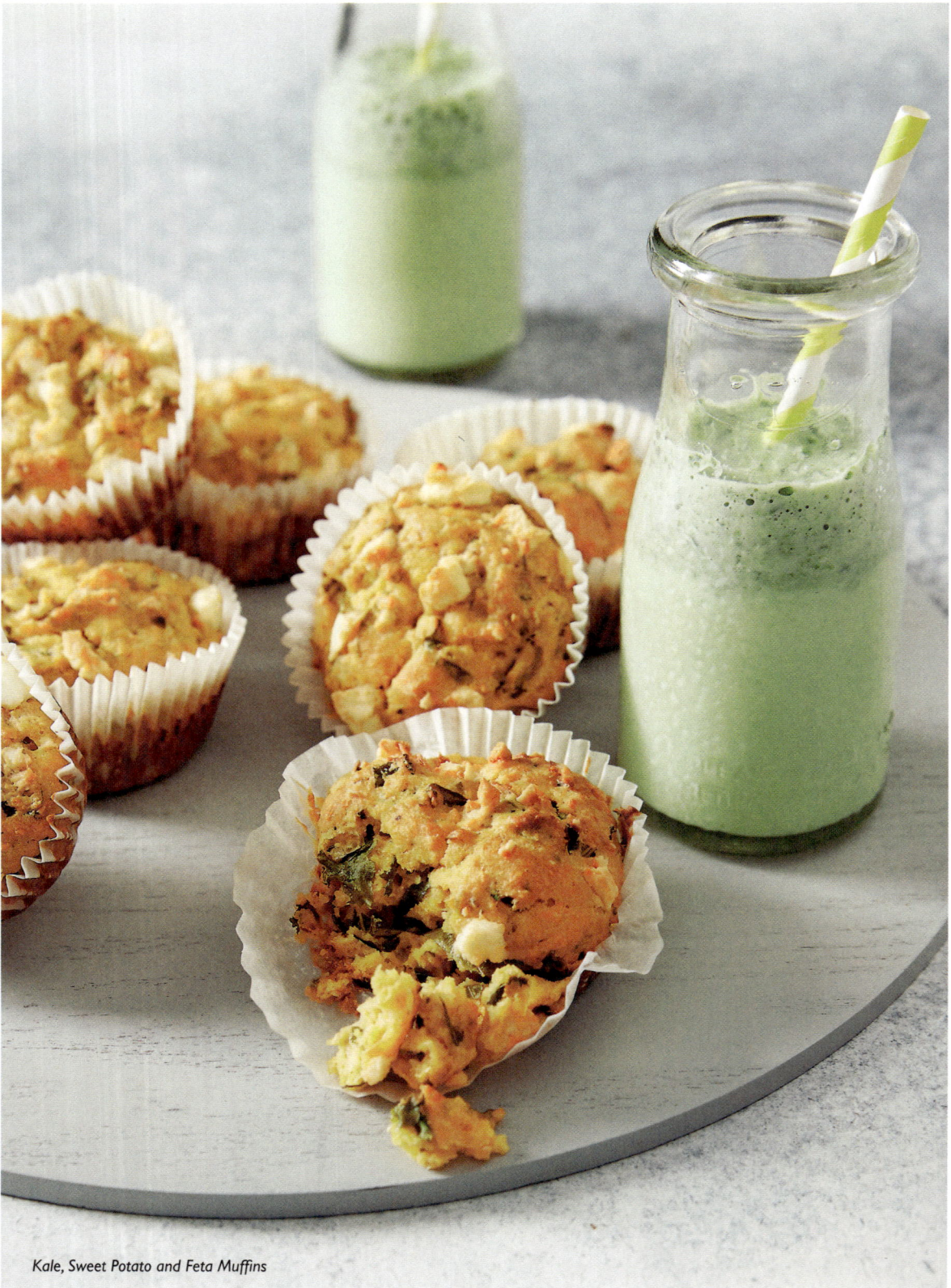

Kale, Sweet Potato and Feta Muffins

KALE, SWEET POTATO AND FETA MUFFINS

MAKES 12
PREP TIME 15 minutes
COOK TIME 40 minutes

200 g (7 oz) sweet potato, peeled and cut into
  2 cm (¾ inch) dice
270 g (9½ oz/2 cups) wholemeal (whole-wheat)
  spelt flour (or gluten-free)
1 teaspoon bicarbonate of soda (baking soda)
salt and pepper
2 kale leaves, stems and spines removed,
  finely chopped
2 tablespoons finely chopped flat-leaf (Italian)
  parsley
125 ml (4 fl oz/½ cup) olive oil
130 g (4½ oz/½ cup) Greek-style yoghurt
3 large eggs, lightly beaten
60 g (2¼ oz) feta cheese

Preheat the over to 180°C (350°F) and line a
12-hole standard (60 ml/¼ cup) muffin tin with
paper cases.

Place the sweet potatoes in a medium saucepan,
cover with cold water and simmer for 12 minutes,
or until tender. Drain, reserving some of the
cooking water, and allow the potato to cool
before putting in a food processor. Add some of
the cooking water then purée the potato, adding
more water, if needed.

Combine the flour, bicarb, salt and pepper, kale
and parsley in a large bowl and make a well in the
centre.

Whisk the oil, yoghurt, eggs and sweet potato
purée together and fold into the dry ingredients
using a wooden spoon until just combined. Don't
overmix. Spoon the mixture into the paper cases
and crumble some feta over each muffin.

Bake for 20–25 minutes, or until a toothpick
inserted into one of the muffins comes out clean.
Allow to cool for 10–15 minutes. Store in an
airtight container in the fridge for up to 3 days.

VEGGIE LETTUCE WRAPS

SERVES 2
PREP TIME 15 minutes

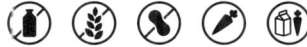

DIPPING SAUCE
2 teaspoons mirin
1 teaspoon soy sauce (or tamari if gluten-free)
2 teaspoons sweet chilli sauce
juice of ½ lime
60 ml (2 fl oz/¼ cup) boiling water

LETTUCE WRAPS
4 large cos (romaine lettuce) leaves
2 tablespoons hummus
½ avocado, sliced
1 carrot, cut into matchsticks
½ telegraph (long) cucumber, cut into
  matchsticks

Combine the dipping sauce ingredients in a small
bowl, mix well, then set aside.

Lay the lettuce leaves out flat, spread each of
them with hummus, then top with avocado, carrot
and cucumber.

Carefully fold the edges of each lettuce leaf in
and roll up; you can secure them with a toothpick
if you like.

Serve with the dipping sauce.

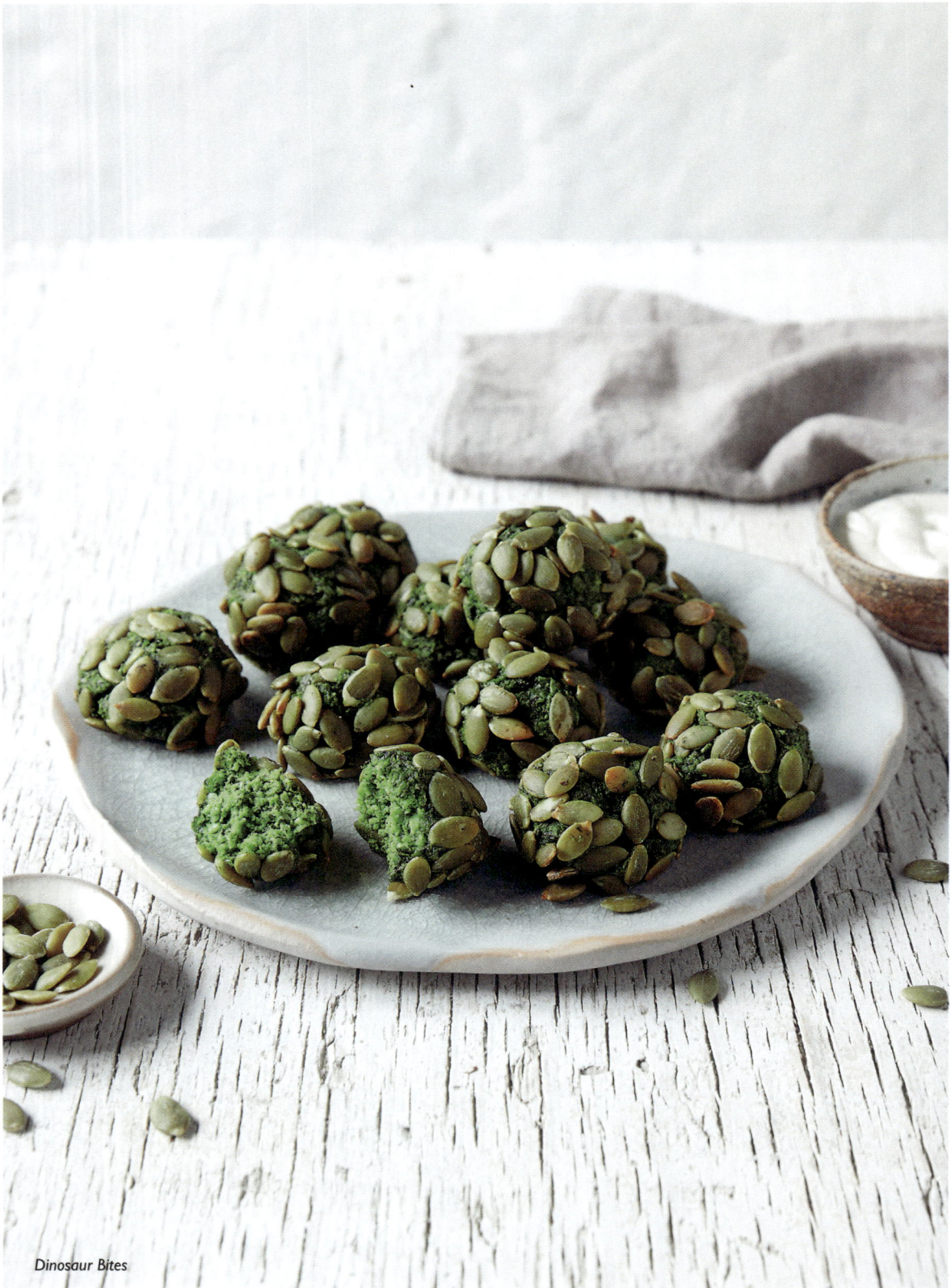

Dinosaur Bites

DINOSAUR BITES

MAKES 12
PREP TIME 15 minutes
COOK TIME 20 minutes

100 g (3½ oz) broad beans, podded
   (thawed and drained, if frozen)
100 g (3½ oz) edamame (soya beans)
   (thawed and drained, if frozen)
100 g (3½ oz) green peas (thawed and
   drained, if frozen)
30 g (1 oz/1 cup) kale, stems and spines
   removed, coarsely chopped
10 g (¼ oz/¼ cup) mint, coarsely chopped
2 spring onions (scallions), sliced
1 egg, beaten
salt and pepper
40 g (1½ oz/¼ cup) pepitas (pumpkin seeds)
1 teaspoon tahini
2 tablespoons dairy-free yoghurt

Preheat the oven to 180°C (350°F). Line a baking
tray with baking paper and set aside.

Combine the beans, edamame, peas, kale, mint,
spring onion, egg, salt and pepper in a food
processor and pulse until combined. Portion the
mixture into 30 g (1 oz) balls, then roll these in
the pepitas to coat completely.

Place the balls on the prepared tray and bake for
20 minutes, or until brown and cooked through.

Combine the tahini and yoghurt in a small bowl
and mix until smooth. Serve the balls drizzled
with the tahini–yoghurt as a snack, or tossed
through a green salad for an extra hit of protein.

YOGHURT, BLUEBERRY AND MUESLI SNACK CUP

SERVES 1
PREP TIME 5 minutes
COOK TIME 3 minutes

1 teaspoon coconut oil
1 teaspoon flaked almonds
2 tablespoons puffed brown rice
70 g (2½ oz/¼ cup) Greek-style yoghurt
40 g (1½ oz/¼ cup) blueberries (fresh or frozen)

Heat the oil in a small frying pan over medium–
high heat, add the almonds and puffed rice and
toast for 2–3 minutes, or until golden. Set aside
to cool.

Place half the yoghurt in a glass, and top with half
the cooled nut mixture and the blueberries.

Spoon over the remaining yoghurt, nut mixture
and blueberries to serve.

PUMPKIN DOUGHNUTS WITH CHOCOLATE FROSTING

MAKES 8 **PREP TIME** 20 minutes **COOK TIME** 20 minutes

1 teaspoon coconut oil, melted
150 g (5½ oz) pumpkin, peeled
    and diced
40 g (1½ oz) unsalted butter
½ teaspoon ground cinnamon
100 g (3½ oz/¾ cup) wholemeal
    (whole-wheat) spelt flour
½ teaspoon baking powder
1 egg
2 tablespoons milk
1 tablespoon maple syrup
½ teaspoon ground turmeric,
    for dusting

FROSTING
50 g (1¾ oz) dark chocolate
    (70%)
2 teaspoons coconut oil
½ avocado, peeled and stone
    removed
½ teaspoon natural vanilla
    extract

Preheat the oven to 150°C (300°F) and lightly grease an eight-hole doughnut tin with coconut oil.

Place the pumpkin in a microwave-safe bowl and cover with plastic wrap. Cook on high for 3 minutes, or until the pumpkin is tender. Alternatively, place the pumpkin in a steamer over a saucepan of boiling water and simmer, covered, for 5–10 minutes, or until tender.

Transfer the pumpkin to a food processor while still warm. Add the butter, cinnamon, flour, baking powder, egg, milk and maple syrup, then blend until smooth.

Spoon or pipe the mixture into the doughnut holes and bake for 10 minutes, or until lightly golden and a toothpick inserted into a doughnut comes out clean. Cool in the tin for 5 minutes then transfer to a wire rack to cool completely.

To make the frosting, put the chocolate and the coconut oil together in a heatproof bowl and microwave for 30 seconds at a time, stirring after each time, until melted and smooth. Alternatively, use the double-boiler method on page 73.

Place the avocado in a food processor and blend until very smooth. Add the melted chocolate mixture and the vanilla, and blend again until smooth and combined.

Use a small spatula to cover the doughnuts with the frosting, then dust lightly with the turmeric. Store in an airtight container in the fridge or freezer.

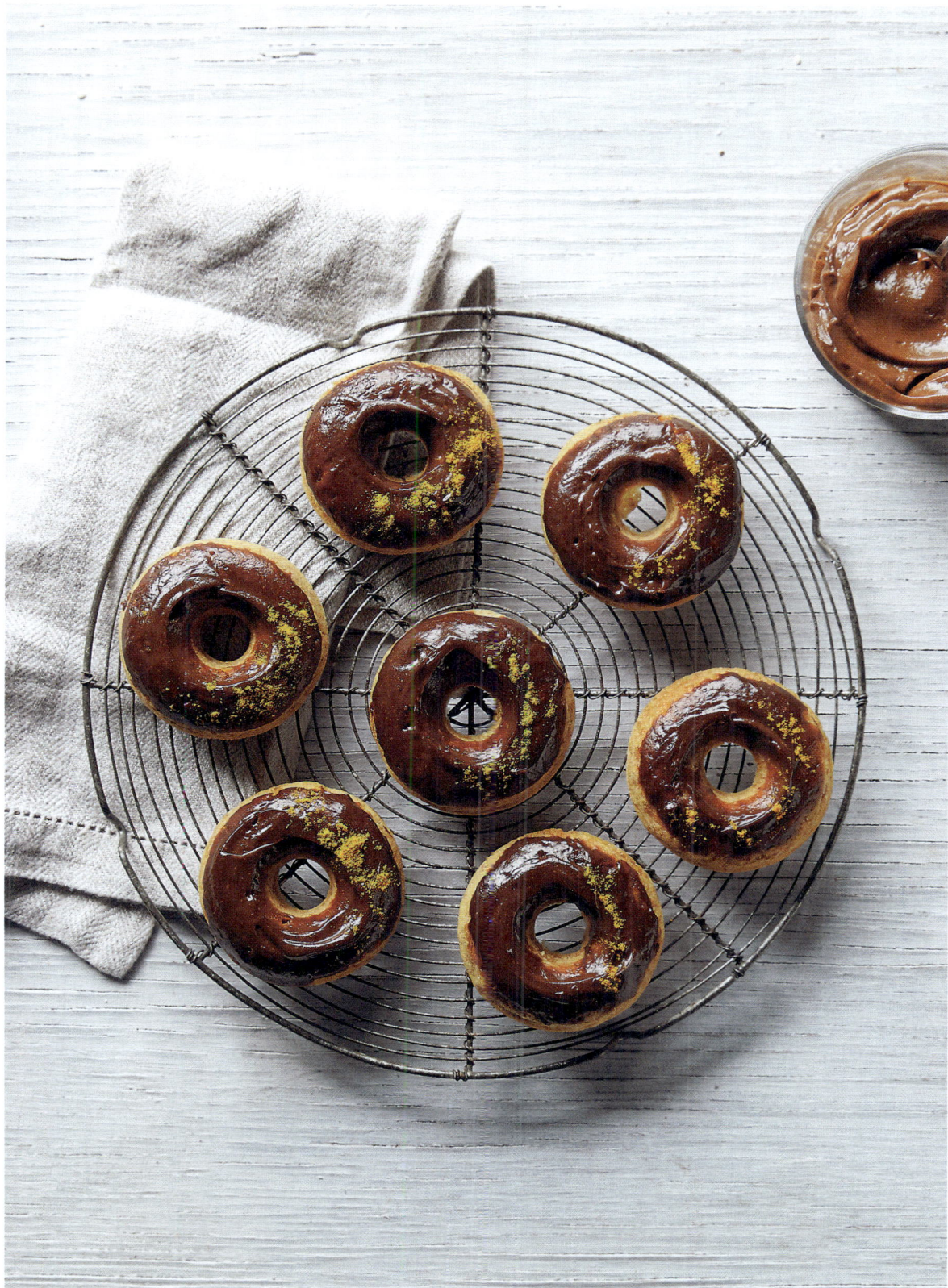

SPELT, OAT AND APPLE MUFFINS

MAKES 12
PREP TIME 10 minutes
COOK TIME 20 minutes

205 g (7¼ oz/1½ cups) spelt flour
100 g (3½ oz/1 cup) rolled (porridge) oats
   plus 1 tablespoon extra, for sprinkling
2 teaspoons baking powder
1 teaspoon mixed spice
1 teaspoon sea salt
1 large apple, cored and diced
100 g (3½ oz/½ cup, lightly packed) brown sugar
2 eggs
95 g (3¼ oz/½ cup) coconut oil, melted
125 ml (4 fl oz/½ cup) milk

Preheat the oven to 180°C (350°F) and line a
12-hole standard (60 ml/¼ cup) muffin tin with
paper cases.

Combine the flour, oats, baking powder, mixed
spice and salt in a medium bowl, then toss the
apple through.

In another medium bowl, whisk the sugar, eggs,
oil and milk together, then gently stir this mixture
through the dry ingredients just to combine.

Divide the batter between the paper cases, sprinkle
over the extra oats and bake for 15–20 minutes,
until a toothpick inserted into one of the muffins
comes out clean. Transfer to a wire rack to cool.
Store in an airtight container for up to 3 days.

OATMEAL, BANANA AND DARK CHOCOLATE COOKIES

MAKES 12 (2 cookies per snack)
PREP TIME 5 minutes
COOK TIME 20 minutes

3 very ripe bananas, mashed
90 g (3¼ oz/⅓ cup) unsweetened apple sauce
200 g (7 oz/2 cups) rolled (porridge) oats
60 ml (2 fl oz/¼ cup) milk
45 g (1⅔ oz/¼ cup) dark chocolate chips

Preheat the oven to 180°C (350°F) and line a
baking tray with baking paper.

Combine the bananas, apple sauce, oats and milk
in a medium bowl. Stir through the chocolate
chips until well combined.

Spoon tablespoon-sized amounts onto the
prepared tray, and flatten with the back of
the spoon.

Bake for 15–20 minutes, or until slightly golden.
Allow to cool on the tray before transferring to
a wire rack to cool completely. Store in an airtight
container for up to 3 days.

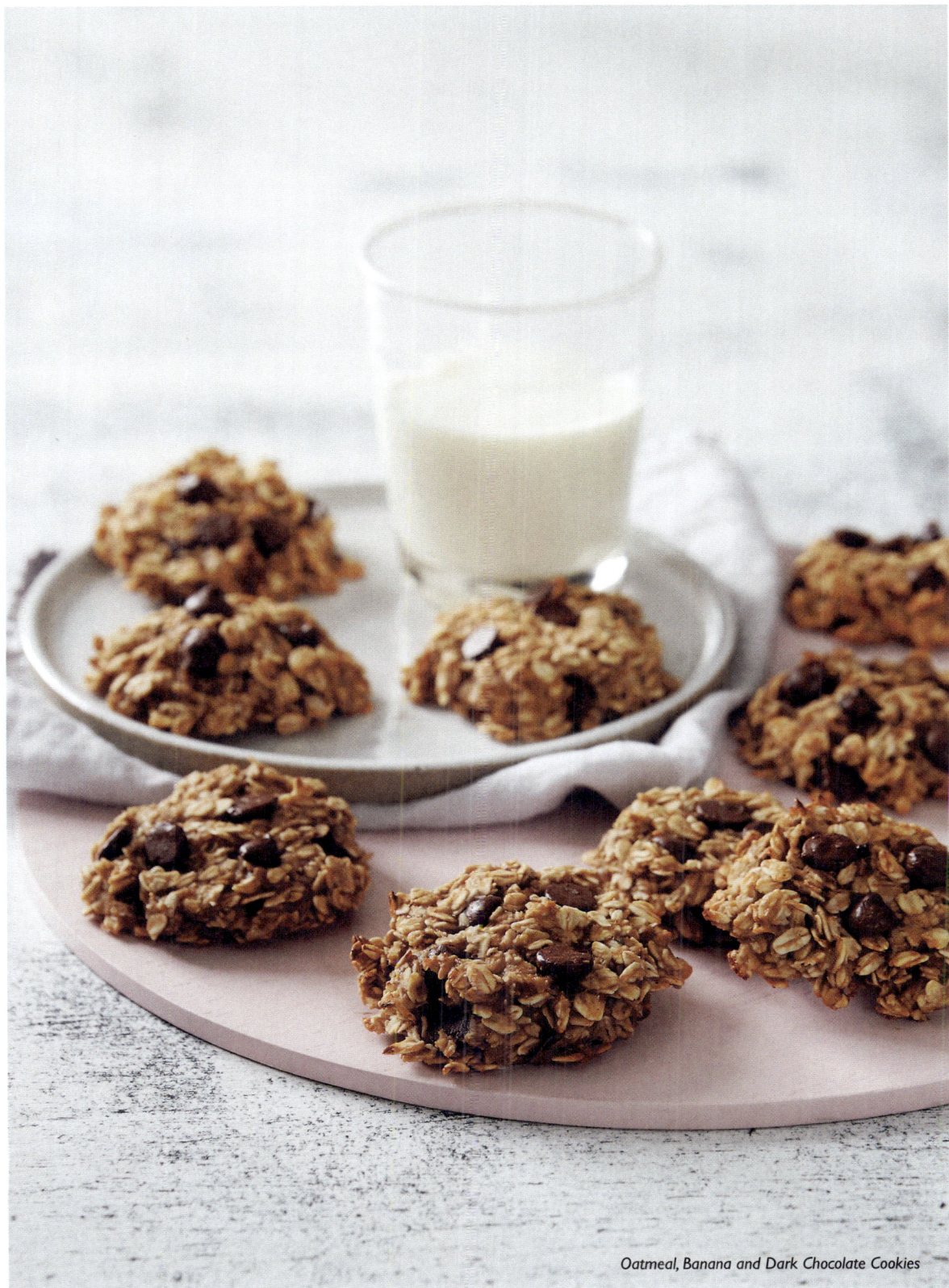

Oatmeal, Banana and Dark Chocolate Cookies

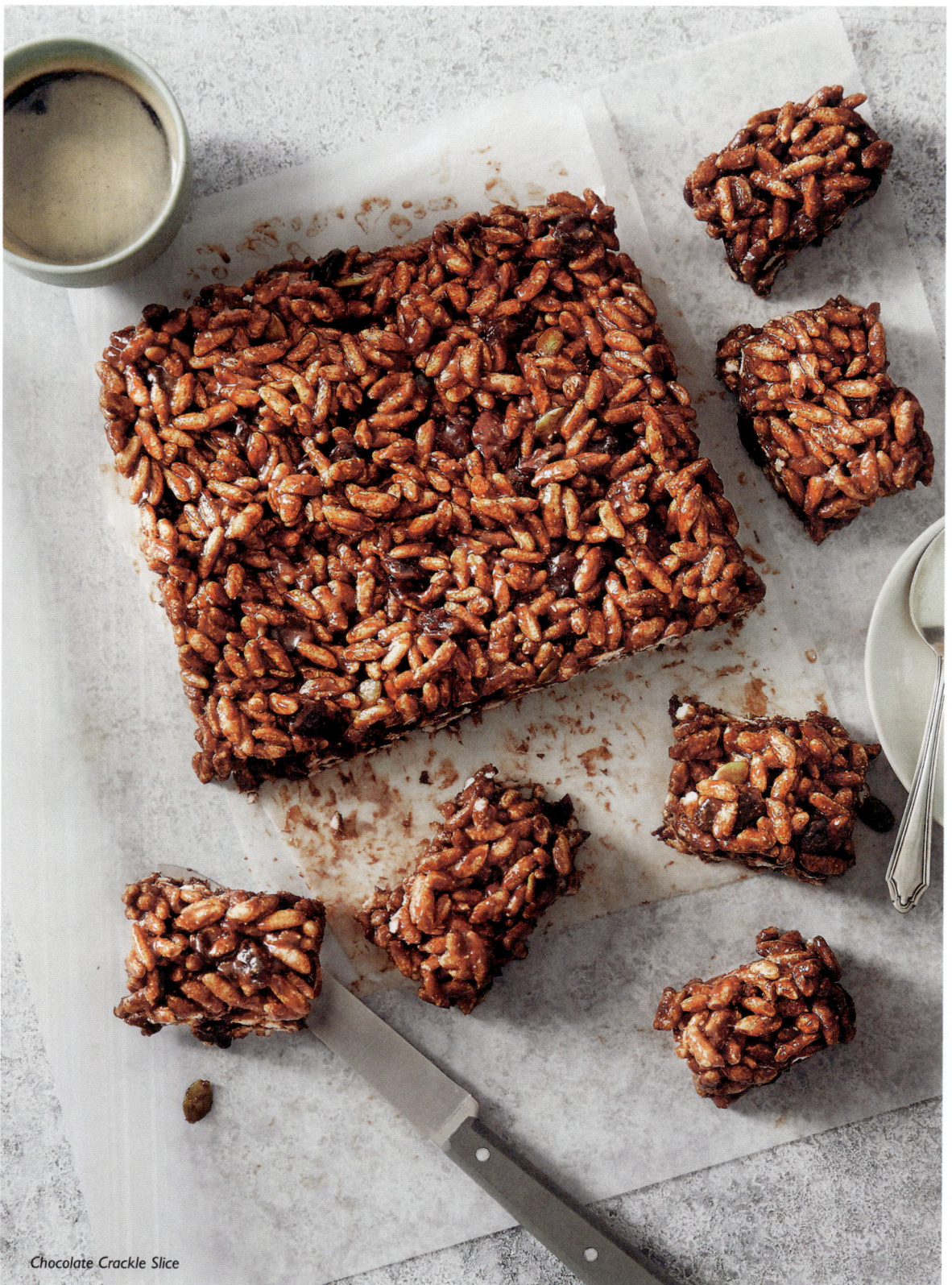

Chocolate Crackle Slice

CHOCOLATE CRACKLE SLICE

MAKES 16
PREP TIME 10 minutes

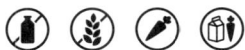

120 g (4½ oz/⅓ cup) rice malt syrup
80 g (2¾ oz/⅓ cup) coconut oil
100 g (3½ oz/⅓ cup) almond butter
3 tablespoons raw cacao powder or sugar-free cocoa powder
pinch of salt
50 g (1¾ oz/⅓ cup) dried cranberries, coarsely chopped
2 tablespoons pepitas (pumpkin seeds)
75 g (2⅔ oz/3 cups) puffed rice

Line a 20 cm (8 inch) square baking tin with baking paper.

Melt the rice malt syrup, coconut oil, almond butter, cacao and salt in a medium saucepan over low heat.

Remove from the heat and stir through the cranberries, pepitas and puffed rice.

Spoon the mixture into the prepared tin, press down into an even layer then refrigerate for 3 hours, or until firm.

Slice into 16 pieces and store in an airtight container for up to a week.

These snacks are family friendly.

I cross my heart the whole family will love them, and it's not because they're full of good stuff that's good for you. These are guaranteed table-trophy snacks. I don't know about your family, but no one in my family has ever said 'no' to a cookie or a slice.

MIXED BERRY SPELT MUFFINS

MAKES 10
PREP TIME 20 minutes
COOK TIME 20 minutes

205 g (7¼ oz/1½ cups) wholemeal (whole-wheat) spelt flour
1½ teaspoons baking powder
55 g (2 oz/¼ cup) coconut oil, melted
60 ml (2 fl oz/¼ cup) maple syrup
1 large egg, lightly beaten
100 ml (3½ fl oz) milk
250 g (9 oz/2 cups) mixed frozen berries
1 tablespoon shredded coconut, to sprinkle

Preheat the oven to 160°C (320°F) and line 10 holes in a 12-hole standard (60 ml/¼ cup) muffin tin with paper cases.

Sift the flour and baking powder into a large bowl, and stir to combine.

Warm the coconut oil and maple syrup together in a small saucepan over low heat to combine. Set aside to cool slightly.

Beat the egg, milk and warm oil mixture together in a small bowl, then add to the dry ingredients, and mix until combined. Gently fold through half of the berries.

Divide the batter between the paper cases then top with the remaining berries and bake for 15 minutes.

Scatter over the coconut and continue to cook for a further 5–7 minutes, or until golden brown and a toothpick inserted into one of the muffins comes out clean.

Remove from the oven, and allow to cool in the tin for a few minutes before transferring to a wire rack to cool completely. Store in an airtight container for up to 3 days.

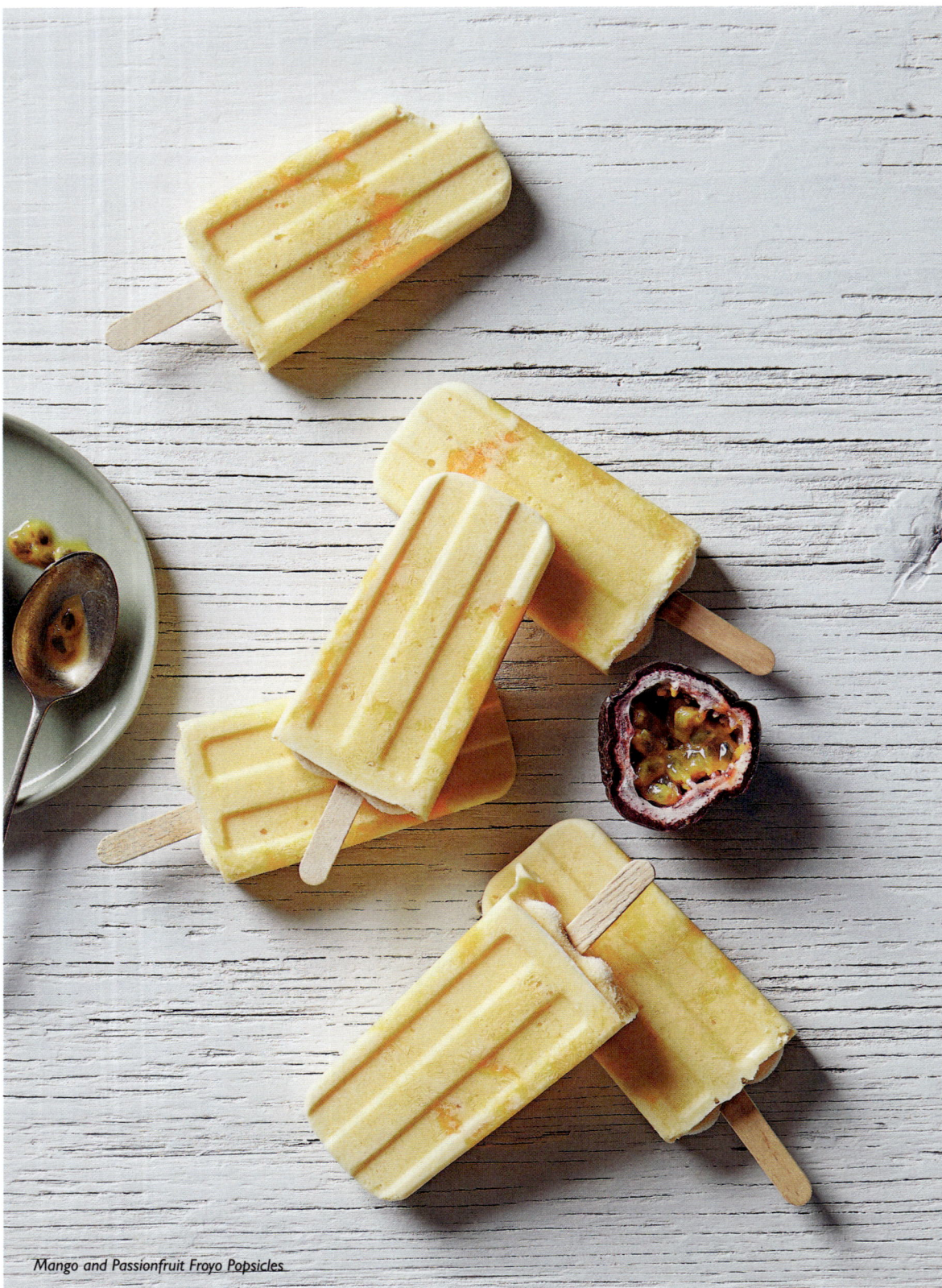

Mango and Passionfruit Froyo Popsicles

PEANUT BUTTER BANANA WITH TOASTED COCONUT

SERVES 1
PREP TIME 5 minutes

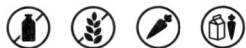

1 small banana
2 teaspoons natural, crunchy peanut butter
2 teaspoons desiccated coconut, toasted

Slice the banana in half lengthways, spread both halves with peanut butter then sprinkle with toasted coconut.

MANGO AND PASSIONFRUIT FROYO POPSICLES

MAKES 6
PREP TIME 5 minutes + overnight freezing

260 g (9¼ oz/1 cup) Greek-style yoghurt
1 tablespoon honey
300 g (10½ oz) mango flesh, fresh or frozen
pulp from 3 passionfruit, seeds removed

Combine the yoghurt, honey and mango in a blender and blitz until smooth.

Spoon 1 tablespoon of the mixture into each popsicle mould, followed by 1 teaspoon of the passionfruit pulp. Repeat until six moulds are full.

Freeze overnight. Enjoy in the sunshine!

RASPBERRY AND CHIA ICY POLES

MAKES 4
PREP TIME 10 minutes

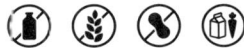

185 g (6½ oz/1½ cups) frozen raspberries
1 tablespoon honey
1 tablespoon chia seeds
90 g (3¼ oz/⅓ cup) coconut cream

Put the raspberries in a blender with 125 ml (4 fl oz/½ cup) water. Add the rest of the ingredients, and blitz until smooth.

Divide the mixture between four icy-pole (popsicle) moulds and place in the freezer for 2–3 hours, or until set.

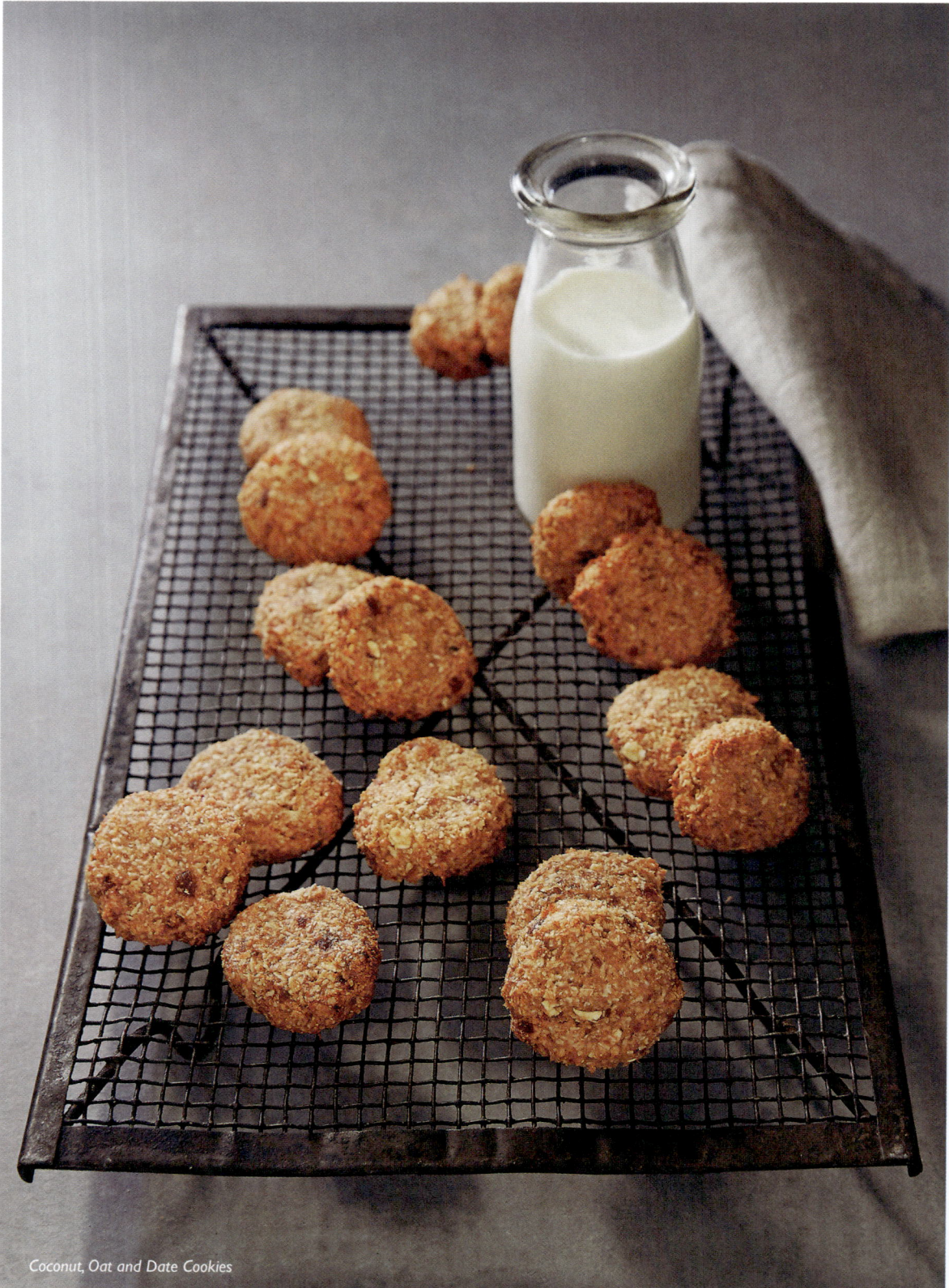

Coconut, Oat and Date Cookies

COCONUT, OAT AND DATE COOKIES

MAKES 16 (2 cookies per snack)
PREP TIME 5 minutes
COOK TIME 15 minutes

160 g (5⅔ oz/1 cup) pitted medjool dates
25 g (1 oz/¼ cup) rolled (porridge) oats
35 g (1¼ oz/¼ cup) wholemeal (whole-wheat) flour
45 g (1⅔ oz/½ cup) desiccated coconut
1 teaspoon baking powder
½ ripe banana
1 tablespoon unsalted butter
1 tablespoon honey
60 ml (2 fl oz/¼ cup) milk

Preheat the oven to 180°C (350°F) and line two baking trays with baking paper.

Blend the dates in a food processor until they form a paste, then add the oats, flour, coconut, baking powder, banana, butter and honey, and pulse until the mixture just comes together.

Add the milk to the mixture 1 tablespoon at a time and pulse until a dough forms.

Roll heaped teaspoons of the mixture into balls and place on the baking trays. Flatten gently with the back of a spoon.

Bake for 12–15 minutes, or until golden. Allow to cool completely on a wire rack, then refrigerate in an airtight container for up to 5 days.

SALTED CARAMEL BLISS BALLS

MAKES 12 (2 balls per snack)
PREP TIME 15 minutes

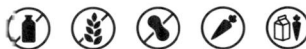

60 g (5⅔ oz/1 cup) pitted medjool dates, coarsely chopped
60 g (2¼ oz/⅔ cup) desiccated coconut
50 g (1¾ oz/½ cup) rolled (porridge) oats (use brown rice or quinoa flakes if gluten-free)
½ teaspoon natural vanilla extract
¼ teaspoon salt

Place the dates in a bowl, cover with boiling water and set aside to soften for 10 minutes. Drain.

Save 1 tablespoon of the dates' soaking water, drain the rest and add the dates to a food processor. Blitz until smooth and caramel-like.

Set 4 tablespoons of the coconut aside, then add the rest to the food processor along with all of the other ingredients. Blitz until the oats break down and the mixture comes together, and add a little reserved liquid from the dates if needed.

Scoop tablespoon amounts of the mixture into 12 balls. Roll the balls in the reserved coconut then store in an airtight container in the fridge for up to 5 days.

CARROT CAKE SLICE

MAKES 16
PREP TIME 10 minutes
COOK TIME 30 minutes

260 g (9¼ oz/1¾ cups) wholemeal
   (whole-wheat) flour
1½ teaspoons baking powder
½ teaspoon bicarbonate of soda (baking soda)
1 teaspoon ground cinnamon
½ teaspoon salt
310 g (11 oz/2 cups) peeled and grated carrots
   (about 3 large)
60 g (2¼ oz/½ cup) coarsely chopped walnuts
85 g (3 oz/½ cup) raisins, tossed in
   1 teaspoon of wholemeal flour
80 ml (2½ fl oz/⅓ cup) olive oil
80 ml (2½ fl oz/⅓ cup) maple syrup
2 eggs
260 g (9¼ oz/1 cup) Greek-style yoghurt
1 teaspoon natural vanilla extract

Preheat the oven to 210°C (410°F). Line a
20 cm (8 inch) square cake tin with baking paper.

Combine the flour, baking powder, bicarb,
cinnamon and salt in a large mixing bowl and
whisk. Stir through the grated carrots, walnuts and
raisins.

In another bowl, mix the oil with the maple syrup,
eggs, yoghurt and vanilla. Add this mixture to the
dry ingredients and stir until just combined.

Transfer the batter to the prepared cake tin and
bake for 30 minutes, or until a skewer inserted
into the centre comes out clean.

Cool completely before slicing into 16 squares.
These will keep at room temperature in an
airtight container for a few days, or you can freeze
them for up to 3 months.

BANANA CHOCOLATE-CHIP LOAF

SERVES 12
PREP TIME 10 minutes
COOK TIME 50 minutes

260 g (9¼ oz/1¾ cup) wholemeal (whole-wheat)
   flour
1 teaspoon ground cinnamon
1 teaspoon bicarbonate of soda (baking soda)
½ teaspoon salt
2 eggs
80 ml (2½ fl oz/⅓ cup) olive oil
1 tablespoon warmed honey
70 g (2½ oz/¼ cup) Greek-style yoghurt
1 teaspoon natural vanilla extract
3 very ripe bananas, mashed
50 g (1¾ oz/⅓ cup) dark chocolate chips

Preheat the oven to 160°C (320°F) and grease
a loaf (bar) tin.

Combine the flour, cinnamon, bicarb and salt in
a medium bowl and set aside.

In a large bowl, beat the eggs, oil, honey, yoghurt
and vanilla until well combined. Gently stir in the
bananas and chocolate chips and then combine
with the flour mixture.

Pour the batter into the tin and bake for
50–55 minutes, or until a skewer inserted
into the centre comes out clean. Cool for
10 minutes before slicing.

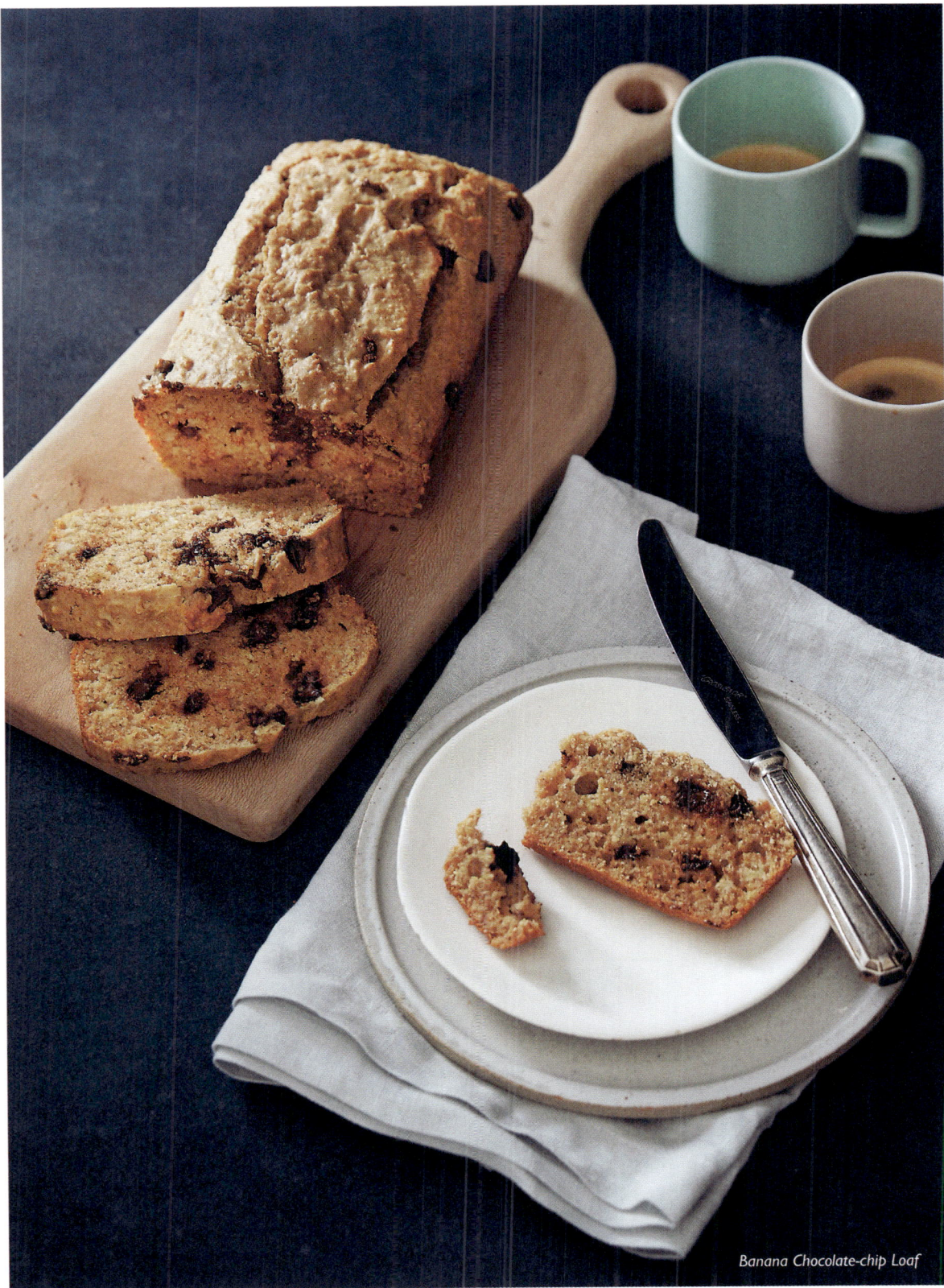

Banana Chocolate-chip Loaf

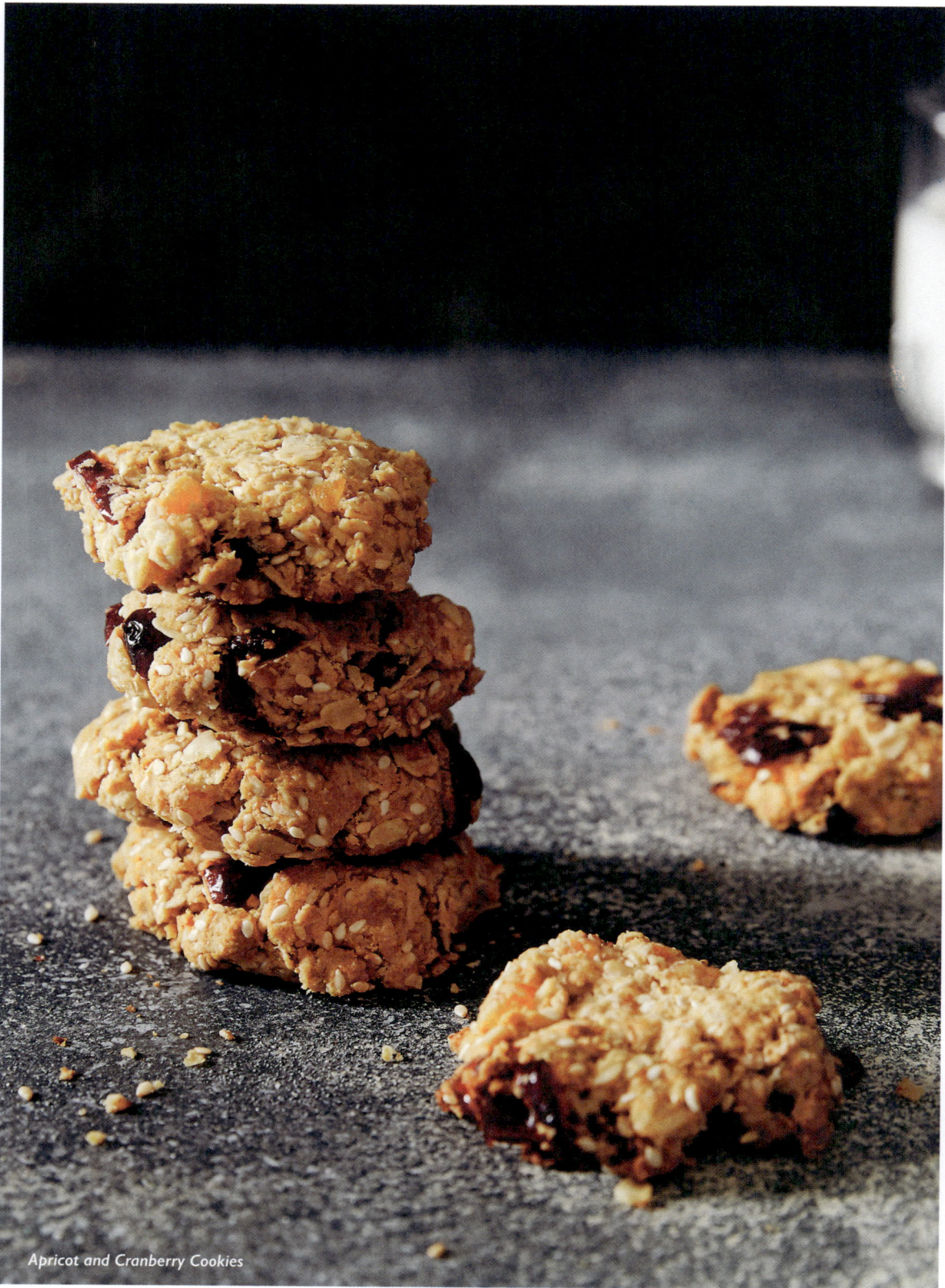

Apricot and Cranberry Cookies

BACK-TO-SCHOOL BLISS BALLS

MAKES 14
PREP TIME 20 minutes

8 medjool dates, pitted
90 g (3¼ oz) rolled (porridge) oats
(or quinoa flakes if gluten-free)
80 g (2¾ oz) desiccated coconut, plus 30 g (1 oz)
extra for rolling
2 tablespoons cocoa powder
1 teaspoon ground cinnamon
2 tablespoons honey
55 g (2 oz/¼ cup) coconut oil, melted

Place the dates in a heatproof bowl and cover
with boiling water to soften. Stand for 10 minutes,
then drain.

Meanwhile, add the oats, coconut, cocoa powder
and cinnamon to a food processor and whizz until
fine. Add the softened dates, honey and coconut
oil, and whizz again until well combined and the
mixture comes together.

Roll tablespoons of the mixture into 14 balls and
coat these in the extra desiccated coconut. Store
any remaining balls in an airtight container in the
fridge for up to 1 week.

APRICOT AND CRANBERRY COOKIES

MAKES 16
PREP TIME 10 minutes
COOK TIME 10 minutes

100 g (3½ oz/1 cup) rolled (porridge) oats
110 g (3¾ oz/¾ cup) wholemeal (whole-wheat)
flour
40 g (1½ oz/¼ cup) sesame seeds
120 g (4¼ oz/⅔ cup) dried apricots, chopped
105 g (3¾ oz/⅔ cup) dried cranberries
100 g (3½ oz) unsalted butter
115 g (4 oz/⅓ cup) honey
1 teaspoon bicarbonate of soda (baking soda)

Preheat the oven to 180°C (350°F). Line two
large baking trays with baking paper.

Combine the oats, flour, sesame seeds, apricots
and cranberries in a large bowl.

Put the butter and honey in a small saucepan with
60 ml (2 fl oz/¼ cup) water and bring to the boil
over a medium heat. Once melted and combined,
stir through the bicarb so mixture starts to foam
up, then immediately remove from the heat. Pour
this mixture over the dry ingredients (while still
hot and foaming) and stir well.

Roll tablespoons of the mixture into 16 balls.
Place 5 cm (2 inches) apart on the lined trays.
Use a fork to flatten slightly. Bake in the oven for
8–10 minutes, or until light golden. Set aside on
the trays for 5 minutes to cool slightly before
transferring to a wire rack to cool completely.
Store in an airtight container.

PUFFED QUINOA CRUNCH BITES

MAKES 12
PREP TIME 20 minutes

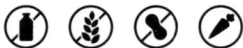

30 g (1 oz/½ cup) puffed quinoa
15 g (½ oz/½ cup) puffed amaranth
45 g (1⅔ oz/¼ cup) buckinis (see note)
20 g (¾ oz/¼ cup) shredded coconut
25 g (1 oz/¼ cup) raw cacao powder
60 ml (2 fl oz/¼ cup) maple syrup
80 ml (2½ fl oz/⅓ cup) melted coconut oil
1 teaspoon freeze-dried raspberries
1 teaspoon pepitas (pumpkin seeds),
  roasted and chopped

Line a 12-hole mini-muffin tin with paper cases (skip this step if using a silicone muffin mould).

In a large bowl, combine the quinoa, amaranth, buckinis, coconut and cacao. Stir to combine then add the maple syrup and melted coconut oil, ensuring the ingredients are evenly distributed.

Divide the mixture between the paper cases, pressing into the bases.

Decorate the tops with freeze-dried raspberries and chopped pepitas. Refrigerate until set.

APRICOT COCONUT ENERGY BARS

MAKES 18
PREP TIME 10 minutes

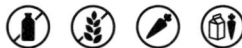

1 tablespoon chia seeds
170 g (6 oz) dried apricots (look for ones
  with no added sugar)
155 g (5½ oz/1 cup) raw cashew nuts
85 g (3 oz/1½ cups) coconut flakes
½ teaspoon salt
55 g (2 oz/¼ cup) coconut oil, melted

Soak the chia seeds in 60 ml (2 fl oz/¼ cup) water for 10 minutes. Meanwhile, line a square 20 cm (8 inch) baking tin with baking paper.

Combine all of the ingredients in a food processor and blitz until a sticky paste forms.

Pour the mixture into the prepared tin and flatten out so the mixture is even.

Place in the freezer for 2–3 hours to set, then cut into 18 bars and store in an airtight container in the fridge for up to a week, or in the freezer for up to 3 months.

Note:

Buckwheat groats are amazing little seeds—they're full of protein, and packed with minerals such as zinc, iron, copper, manganese, magnesium and B vitamins. Buckinis are activated buckwheat groats. Activating them unlocks all their nutrients so we can better absorb them, and it makes them easier to digest. They can be eaten raw, or cooked, and you can buy them from health food stores, or online. If you've got the time and the inclination, it's easy to make your own.

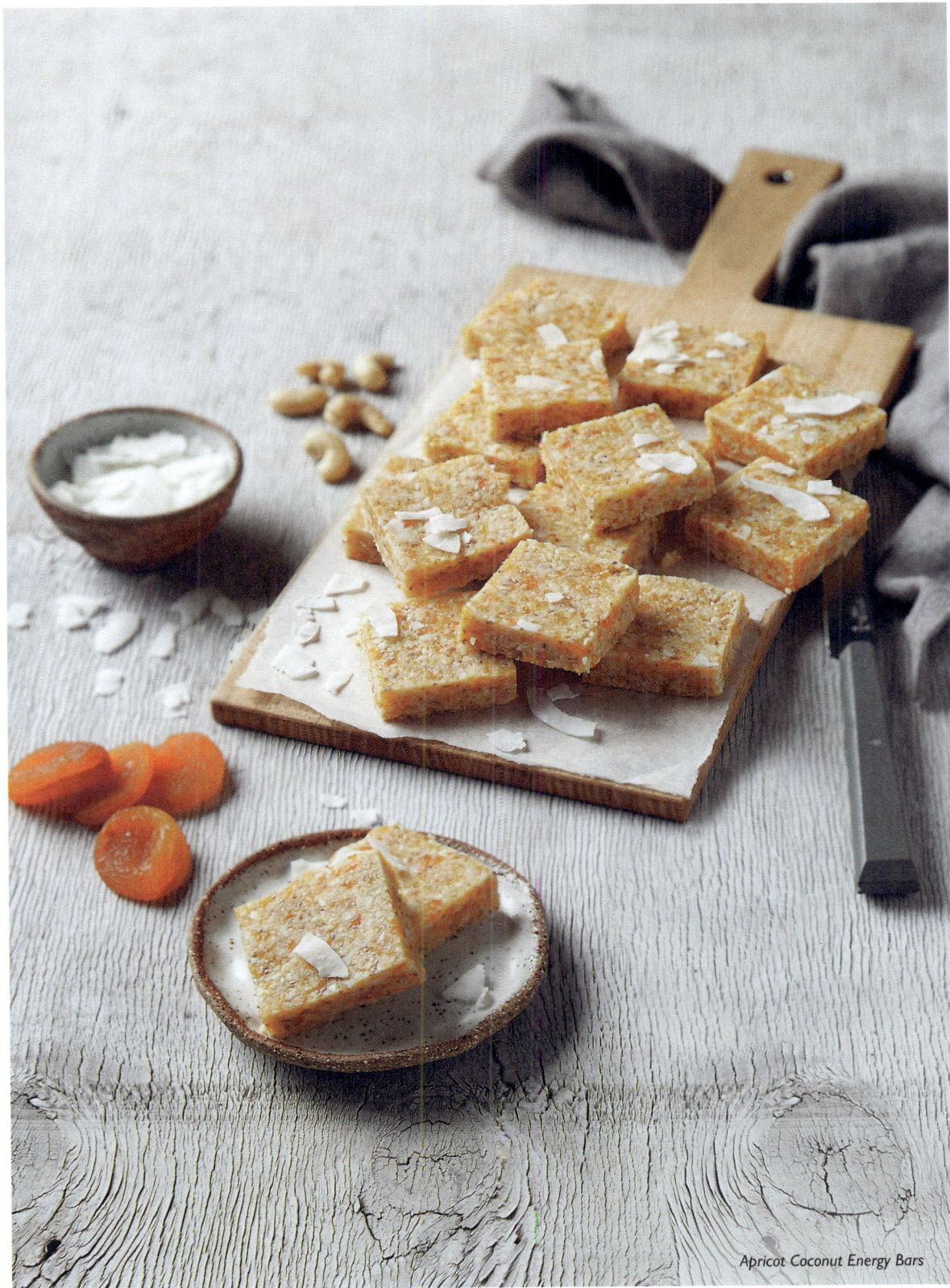

Apricot Coconut Energy Bars

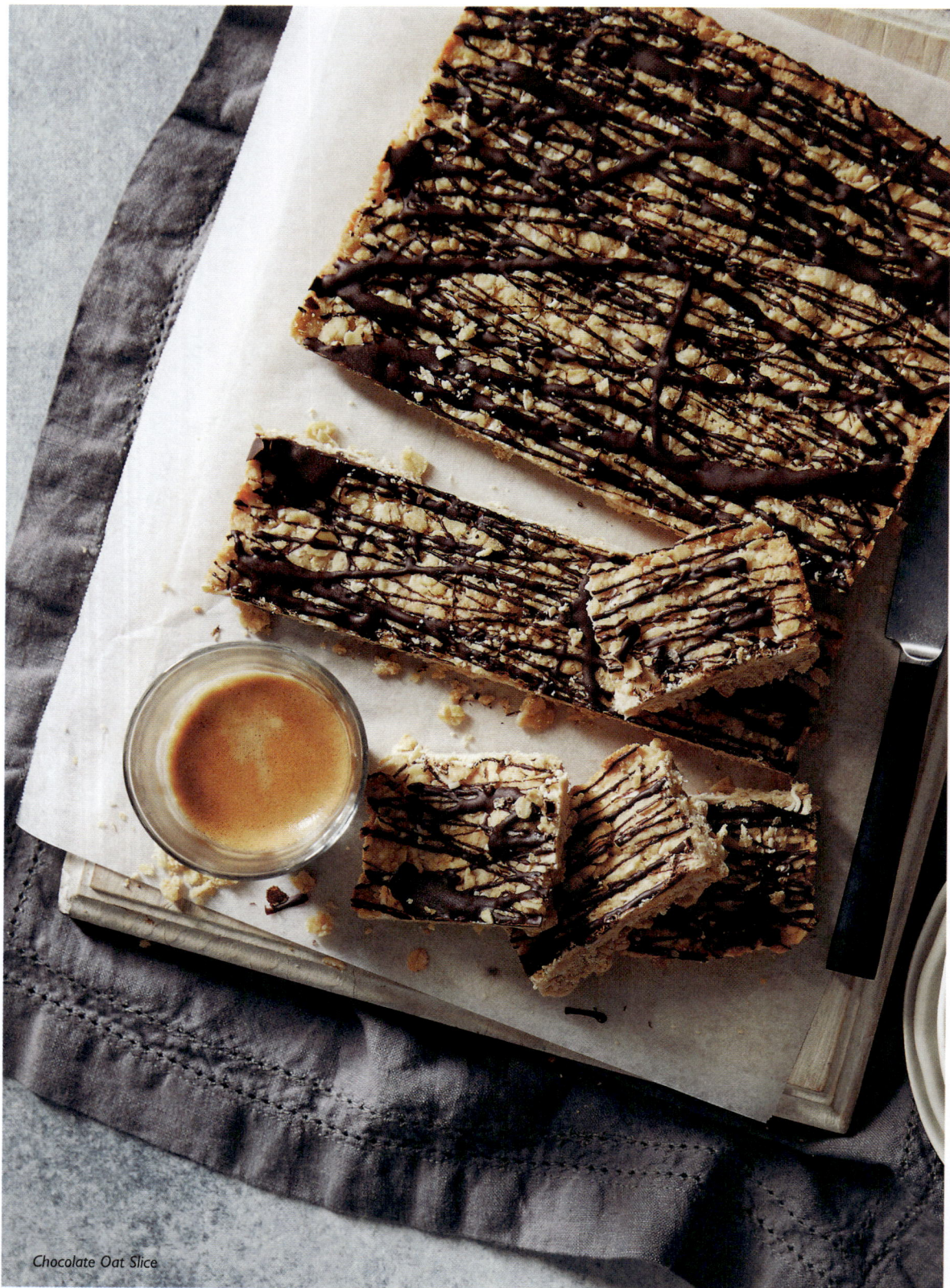

Chocolate Oat Slice

CHOCOLATE OAT SLICE

MAKES 16
PREP TIME 15 minutes
COOK TIME 30 minutes

150 g (5½ oz/1 cup) wholemeal (whole-wheat)
  flour (or gluten-free if needed)
100 g (3½ oz/1 cup) rolled (porridge) oats
  (use brown rice or quinoa flakes if gluten-free)
20 g (¾ oz/¼ cup) shredded coconut
130 g (4½ oz) unsalted butter
90 g (3¼ oz/¼ cup) honey
½ teaspoon bicarbonate of soda (baking soda)
100 g (3½ oz) dark chocolate (70%)

Preheat the oven to 180°C (350°F) and line a
square 20 cm (8 inch) baking tin with baking
paper.

Put the flour, oats and coconut in a large mixing
bowl and combine.

Melt the butter and honey together in a small
saucepan over low heat—continuously stirring to
combine. Remove from the heat then stir through
the bicarb until the mixture doubles in size.

Add the hot honey mixture to the dry ingredients
and gently mix together. Pour into the prepared
tin and bake for 25–30 minutes, or until cooked
through. Cool in the tin.

Meanwhile melt the chocolate in a heatproof
bowl and microwave for 30 seconds at a time,
stirring in between, until melted and smooth.
Alternatively, use the double-boiler method on
page 73.

Drizzle the melted chocolate all over the cooled
slice. Once hardened, slice into 16 pieces. Store
in an airtight container in the fridge for 5 days, or
freeze for up to 3 months.

SPELT BLUEBERRY MUFFINS

MAKES 10
PREP TIME 20 minutes
COOK TIME 20 minutes

205 g (7¼ oz/1½ cups) wholemeal (whole-
  wheat) spelt flour
1½ teaspoons baking powder
1 egg
100 ml (3½ fl oz) milk
55 g (2 oz/¼ cup) coconut oil, melted
2 tablespoons rice malt syrup
200 g (7 oz) blueberries (fresh or frozen)
2 tablespoons pepitas (pumpkin seeds)
2 teaspoons linseeds (flaxseeds)
2 tablespoons rolled (porridge) oats

Preheat the oven to 160°C (320°F) and line
10 holes of a 12-hole standard (60 ml/¼ cup)
muffin tin with paper cases.

Sift the flour and baking powder into a large bowl,
and stir to combine.

Put the egg in a bowl with the milk, coconut
oil and rice malt syrup and mix until everything
is well combined. Add this mixture to the dry
ingredients, and stir until combined, then add the
blueberries to the batter and gently fold through.

Mix the pepitas, linseeds and oats in a bowl.
Divide the muffin mixture between the 10 muffin
holes. Sprinkle with the seed mix, then bake in the
oven for 20 minutes, or until golden brown and a
toothpick inserted into one of the muffins comes
out clean.

Allow to cool in the tin for a few minutes before
transferring to a wire rack to cool completely.
Store in an airtight container for up to 3 days.

SNACKS FOR SPECIAL DIETS

Finding healthy options can be a minefield when you're an omnivore, let alone if you've got special dietary requirements. Spoiler alert (sorry!): many muesli bars, fat-free yoghurts, packaged muffins and slices won't satisfy your hunger. These foods can be high in sugar and will cause your energy to spike and then crash soon after. This can lead to excessive hunger, weight gain and sugar cravings.

Whatever diet you follow, prepping ahead is going to be your biggest ally. Spend an hour or so making snacks in order to stay on top of the 168 hours in the week. It's worth it.

Up your snack game by prepping like a boss

1. SET ASIDE SOME TIME

You don't need to spend hours in the kitchen but you do need to dedicate a little time to preparing your snacks. Sunday is my prep day due to my schedule, but choose whichever day suits you and your lifestyle best. And don't forget to have fun. If you enjoy preparing food you'll love eating it, too.

2. MAKE A PLAN

Write a list and go to the shops with a plan of attack—just like you would with your main grocery list. Knowing exactly what you need to buy helps prevent you from buying unhealthy, packaged snacks and overspending on crap.

3. BUY IN BULK

Sometimes, buying bigger portions of ingredients is cheaper. So when it comes to recipe staples like quinoa, oats, flour or frozen berries, buying more can save you money—win! It also ensures your pantry is filled with good, wholesome ingredients, and you won't run out of food as quickly.

4. COOK UP A BATCH

Don't just prep snacks for a day or two, make enough to keep you going through the week. (Trust me, you'll thank yourself mid-week when you don't need to do any extra cooking.) You can also freeze a batch of snacks for the following week, saving you even more time.

5. WASTE NOT, WANT NOT

Use what you already have floating around in your kitchen. If your recipe calls for spinach but you only have kale, swap it in and give yourself a pat on the back for not wasting those delicious greens. If you have fruit that's too ripe to eat fresh (like bananas or avocados) find a snack recipe you can use them in.

6. LEARN HOW TO READ LABELS

Become a grocery-shopping guru with a lesson on how to read labels. Learn what to look out for, what 'fat-free' really means and how to spot all the different names for sugar—there are loads!

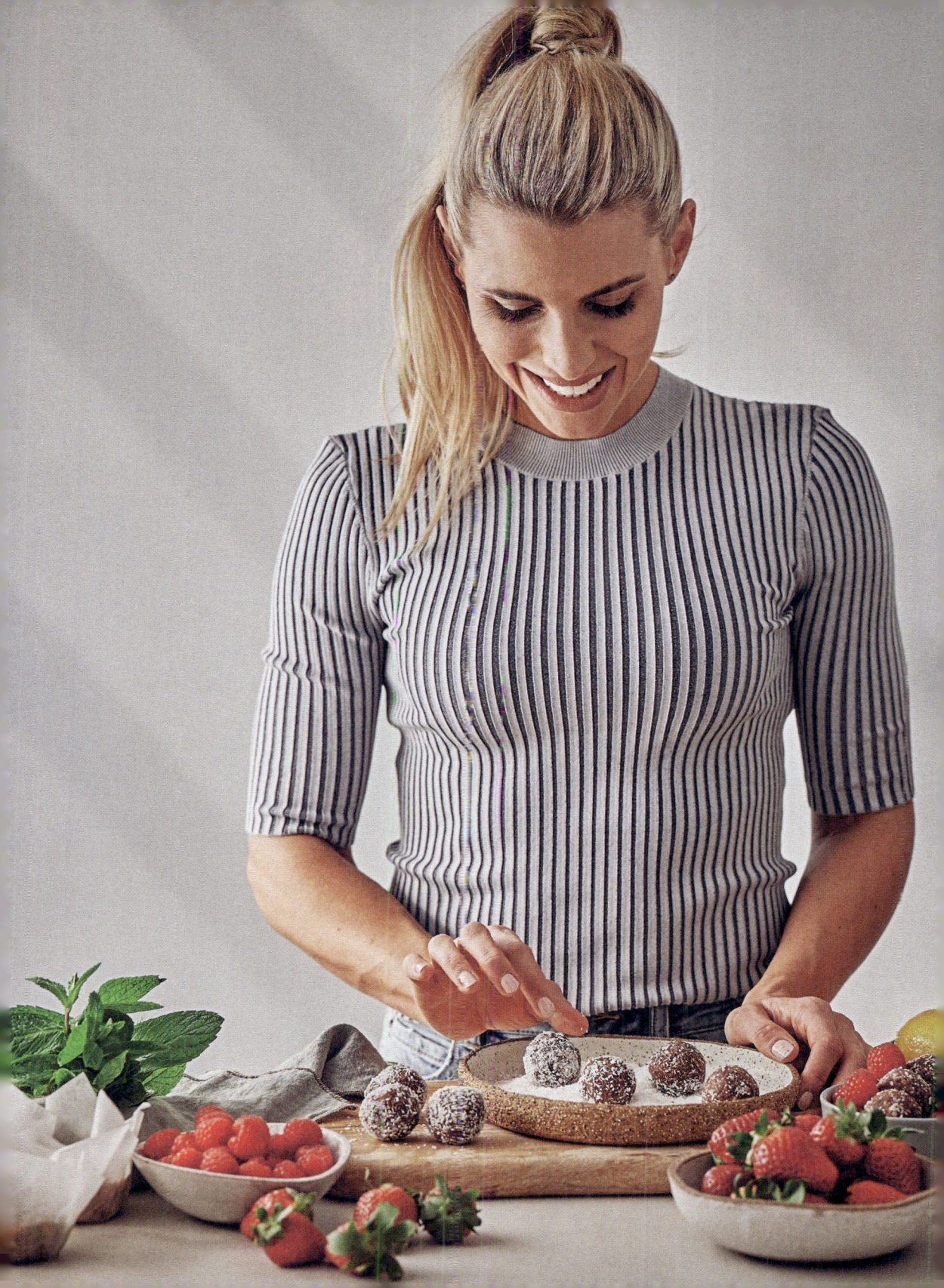

SPICED CAULIFLOWER BITES

SERVES 2
PREP TIME 10 minutes
COOK TIME 30 minutes

40 g (1½ oz/¼ cup) rice flour
1 teaspoon smoked paprika
½ teaspoon ground turmeric
½ head cauliflower, cut into florets
salt and pepper
90 g (3¼ oz/⅓ cup) tzatziki (page 106), to serve

Preheat the oven to 200°C (400°F) and line a baking tray with baking paper.

Place the rice flour, paprika and turmeric in a large bowl. Season well with salt and pepper and whisk to combine. Toss the cauliflower in the seasoned flour and transfer to the baking tray. Bake for 25–30 minutes, or until golden and cooked.

Serve the cauliflower bites hot, in a large bowl with tzatziki on the side.

CHEESY BROCCOLI QUINOA BITES

MAKES 10 (2 bites per snack)
PREP TIME 10 minutes
COOK TIME 30 minutes

100 g (3½ oz/½ cup) white quinoa, rinsed
500 g (1 lb 2 oz) broccoli, coarsely chopped
65 g (2⅓ oz) parmesan cheese, coarsely grated
3 large eggs
1 spring onion, sliced
1 teaspoon dried oregano

Preheat the oven to 180°C (350°F) and line a 12-hole standard (60 ml/¼ cup) muffin tin with 10 paper cases.

Place the quinoa and 250 ml (9 fl oz/1 cup) salted water in a small saucepan and bring to the boil. Simmer, covered, for 15 minutes, or until cooked, then remove from the heat and stand covered for 5 minutes.

Place the broccoli in a food processor and blitz to a rice consistency.

Combine the quinoa, broccoli, parmesan, eggs, spring onion and oregano in a large bowl.

Spoon the mixture into the 10 paper cases and bake for 15 minutes, or until golden and crisp. Once cool, these can be kept in an airtight container in the fridge for up to 5 days.

If you're coeliac or just feel better ditching the gluten, the snacks in this section are free from the big three: wheat, barley and rye. But don't let that fool you; they're seriously satisfying and bursting with flavour.

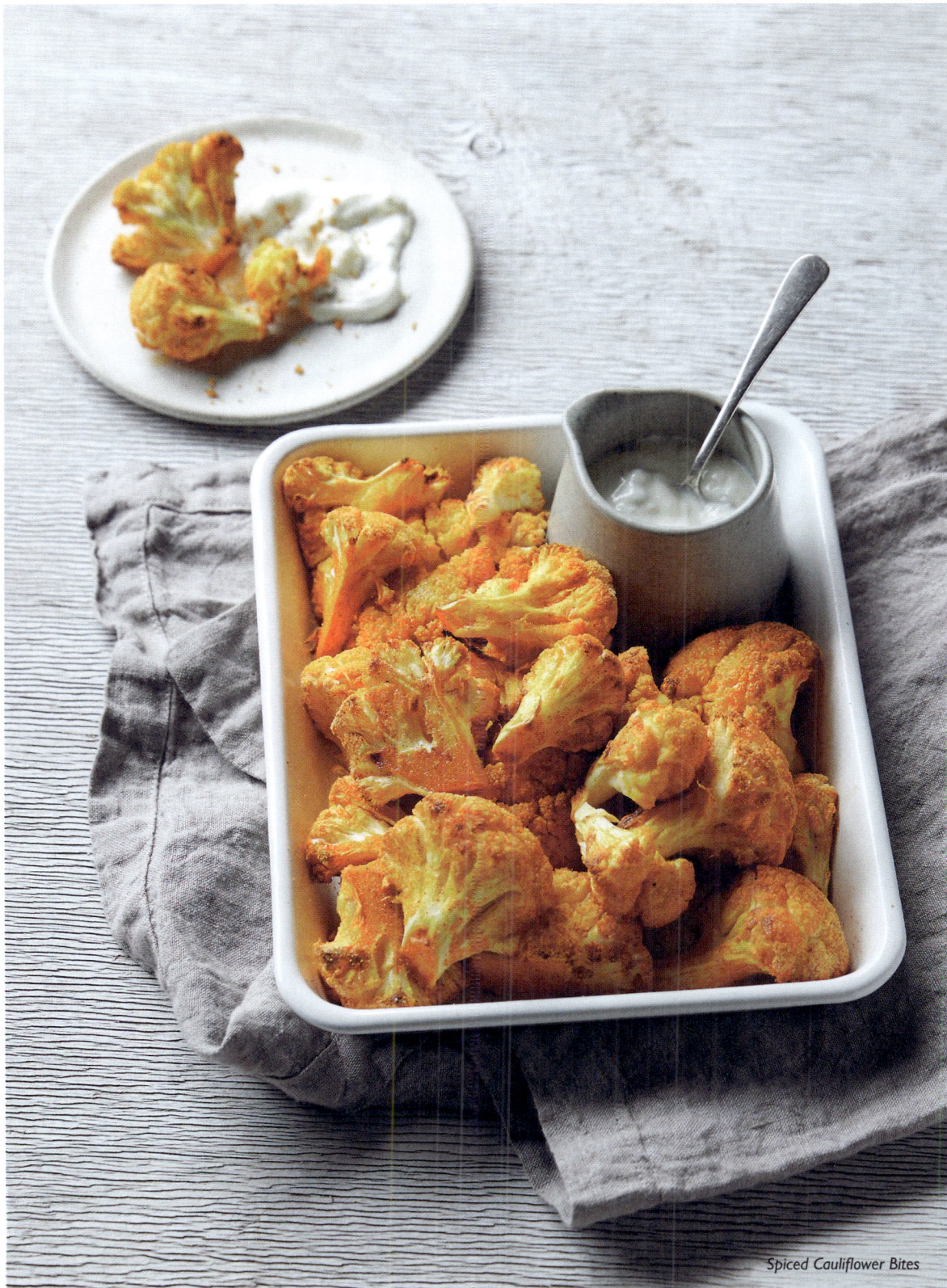

Spiced Cauliflower Bites

KIMCHI PIKELETS

MAKES 8
PREP TIME 15 minutes + 20 minutes chilling time
COOK TIME 10 minutes

60 g (2¼ oz/½ cup) chickpea flour (besan)
½ teaspoon baking powder
½ teaspoon sea salt flakes
80 ml (2½ fl oz/⅓ cup) kimchi liquid, plus extra
150 g (5½ oz) kimchi, squeezed and finely
   chopped
2 spring onions (scallions), thinly sliced,
   plus extra to garnish
2 tablespoons extra virgin olive oil
130 g (4½ oz/½ cup) dairy-free yoghurt
1 Lebanese (short) cucumber, deseeded and
   finely diced
zest and juice of ½ lemon
salt and pepper, to taste
1 teaspoon black sesame seeds

Combine the flour, baking powder and salt in a
large bowl and stir to combine. Add the kimchi
liquid and whisk to form a smooth, thick batter.
Fold through the chopped kimchi, spring onions
and some extra kimchi liquid, if needed. Place the
bowl, covered, in the fridge for at least 20 minutes.

Heat the oil in a large, non-stick frying pan over
medium heat. Drop heaped tablespoons of the
chilled batter into the pan, spreading them out
using the back of a spoon. Cook for 2 minutes on
each side, or until cooked through. Repeat with
the remaining batter, greasing the pan between
each batch.

Combine the yoghurt, cucumber, lemon zest and
juice in a small bowl and season to taste.

Serve the pikelets with yoghurt sauce and sprinkle
with sesame seeds.

PARMESAN AND ROSEMARY CRISPS

SERVES 2
PREP TIME 5 minutes
COOK TIME 7 minutes

50 g (1¾ oz/½ cup) finely grated parmesan
   cheese
1 rosemary sprig, leaves picked and finely
   chopped
⅛ teaspoon paprika
black pepper, to taste

Preheat the oven to 180°C (350°F) and line a
baking tray with baking paper.

Toss the parmesan and rosemary together and
place tablespoons of the mixture on the prepared
baking tray, allowing room for the cheese to
spread while cooking. Sprinkle over the paprika
and season with pepper.

Bake for 7 minutes, or until melted and golden.
Remove from the oven and allow to cool for a
minute, then transfer the crisps to a wire rack
until completely cool.

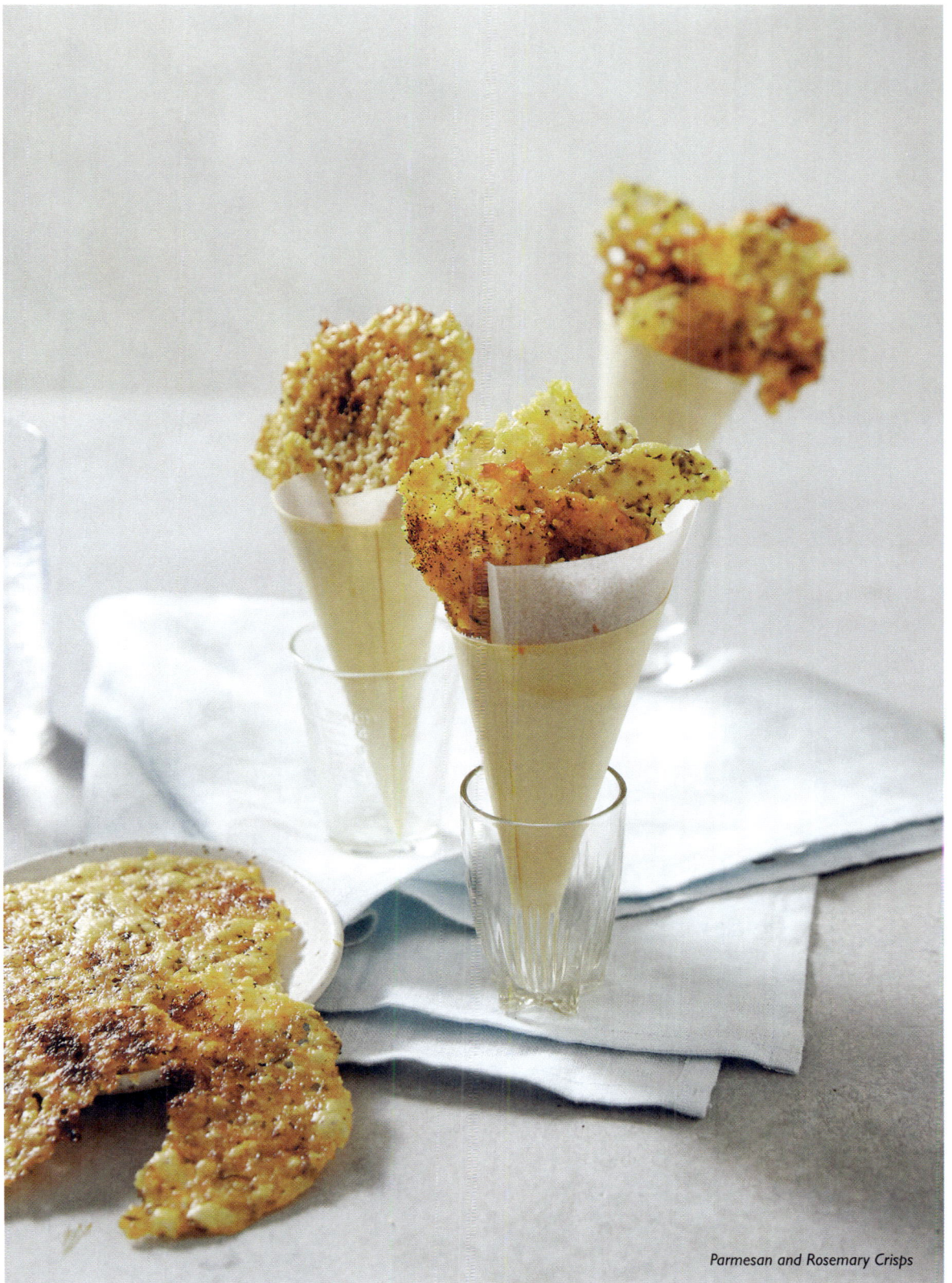

Parmesan and Rosemary Crisps

CARROT, MAPLE AND SEED MUFFINS

MAKES 12
PREP TIME 10 minutes
COOK TIME 20 minutes

210 g (7½ oz/1½ cups) gluten-free flour
1 teaspoon baking powder
½ teaspoon ground ginger
3 large eggs
70 g (2½ oz/¼ cup) Greek-style yoghurt
1 teaspoon natural vanilla extract
60 ml (2 fl oz/¼ cup) maple syrup
150 g (5½ oz) unsalted butter, melted
2 carrots, finely grated

TOPPING
2 teaspoons linseeds (flaxseeds)
3 teaspoons pepitas (pumpkin seeds)
3 teaspoons sunflower seeds

Preheat the oven to 180°C (350°F) and line a 12-hole standard (60 ml/¼ cup) muffin tin with paper cases.

Place all of the dry ingredients in a large mixing bowl and stir to combine.

Place the eggs, yoghurt and vanilla in a small mixing bowl and mix until smooth. Add the maple syrup and melted butter, and stir again to combine.

Add the egg mixture to the dry ingredients, and mix well to combine. Then gently fold through the grated carrot.

Spoon the batter into the prepared muffin tin.

Place the seeds for the topping in a small bowl and combine. Sprinkle them over the muffins then place in the oven to bake for 20 minutes, or until a toothpick inserted in the centre of one of the muffins comes out clean.

Allow the muffins to cool in the tin for a few minutes before removing and transferring to a wire rack to cool completely. Store in an airtight container for up to 3 days.

CHOCOLATE BROWNIE PROTEIN BALLS

MAKES 8
PREP TIME 10 minutes
COOK TIME 2 minutes

3 tablespoons peanut butter
   (or other nut butter)
2 tablespoons coconut oil
2 tablespoons honey
3 tablespoons almond meal
2 tablespoons protein powder
2 tablespoons raw cacao powder,
   plus extra for dusting (optional)

Heat the nut butter, coconut oil and honey in a small saucepan over medium–low heat until melted and combined, then stir through 2 tablespoons water.

Mix the almond meal, protein powder and cacao together in a medium bowl, and stir through the wet ingredients.

With clean damp hands, roll into eight balls and lightly dust with cacao powder, if coating. Refrigerate until set, and then store in an airtight container for up to 5 days.

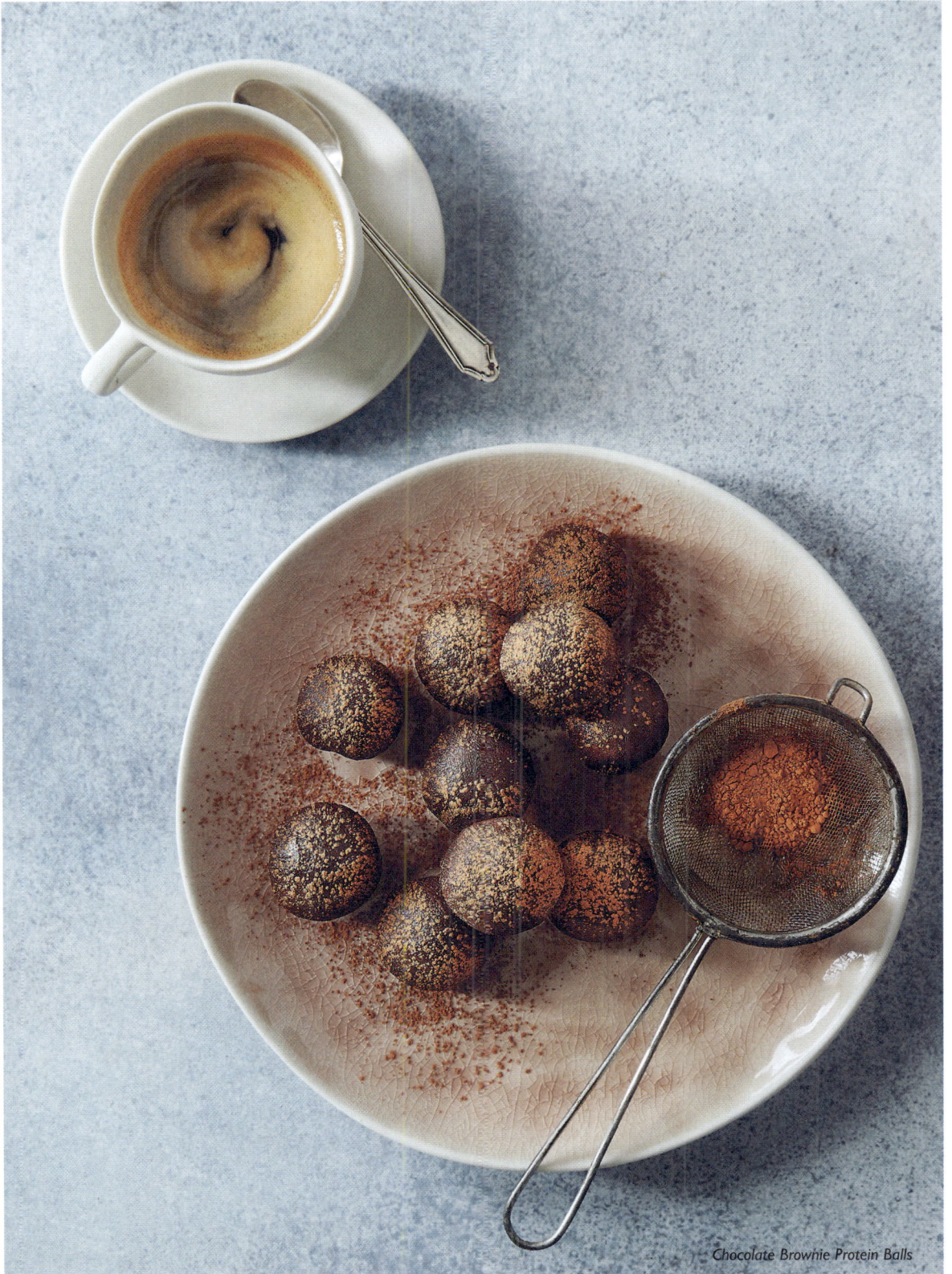

Chocolate Brownie Protein Balls

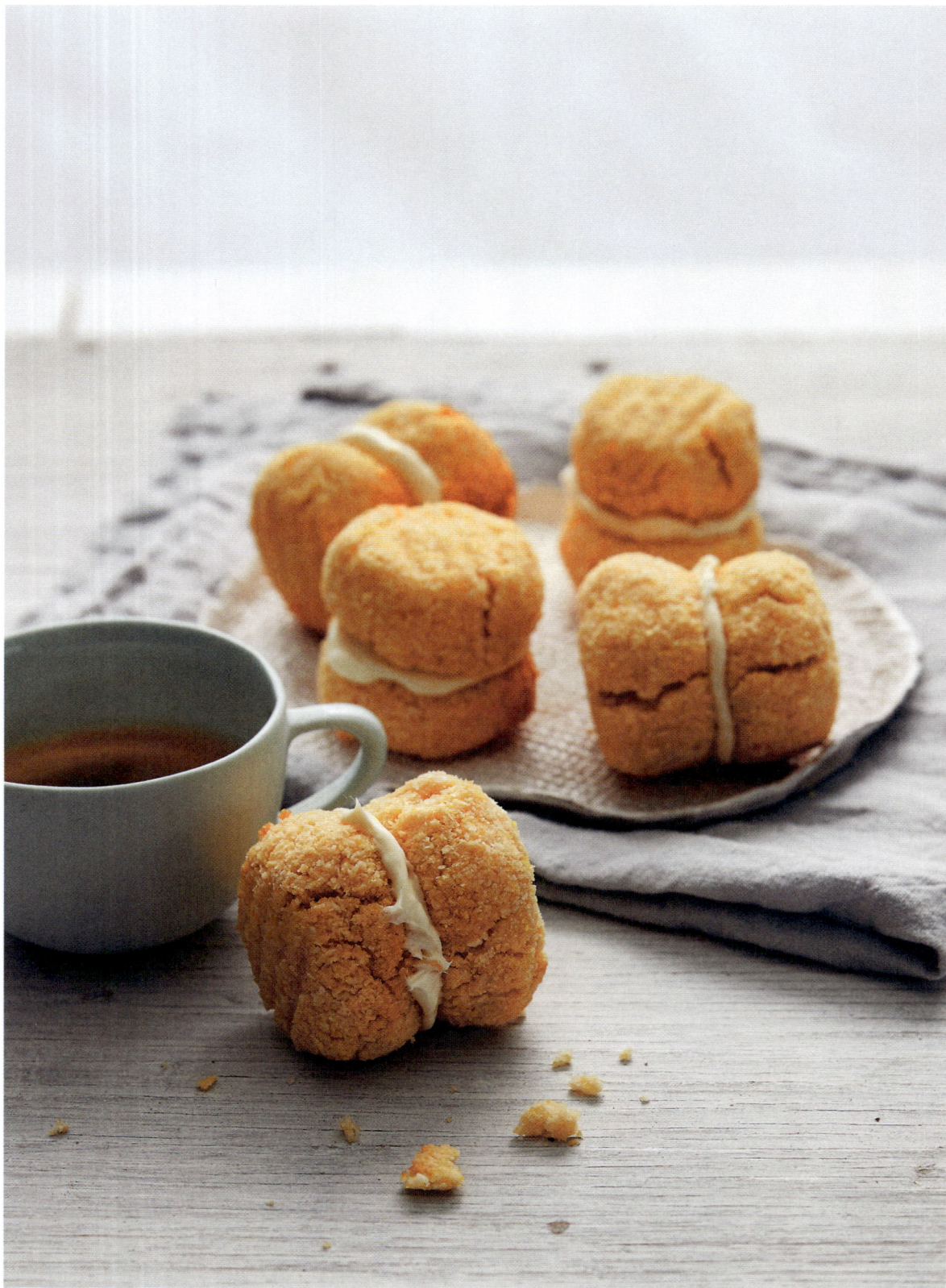

ORANGE-SCENTED YOYOS WITH HONEY CREAM

MAKES 8
PREP TIME 15 minutes
COOK TIME 12 minutes

180 g (6¼ oz/2 cups) desiccated coconut
50 g (1¾ oz/¼ cup) polenta (cornmeal)
35 g (1¼ oz/¼ cup) gluten-free flour
60 ml (2 fl oz/¼ cup) maple syrup
2 large eggs
1 teaspoon natural vanilla extract
zest of ½ orange
60 g (2¼ oz) cream cheese, at room
   temperature
1 teaspoon honey

Preheat the oven to 160°C (320°F). Line a baking tray with baking paper.

Place the coconut, polenta, flour, maple syrup, eggs, vanilla and orange zest in a food processor with 60 ml (2 fl oz/¼ cup) water, and blend until combined. Add a little more water if necessary to bring the mixture together.

Press the mixture together and roll into 16 smooth balls. Place these on the prepared baking tray, flattening slightly with a fork and smoothing out any big cracks with your finger.

Bake for 12 minutes, or until lightly golden, then transfer to a wire rack to cool completely.

Mix the cream cheese and honey in a bowl until smooth and combined. Sandwich two cookies together with ½ teaspoon of the cheese mixture, and repeat until you have eight yoyos.

Serve one as a snack and store the rest in an airtight container in the fridge.

GRILLED PINEAPPLE SKEWERS AND VANILLA YOGHURT

SERVES 2
PREP TIME 5 minutes + 15 minutes soaking time
COOK TIME 5 minutes

95 g (3¼ oz/⅓ cup) Greek-style yoghurt
1 teaspoon natural vanilla extract
500 g (1 lb 2 oz) pineapple, peeled and
   cut into 4 wedges
¼ teaspoon ground cinnamon

YOU'LL ALSO NEED
4 wooden skewers, soaked in water for
   15 minutes

Preheat a grill pan to medium–high heat.

Combine the yoghurt and vanilla in a bowl and set aside.

Thread the pineapple wedges onto the pre-soaked skewers and dust with the cinnamon.

Grill the skewers for 2 minutes on each side, or until golden, and serve with the vanilla yoghurt.

CHEWY AMARETTI

MAKES 20
PREP TIME 20 minutes
COOK TIME 12 minutes

2 eggs, separated
50 ml (1⅔ fl oz) maple syrup
2 drops natural almond essence
200 g (7 oz/2 cups) almond meal
zest of 1 lemon
35 g (1¼ oz/⅓ cup) flaked almonds

Preheat the oven to 150°C (300°F). Line a baking tray with baking paper.

Beat the egg yolks, maple syrup and almond essence together in a large bowl. Add the almond meal and lemon zest, and mix to combine.

In a separate bowl, whisk the egg whites until soft peaks form. Fold a third of the egg whites into the almond mixture to loosen it. Fold through the remaining egg whites until just combined, then portion the mixture into 20 balls. Place these on a large plate and put in the fridge to chill for 20 minutes.

Remove the balls from the fridge and roll them in the flaked almonds, pressing the almonds gently into the dough. Place on the prepared tray and bake for 12 minutes, or until slightly golden.

Allow to cool on a wire rack, then store in an airtight container for up to 1 week.

PLUM CLAFOUTIS

SERVES 6
PREP TIME 12 minutes
COOK TIME 30 minutes

1 teaspoon coconut oil
100 g (3½ oz/1 cup) almond meal
1 teaspoon ground cinnamon
2 whole eggs
250 ml (9 fl oz/1 cup) almond milk
2 tablespoons maple syrup
finely grated zest of 1 orange
3 plums, halved and stones removed
100 g (3½ oz) coconut yoghurt,
    to serve (optional)

Preheat the oven to 160°C (320°F). Generously grease a 750 ml (26 fl oz/3 cup) capacity baking dish with the coconut oil and set aside.

Combine the rest of the ingredients except the plums and yoghurt in a blender. Blitz for two minutes, or until the batter is very smooth.

Pour the batter into the prepared baking dish and evenly distribute the plums, cut side up. Bake for 25–30 minutes, or until firm to touch and lightly browned in colour.

Serve warm, with coconut yoghurt, if you like.

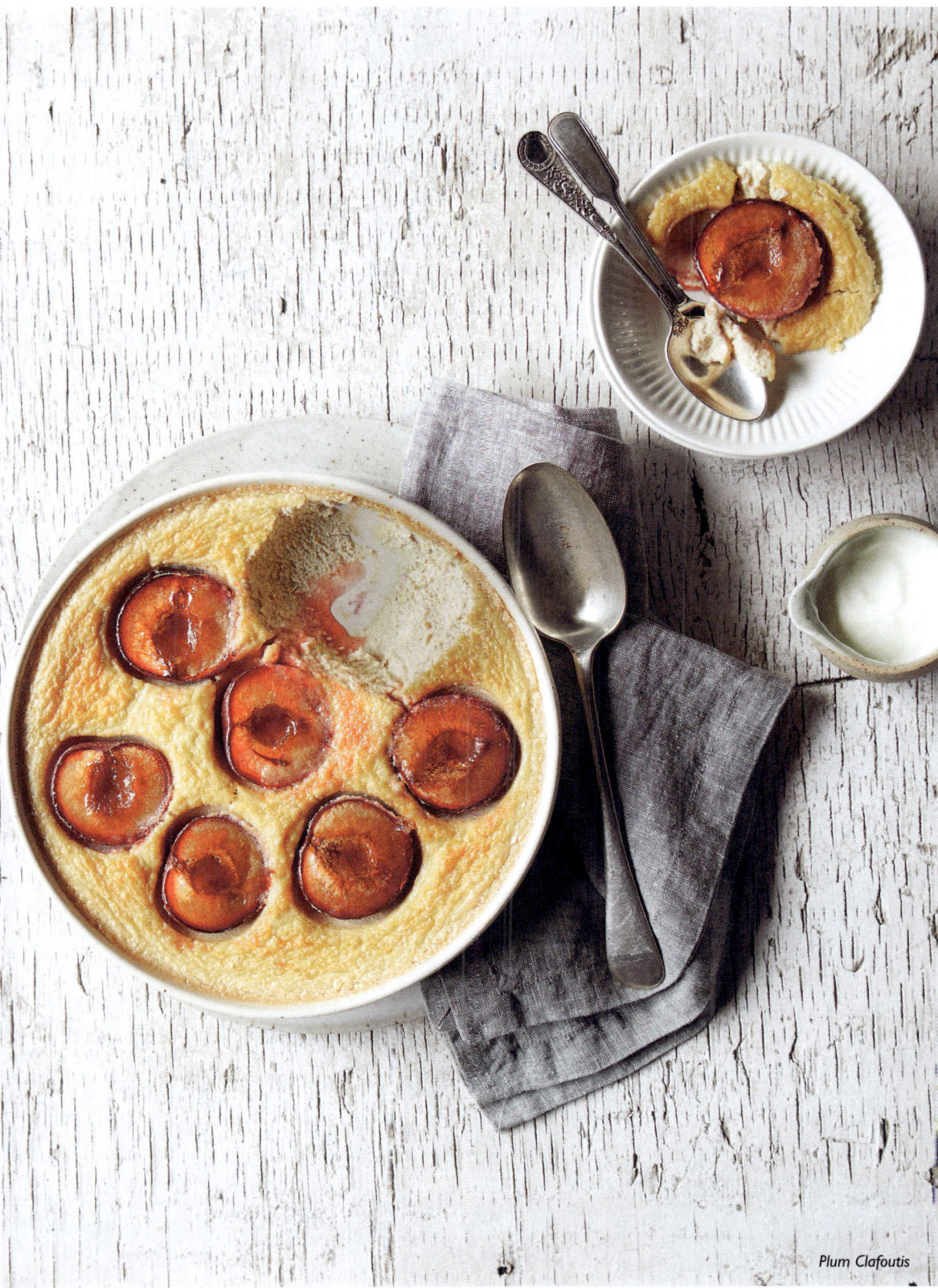

Plum Clafoutis

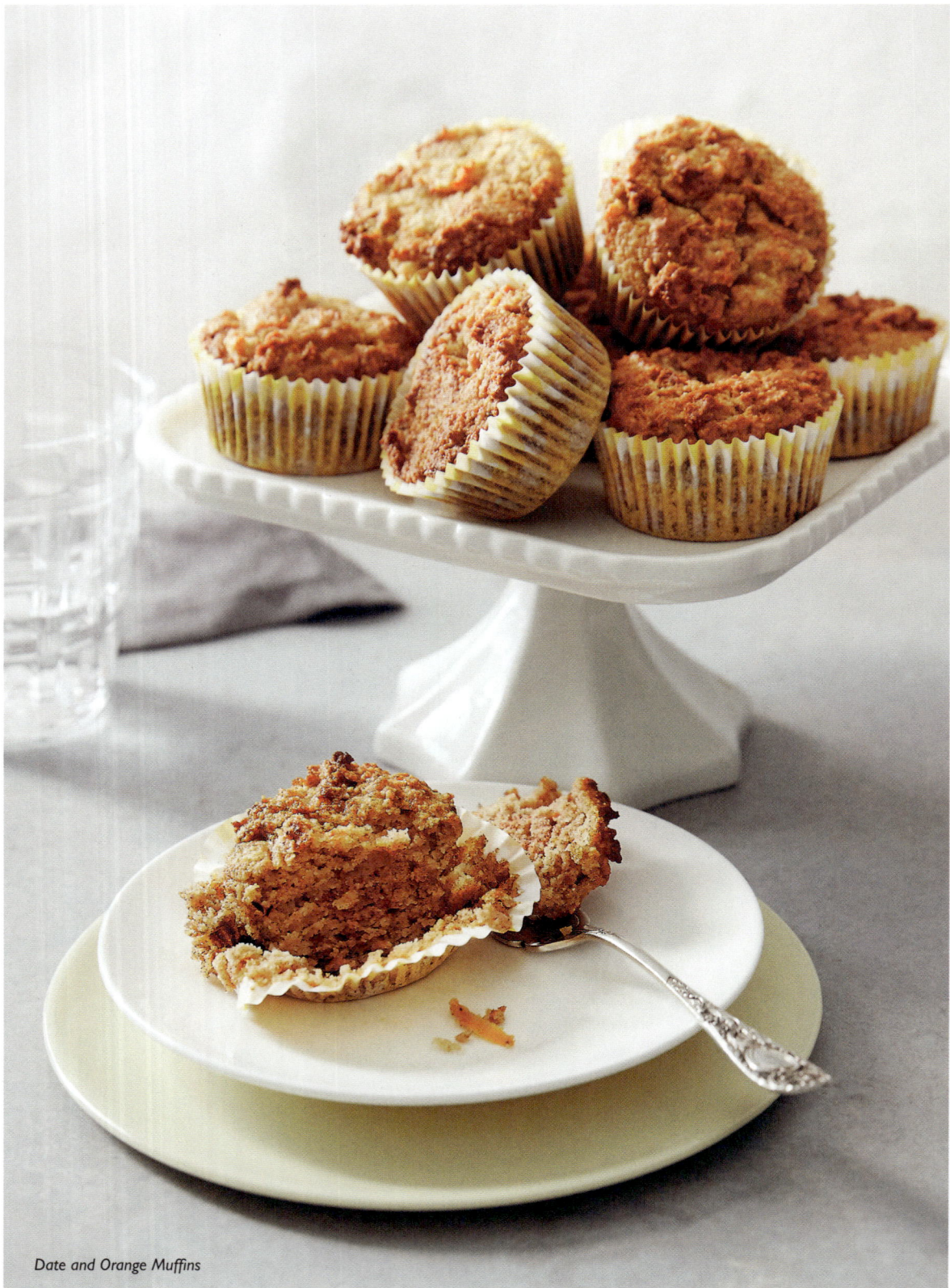

Date and Orange Muffins

DATE AND ORANGE MUFFINS

MAKES 12
PREP TIME 10 minutes
COOK TIME 20 minutes

40 g (1½ oz/¼ cup) pitted medjool dates
150 g (5½ oz/1½ cups) almond meal
1 teaspoon bicarbonate of soda (baking soda)
¼ teaspoon salt
zest and juice of 1 orange
3 large eggs, whisked
40 g (1½ oz) melted butter

Place the dates in a heatproof bowl and cover with boiling water. Leave to soak for 10 minutes.

Preheat the oven to 175°C (345°F) and line a 12-hole standard (60 ml/¼ cup) muffin tin with paper cases.

Combine the almond meal, bicarb, salt and zest in a medium bowl.

Drain and roughly chop the dates, then stir them into the dry ingredients.

Mix the orange juice, eggs and butter together, then add to the dry ingredients and mix until just combined.

Spoon the batter into the paper cases and bake for 20 minutes, or until a toothpick inserted into one of the muffins comes out clean.

Cool on a wire rack.

BLUEBERRY AND LEMON YOGHURT FOOL

SERVES 2
PREP TIME 10 minutes
COOK TIME 5 minutes

1 teaspoon shredded coconut
155 (5½ oz/1 cup) frozen blueberries
zest of 1 lemon
1 teaspoon honey
130 g (4½ oz/½ cup) Greek-style yoghurt
1 teaspoon natural vanilla extract

Place the coconut in a small saucepan over medium heat and toast for 1–2 minutes or until lightly golden, then transfer to a plate and set aside.

Place the blueberries, half the lemon zest and the honey in the same saucepan over medium heat. Bring to a simmer, crush the blueberries with a fork and cook until smooth (about 2–3 minutes).

Transfer the berries to a bowl and place in the fridge to chill for 5 minutes.

Combine the yoghurt, remaining lemon zest and the vanilla in a bowl.

When ready to serve, use a tablespoon to alternate layering yoghurt and berry purée into two glasses or bowls. Top with the toasted coconut to serve.

SWEET AND SAVOURY SNACK BARS

MAKES 12
PREP TIME 15 minutes
COOK TIME 25 minutes

100 g (3½ oz) honey
50 g (1¾ oz) butter, chopped
50 g (1¾ oz/2 cups) puffed rice
75 g (2⅔ oz/½ cup) sunflower seeds
2 tablespoons desiccated coconut
1 tablespoon sesame seeds
½ teaspoon paprika
¼ teaspoon chilli flakes
75 g (2⅔ oz/½ cup) pepitas (pumpkin seeds)
¼ teaspoon salt

Preheat the oven to 160°C (320°F) and line a 20 cm (8 inch) square baking tin with baking paper.

Warm the honey and butter together in a small saucepan over medium–low heat until melted.

Combine the dry ingredients in a large bowl and pour over the honey and butter, mixing well.

Transfer to the prepared tin, press down firmly and bake for 20 minutes, or until golden. Cool in the tin before cutting into 12 pieces. Once completely cool, store in an airtight container.

QUICK BANANA PIKELETS WITH HONEY YOGHURT

SERVES 4
PREP TIME 10 minutes
COOK TIME 5 minutes

3 tablespoons gluten-free flour
¼ teaspoon ground cinnamon
⅛ teaspoon baking powder
2 large eggs
1 large banana, well mashed
1 teaspoon olive oil
130 g (4½ oz/½ cup) Greek-style yoghurt
1 teaspoon honey

Combine the flour, cinnamon and baking powder in a medium bowl.

Whisk the eggs and banana until well combined and the mixture is a little frothy. Gently stir through the flour mixture.

Heat the oil in a small frying pan over medium heat. Spoon 2 tablespoons of mixture per pikelet and cook each one for 1–2 minutes, or until bubbles start to form on the surface. Carefully flip and cook for a further 1–2 minutes.

Combine the yoghurt and honey in a small bowl, and serve with the pikelets.

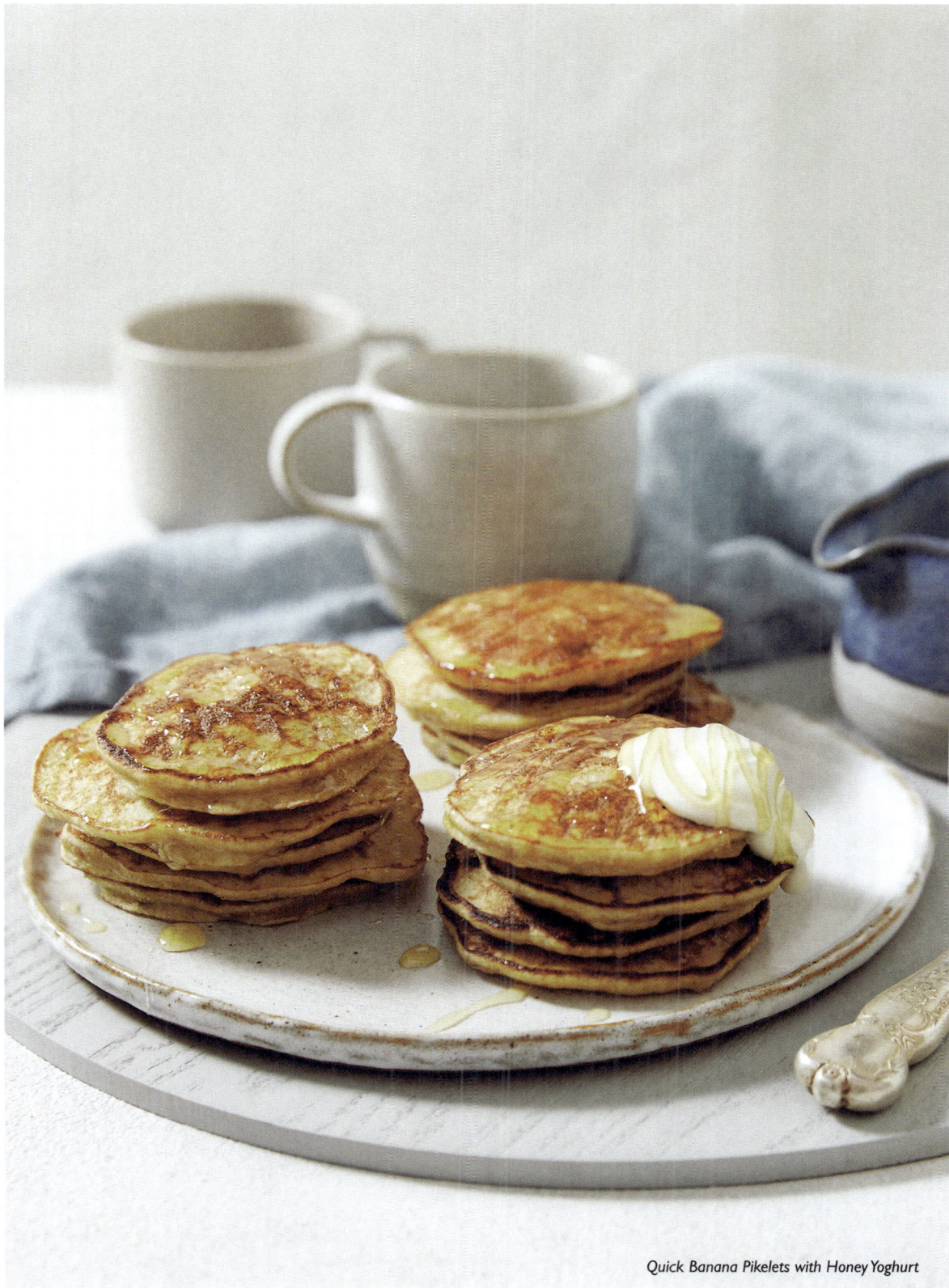

Quick Banana Pikelets with Honey Yoghurt

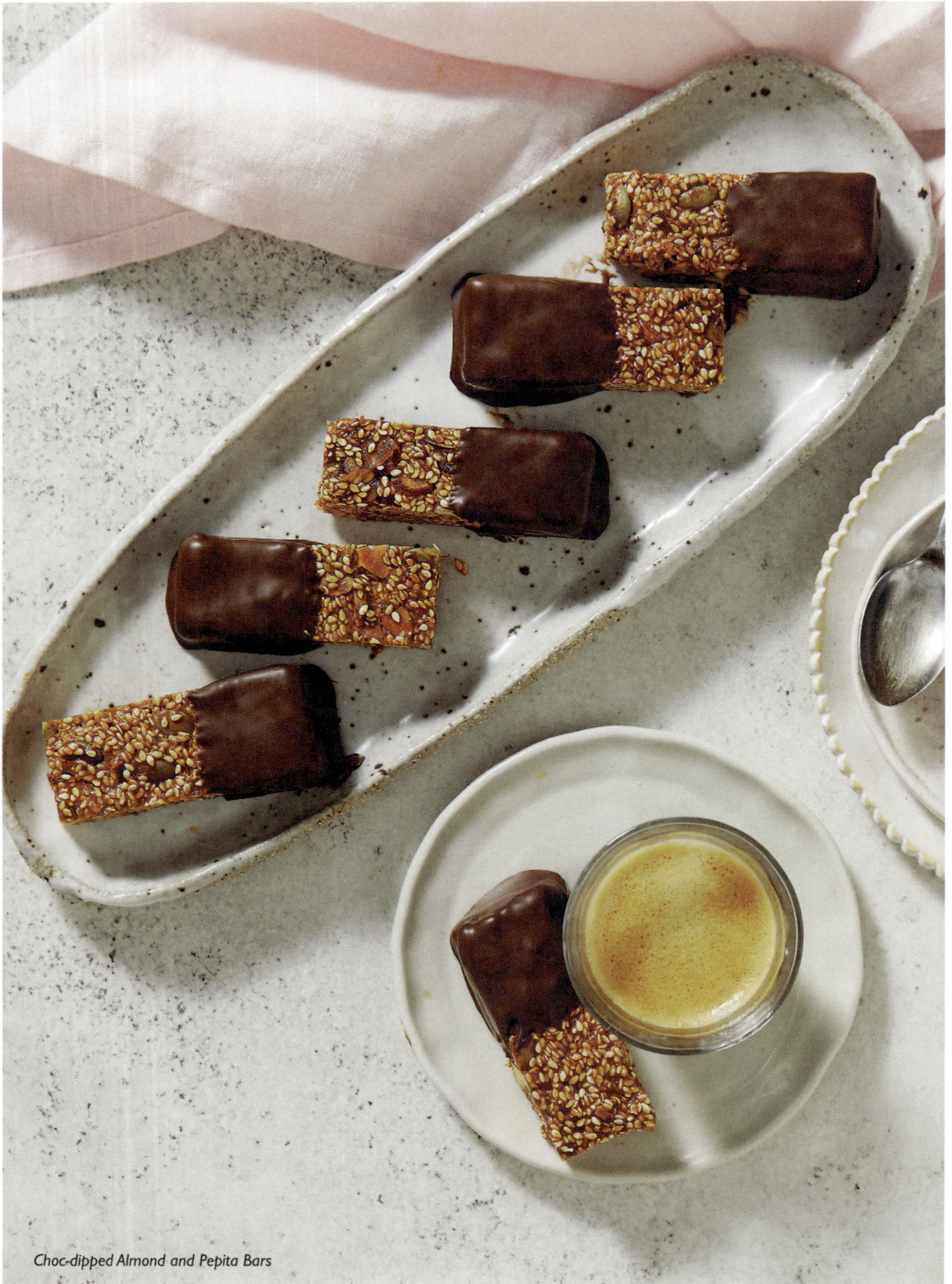

Choc-dipped Almond and Pepita Bars

CHOC-DIPPED ALMOND AND PEPITA BARS

MAKES 16
PREP TIME 15 minutes
COOK TIME 30 minutes

145 g (5¼ oz/1 cup) white sesame seeds
75 g (2⅔ oz/½ cup) pepitas (pumpkin seeds)
155 g (5½ oz/1 cup) coarsely chopped almonds
70 g (2½ oz/¼ cup) natural, crunchy peanut
    butter
175 g (6 oz/½ cup) honey
¼ teaspoon salt
50 g (1¾ oz) dark chocolate (70%)

Preheat the oven to 180°C (350°F) and line an 18 cm (7 inch) square cake tin with baking paper. Line a baking tray with baking paper and place in the freezer.

Toss the seeds and almonds in a large bowl.

Heat the peanut butter, honey and salt in a small saucepan over medium heat, stirring, until combined and melted together.

Pour the warm honey mixture into the bowl of seeds and nuts, and mix through, ensuring all are well coated. Transfer to the prepared tin and press the mixture firmly down with a spatula.

Bake for 25 minutes, or until dark golden. Cool completely in the tin then place in the freezer until completely firm. Cut into 16 bars.

Meanwhile melt the chocolate in a heatproof bowl and microwave for 30 seconds at a time, stirring in between, until melted and smooth. Alternatively, use the double-boiler method on page 73.

Dip the bars in the chocolate, allowing any excess chocolate to drip off, then place on the chilled baking tray and refrigerate until set.

Store in an airtight container in the fridge.

YOGHURT PANNA COTTA POTS

SERVES 6
PREP TIME 15 minutes
COOK TIME 5 minutes

115 g (4 oz/⅓ cup) honey
finely grated zest of 1 lemon
125 ml (4 fl oz/½ cup) lemon juice
    (about 2–3 lemons)
3 teaspoons agar-agar
520 g (1 lb 2¼ oz/2 cups) Greek-style yoghurt
125 g (4½ oz) fresh blueberries, to serve

Combine the honey, lemon zest and juice, and the agar-agar in a small saucepan and bring to the boil. Reduce the heat to low and simmer for 2 minutes, or until the agar-agar has dissolved.

Remove the honey mixture from the heat and pour into a large bowl. Add the yoghurt, then whisk to combine. Strain the mixture through a fine mesh sieve then pour into six serving glasses. Refrigerate, uncovered, for at least 3 hours, or until set.

Serve the yoghurt pots with the fresh blueberries. You can either invert the pots onto plates for dessert, or serve them in their glasses for an easily transportable snack.

ZUCCHINI AND POLENTA FRITTATAS

MAKES 12
PREP TIME 15 minutes
COOK TIME 30 minutes

1 teaspoon olive oil
1 red capsicum (pepper), diced
1 teaspoon ground cumin
½ teaspoon smoked paprika
500 ml (9 fl oz/2 cups) low-FODMAP stock
   (I like the Massel brand)
50 g (1¾ oz/¼ cup) polenta (cornmeal)
6 eggs, beaten
60 g (2¼ oz/½ cup) cheddar cheese, grated
1 zucchini (courgette), grated
salt and pepper
70 g (2½ oz/¼ cup) low-FODMAP tomato
   chutney

Preheat the oven to 220°C (425°F). Line a 12-hole standard (60 ml/¼ cup) muffin tin with paper cases (skip this step if using a silicone muffin mould).

Heat the oil in a large saucepan. Sauté the capsicum in a large saucepan over medium heat with the cumin and paprika until softened and fragrant. Add the stock and bring to the boil, then lower the heat to a simmer. Add the polenta in a slow and steady stream, stirring continuously. Reduce the heat to low and cook, stirring occasionally, for 10 minutes, then remove from the heat and set aside.

Combine the eggs, cheddar and zucchini in a large bowl. Stir through the polenta mixture and season to taste. Divide the batter between the paper cases, then transfer to the oven and cook for 12 minutes, or until golden brown and cooked through.

Serve the frittatas with a side of tomato chutney.

PINWHEEL OMELETTE

SERVES 2
PREP TIME 15 minutes
COOK TIME 10 minutes

4 eggs, lightly beaten
½ red capsicum (pepper), finely chopped
2 spring onions (scallions), green parts only,
   sliced
½ teaspoon sea salt
black pepper, to taste
1 teaspoon olive oil
1 sheet nori

Combine the eggs, capsicum, spring onion, salt and pepper in a medium bowl, and whisk to combine.

Heat the oil in a 20 cm (8 inch) frying pan over medium heat. Add a third of the mixture to the pan, swirling so the mixture covers the base. Allow to cook for a minute or so until set around the edges, then roll the omelette up a couple of times, so it is sitting, half-rolled, in the centre of the pan.

Pour another third of the mixture into the pan so it pools around the unrolled section of omelette. Swirl to cover as much of the base as possible. Allow this layer to cook until the edges start to set.

Place the sheet of nori on the top of the unrolled section, then roll the omelette until most of the second layer is rolled up. Slide the omelette back across the pan a little, add the remaining mixture and allow that to cook until the edges are crispy. Gently finish rolling your omelette then cook for a further 30 seconds on all sides.

Carefully transfer the omelette to a cutting board and allow to cool for 10 minutes before slicing. Trim the edges, then slice into 2 cm (¾ inch) portions.

Serve the omelette as a protein-packed snack, or put into a lunch box.

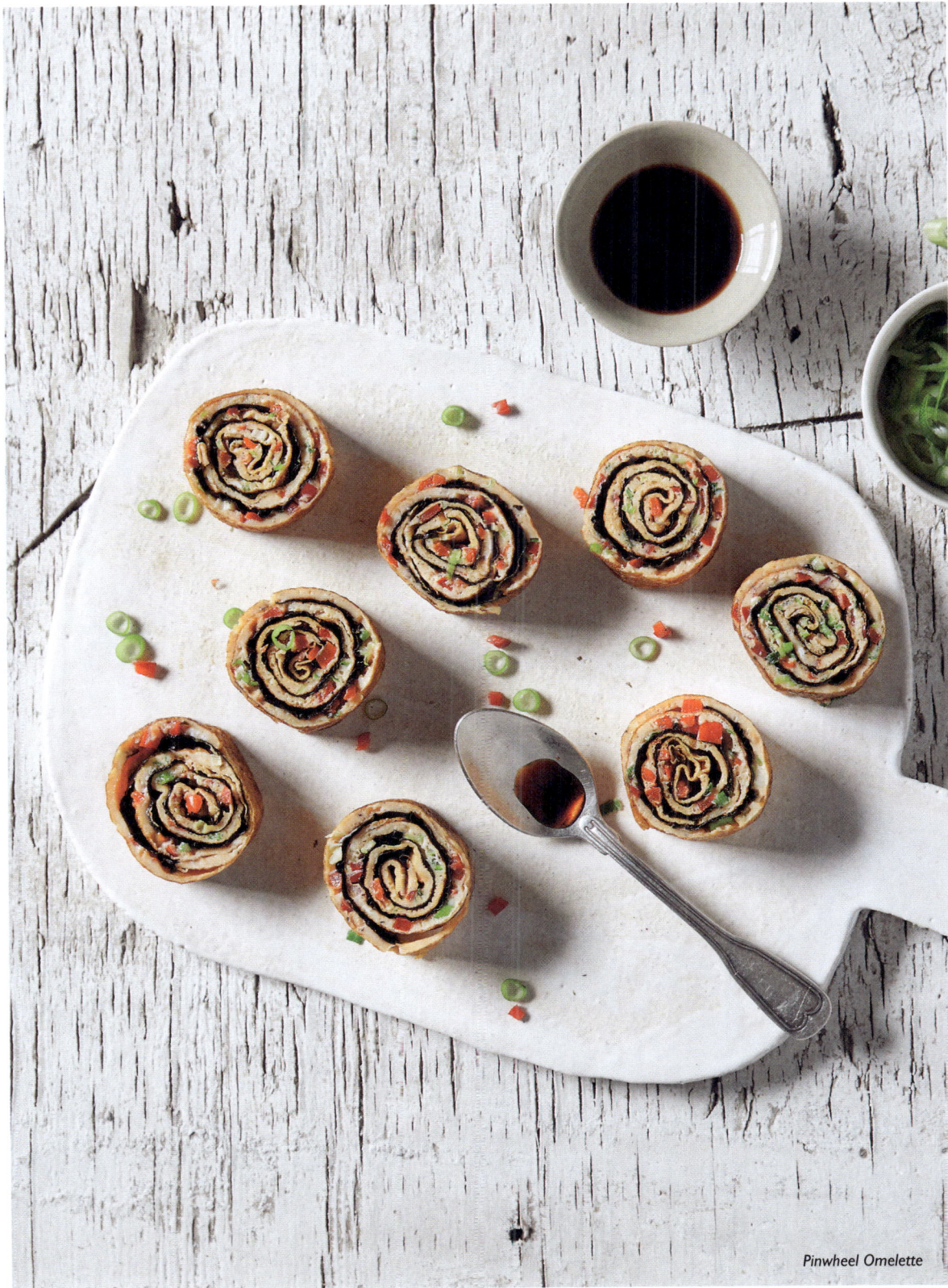

Pinwheel Omelette

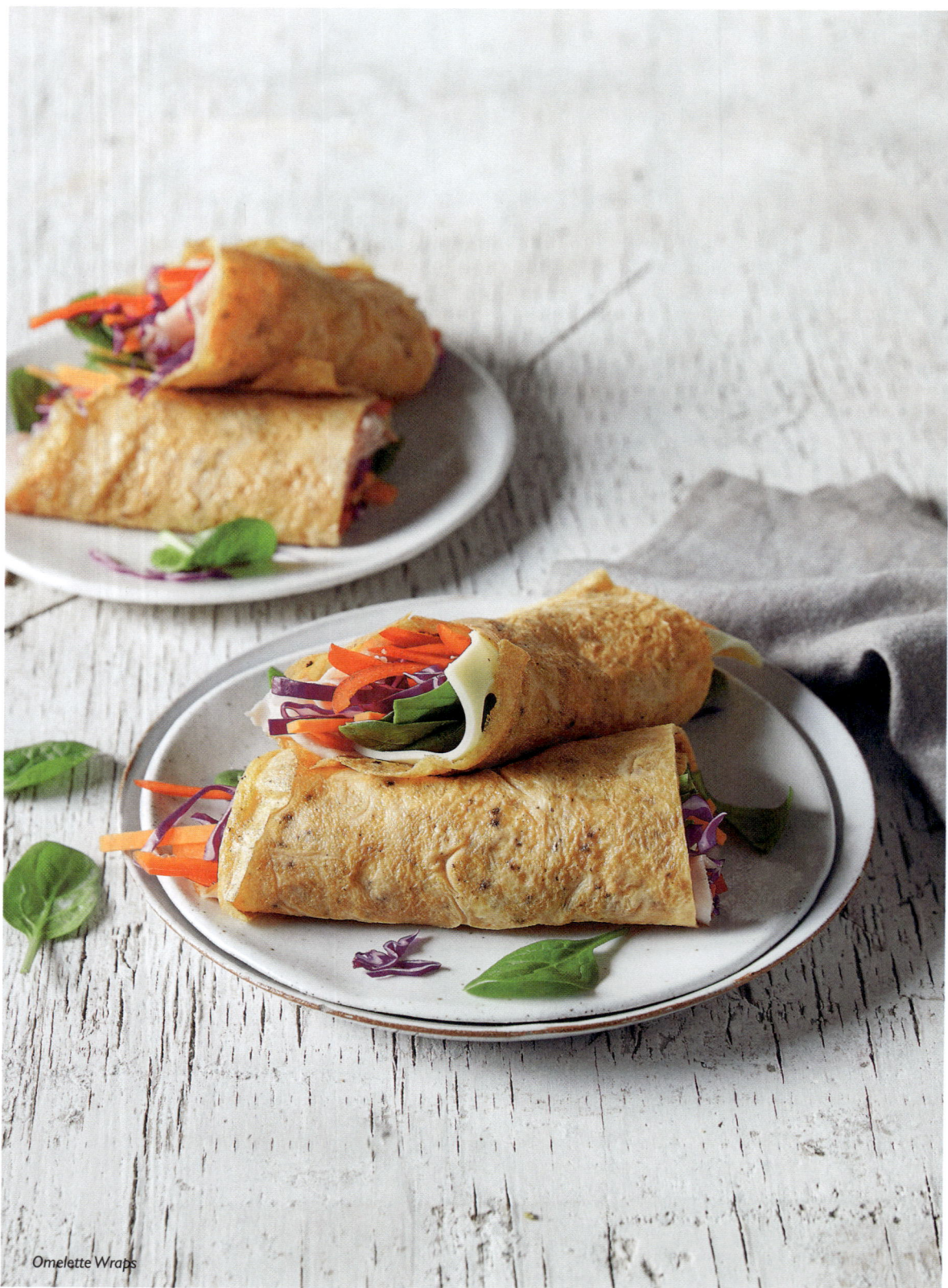

Omelette Wraps

OMELETTE WRAPS

SERVES 2
PREP TIME 15 minutes
COOK TIME 10 minutes

3 eggs
salt and pepper
olive oil spray, to grease
25 g (1 oz/½ cup) baby spinach leaves
40 g (1½ oz/½ cup) finely shredded purple
  cabbage
½ carrot, cut into matchsticks
½ red capsicum (pepper), cut into matchsticks
150 g (5½ oz) shaved ham off the bone (see tip)
2 slices Swiss cheese

Put the eggs, salt and pepper in a jug and whisk
to combine.

Spray a 20 cm (8 inch) frying pan with a fine
mist of cooking oil and place over medium heat.
Pour in half the egg mixture and swirl around the
pan to cover the base. Cook until the edges turn
golden brown and crispy, then carefully turn over
using a spatula. Continue to cook for a further
30 seconds then transfer to a cutting board.

Repeat step 2 with the remaining mixture and
place that omelette next to the other one on
the board to cool while you prep the fillings.

Top the omelette 'wraps' with the remaining
ingredients. Roll each of them up tightly, leaving
the ends open. Serve immediately or refrigerate
for lunch boxes.

ROASTED CARROT HUMMUS

SERVES 4
PREP TIME 5 minutes
COOK TIME 20 minutes

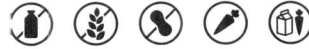

1 teaspoon olive oil
3 carrots, trimmed and coarsely chopped,
  plus 1 carrot, cut into matchsticks
1 teaspoon ground cumin
400 g (14 oz) tinned chickpeas, drained and
  rinsed
1 tablespoon tahini
2 tablespoons lemon juice
salt and pepper
1 pitta bread (gluten-free if needed), warmed
8 radishes, halved

Preheat the oven to 200°C (400°F) and line a
baking tray with baking paper.

Drizzle the oil over the chopped carrot, toss with
cumin and bake for 20 minutes, or until cooked
through. Allow to cool slightly.

Add the warm carrot to a food processor with
the chickpeas, tahini, lemon juice and 60 ml
(2 fl oz/¼ cup) water and pulse to your desired
consistency—add extra water if needed. Taste
and adjust the seasoning.

Serve the hummus with the warm pitta bread,
radishes and carrot sticks.

Tip:
When buying ham, it's always good to check the label and ensure the ham has no
honey or high-fructose corn syrup added to it.

SEA SALT ZUCCHINI CRISPS WITH ROASTED CAPSICUM HUMMUS

SERVES 4
PREP TIME 10 minutes
COOK TIME 20 minutes

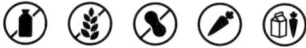

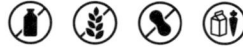

(◯) (◯) (◯) (◯) (◯)

1 red capsicum (pepper), deseeded and quartered
1 garlic clove
2 zucchini (courgettes), thinly sliced
1 teaspoon olive oil
salt and pepper
2 × 125 g (4½ oz) tins chickpeas, rinsed
2 teaspoons tahini
2 tablespoons lemon juice
½ teaspoon ground cumin

Preheat the oven to 210°C (410°F) and line two baking trays with baking paper.

Place the capsicum and garlic on one baking tray and roast for 15 minutes, until the edges of the capsicum are starting to blister. Set aside to cool slightly, then peel the garlic clove.

Meanwhile, press the zucchini between two sheets of paper towel to remove any excess moisture, then place on the other tray. Lightly brush with the olive oil, sprinkle with salt and, bake for 10 minutes then turn over and bake for another 10 minutes, or until golden. Allow to cool on the tray.

Blend the roasted capsicum and garlic with the chickpeas, tahini, lemon juice and cumin to a rough paste, adding extra lemon juice if the mixture is too thick. Adjust the seasoning and serve with the zucchini crisps.

SALTED CHOCOLATE QUINOA COOKIES

MAKES 16
PREP TIME 20 minutes
COOK TIME 20 minutes

(◯) (◯) (◯) (◯)

80 g (2¾ oz) quinoa flakes
2 tablespoons cocoa powder
80 g (2¾ oz) gluten-free flour
½ teaspoon baking powder
45 g (1⅔ oz/½ cup) desiccated coconut
50 g (1¾ oz) coconut oil, melted
60 ml (2 fl oz/¼ cup) maple syrup
2 large eggs
25 g (1 oz) dark chocolate (70%), coarsely chopped
1 teaspoon sea salt

Preheat the oven to 160°C (320°F) and line a baking tray with baking paper.

Place the quinoa flakes, cocoa powder, flour, baking powder, coconut, coconut oil, maple syrup, eggs and chocolate in a large bowl and mix well to combine.

Using wet hands, roll the mixture into walnut-sized balls and place these on the baking tray. Flatten the tops slightly and sprinkle with the sea salt.

Bake the cookies for 20 minutes then cool on the tray for 5 minutes before transferring to a wire rack to cool completely.

Store in an airtight container for up to 5 days. These cookies can also be frozen for up to 1 month.

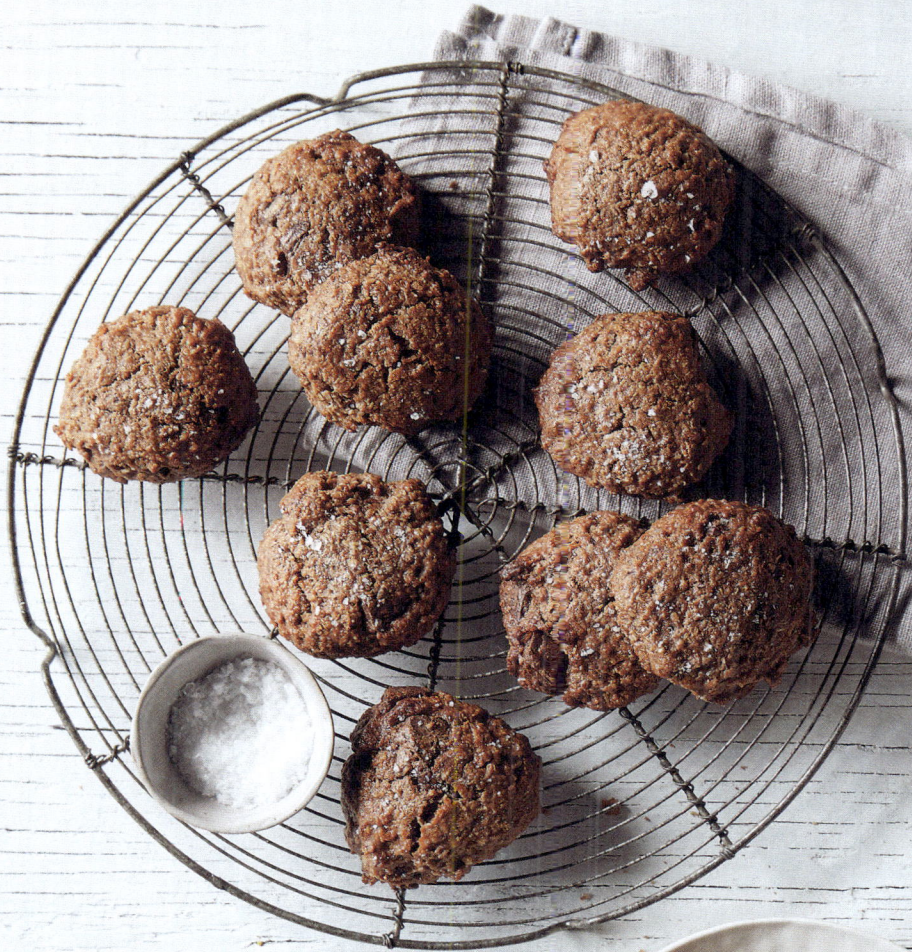

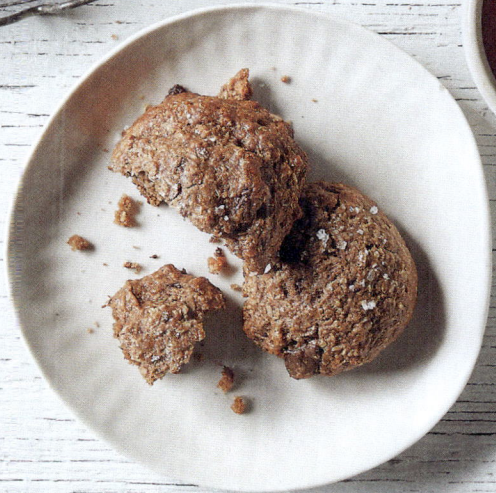

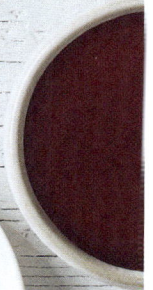

Salted Chocolate Quinoa Cookies

JUST BECAUSE YOU SUFFER FROM DIGESTIVE ISSUES DOESN'T MEAN YOU SHOULD MISS OUT. THESE GORGEOUS GUT-LOVING SNACKS ARE NOURISHING AND GENTLE ON SENSITIVE TUMMIES.

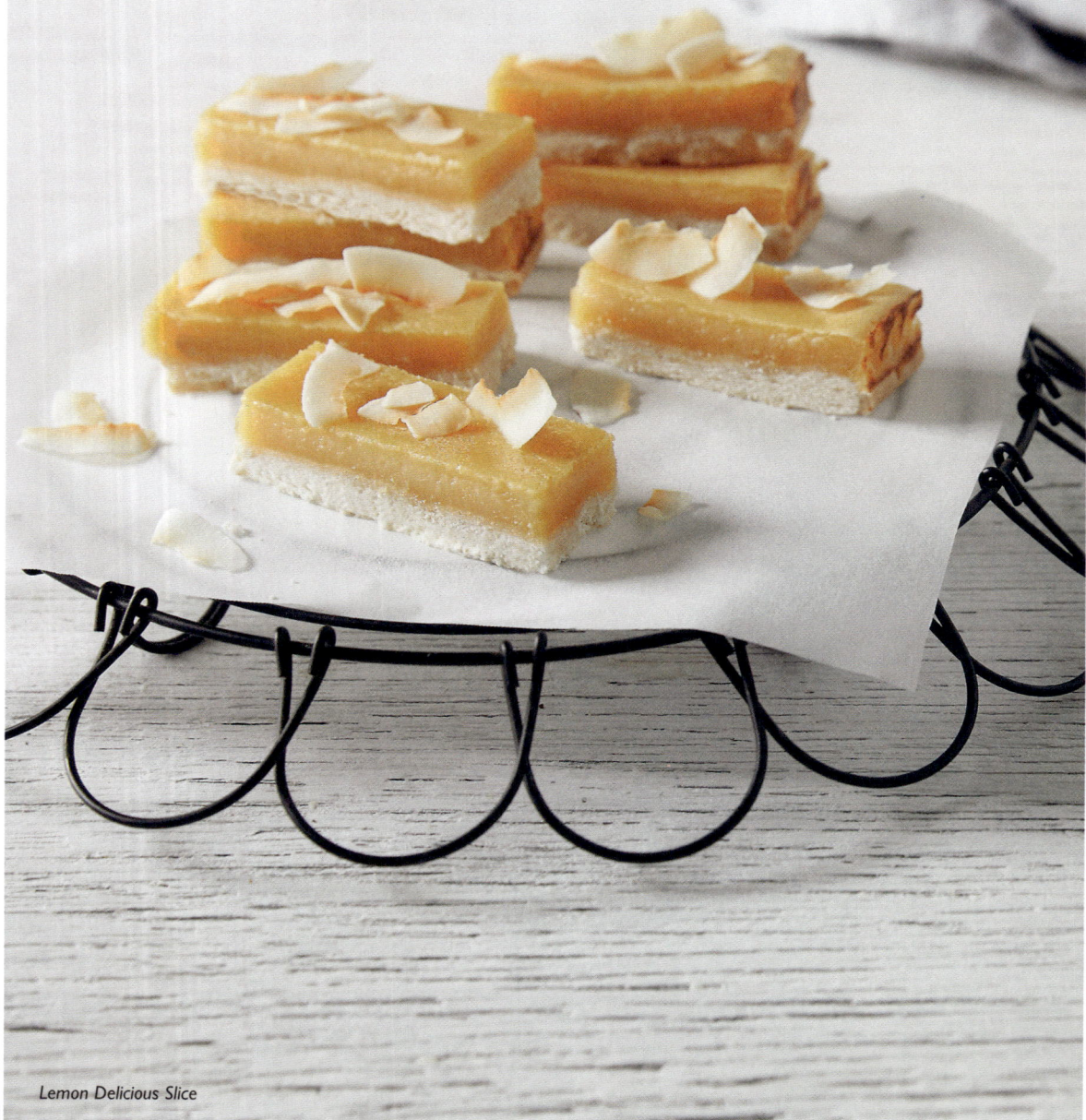

Lemon Delicious Slice

LEMON DELICIOUS SLICE

MAKES 18
PREP TIME 10 minutes
COOK TIME 30 minutes

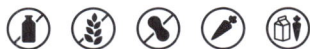

BASE
170 g (6 oz/1 cup) gluten-free flour
90 g (3¼ oz) brown rice flour
1 teaspoon cornflour (cornstarch)
95 g (3¾ oz/½ cup) coconut oil, melted
2 tablespoons maple syrup

TOPPING
4 eggs
125 ml (4 fl oz/½ cup) lemon juice
    (about 3 lemons)
150 ml (5 fl oz/½ cup) maple syrup
30 g (1 oz/¼ cup) gluten-free flour
3 tablespoons flaked coconut, toasted

Preheat the oven to 170°C (340°F). Line a square 20 cm (8 inch) baking tin with baking paper.

Combine the flours for the base in a large mixing bowl. Add the coconut oil and maple syrup, and combine until you have a smooth dough. The dough should be soft and a little tacky.

Press the dough into the base of the prepared tin and bake for 15 minutes, or until cooked through.

Combine all of the topping ingredients except the coconut in a large bowl and whisk well to combine. Pour this mixture over the baked crust and return to the oven for 15 minutes, or until the lemon topping has set. Allow to cool completely before portioning into 18 pieces.

BANANA POPS

SERVES 4 (2 per snack)
PREP TIME 10 minutes
COOK TIME 2 minutes

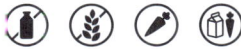

2 tablespoons chopped peanuts
50 g (1¾ oz) dark chocolate melts
2 teaspoons coconut oil
2 bananas (not overly ripe), quartered

YOU'LL ALSO NEED
8 wooden toothpicks

Place the peanuts in a small shallow bowl.

Melt the chocolate in a heatproof bowl and microwave for 30 seconds at a time, stirring after each time, until melted and smooth. Alternatively, use the double-boiler method on page 73.

Insert a toothpick into each piece of banana, and roll it in the melted chocolate first, allowing any excess to drip off before rolling in the peanuts. Place these banana pops onto a plate and place in the freezer for 30 minutes to set the chocolate and freeze the banana before eating.

YOU CAN STILL ENJOY BANANAS ON A LOW–FODMAP DIET PROVIDED THE BANANAS ARE NOT OVERLY RIPE AND YOU KEEP PORTION SIZES SMALL.

VEGAN PASTELI

MAKES 20
PREP TIME 5 minutes
COOK TIME 15 minutes

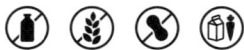

115 g (4 oz/¾ cup) white sesame seeds
115 g (4 oz/¾ cup) black sesame seeds
185 ml (6 fl oz/¾ cup) maple syrup
225 g (8 oz/¾ cup) brown rice syrup

Preheat the oven to 170°C (340°F).

Place the sesame seeds on a baking tray and toast in the oven for 4–5 minutes until golden and aromatic.

Combine both syrups in a saucepan and bring to the boil over medium–high heat. Allow the mixture to boil for 5 minutes before adding the toasted sesame seeds and reducing the heat to medium.

Continue to stir the mixture for a further 10 minutes, then remove from the heat and set aside to cool slightly.

Pour the warm mixture onto a sheet of greased baking paper, top with another sheet of greased baking paper and use a rolling pin to roll the mixture out flat to a thickness of 5 mm (¼ inch).

Remove the top sheet of paper, and leave the pasteli to cool before slicing into 20 pieces.

Store the pasteli between sheets of baking paper in the fridge for up to 3 days, or in the freezer.

CHEESY KALE CHIPS

SERVES 6
PREP TIME 20 minutes
COOK TIME 45 minutes

1 bunch (200 g/7 oz) curly kale

SEASONING
120 g (4¼ oz/¾ cup) cashew nuts
1 red chilli, seeds removed
1 small red capsicum (pepper), deseeded and
   stalk removed
25 g (1 oz/⅓ cup) nutritional yeast
2 tablespoons extra virgin olive oil
1 tablespoon lemon juice
½ teaspoon sea salt flakes
¼ teaspoon cayenne pepper
¼ teaspoon garlic powder
¼ teaspoon onion powder

Preheat the oven to 120°C (235°F). Line a baking tray with baking paper.

Blend all of the seasoning ingredients to a paste in a food processor—add more lemon juice if needed.

Strip the kale leaves from their stems, and discard the stems. Wash and dry the leaves thoroughly then tear into pieces. Toss the kale through the seasoning paste then arrange in a single layer on the baking tray. Bake for 45 minutes, or until dried out and crisp. Alternatively, you can dehydrate your chips overnight at 50°C (120°F). Store in an airtight container for up to 3 days.

ROASTED CAPSICUM AND CASHEW DIP
WITH PITTA BREAD

SERVES 6 **PREP TIME** 10 minutes **COOK TIME** 25 minutes

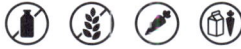

2 large red capsicums (peppers), deseeded and coarsely chopped
1 red onion, coarsely chopped
3 garlic cloves, unpeeled
2 teaspoons olive oil
salt and pepper
155 g (5½ oz/1 cup) raw cashew nuts
2 small wholemeal (whole-wheat) (or gluten-free if needed) pitta breads
1 tablespoon apple cider vinegar
¼ teaspoon dried chilli flakes

Preheat the oven to 200°C (400°F) and line a baking tray with baking paper.

Place the capsicum, onion and garlic on the baking tray and rub with olive oil. Season with salt and pepper and roast for 20 minutes. Scatter over the cashews and roast for a further 5 minutes, or until the nuts are golden and toasted.

Meanwhile, split the pitta breads in half and cut each piece into triangles. Place these on another baking tray and bake in the oven for 5–8 minutes, or until crisp and golden. Set aside to cool.

Squeeze the garlic out of its skin and transfer to a food processor along with the roasted capsicum, onion and nuts. Add the vinegar, chilli flakes and 60 ml (2 fl oz/¼ cup) water, and blend until smooth. Add extra water 1 tablespoon at a time if the mixture is too thick.

Serve the dip with the crispy pitta bread and store any leftover dip in the fridge for up to 5 days.

One hundred per cent dairy and animal free, my vegan snacks will satisfy every craving. Made with yummy nuts and seeds, fruit and vegetables, these snacks are good for you and the planet, too.

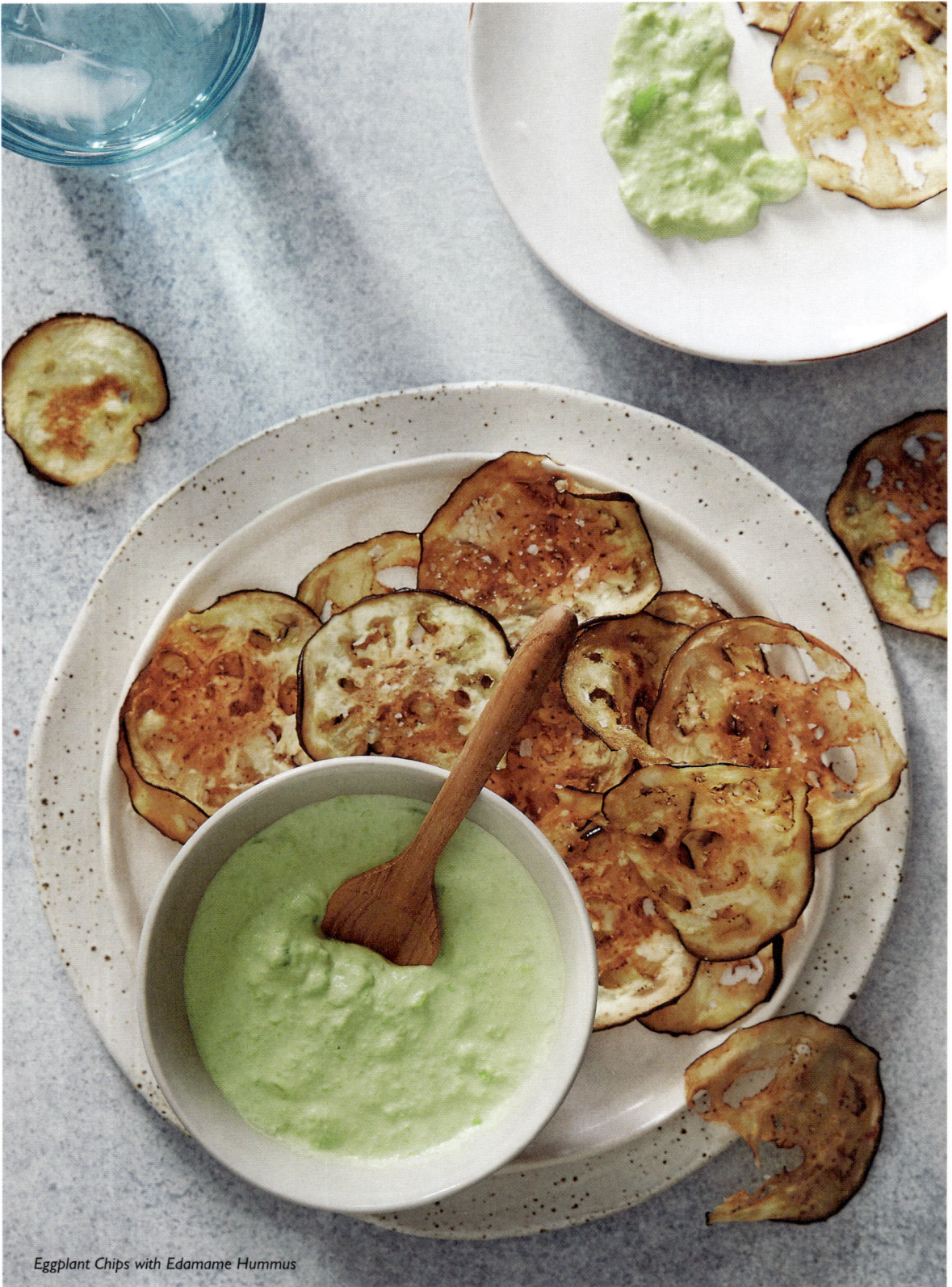

Eggplant Chips with Edamame Hummus

EGGPLANT CHIPS WITH EDAMAME HUMMUS

SERVES 2
PREP TIME 10 minutes
COOK TIME 20 minutes

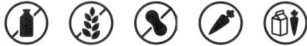

EGGPLANT CHIPS
1 Lebanese eggplant (aubergine), thinly sliced
½ teaspoon salt
1 teaspoon olive oil

EDAMAME HUMMUS
2 tablespoons tahini
1 teaspoon olive oil
juice of ½ lemon
1 garlic clove, peeled
30 g (1 oz/½ cup) edamame (soya beans),
    podded (thawed and drained if using frozen)

Preheat the oven to 200°C (400°F) and line a baking tray with baking paper.

Place a few sheets of paper towel on your work surface and put the eggplant slices on top. Sprinkle the salt over the eggplant, lay a few more sheets of paper towel on top and leave to sit for 10 minutes—this will help to draw out any excess moisture.

Pat the water and salt from the eggplant then transfer the slices to the prepared tray and brush with the olive oil. Bake for 12 minutes, then remove from the oven, turn over the slices and bake for a further 10–12 minutes, or until golden and crisp.

Meanwhile, place all of the hummus ingredients in a food processor and blitz until smooth, adding water 1 tablespoon at a time, if needed.

Serve the edamame hummus with the eggplant chips.

ZUCCHINI AND CORN FRITTERS

MAKES 6
PREP TIME 15 minutes
COOK TIME 12 minutes

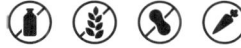

200 g (7 oz/1 cup) corn kernels
120 g (4¼ oz) grated zucchini (courgette)
1 jalapeño (fresh), finely chopped
2 spring onions (scallions), thinly sliced
1 teaspoon ground cumin
½ teaspoon cayenne pepper
small handful of coriander (cilantro), chopped
2 tablespoons cornflour (cornstarch)
2 tablespoons chickpea flour (besan)
½ teaspoon baking powder
salt and pepper
2 tablespoons olive oil, plus extra for frying
lemon wedge, to serve

Combine all of the ingredients except the lemon wedge in a large bowl and mix to combine.

Heat the extra olive oil in a large non-stick frying pan over medium heat. Using damp hands, divide the mixture into six fritters. Fry two fritters at a time until they are golden brown and cooked through, approximately 3 minutes on each side. Repeat with the remaining mixture, greasing the pan between each batch.

Serve the fritters warm, with a squeeze of fresh lemon.

TERIYAKI TOFU AND QUINOA SUSHI

SERVES 3 (4 pieces per person)   **PREP TIME** 15 minutes + marinating time   **COOK TIME** 15 minutes

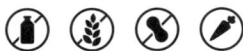

100 g (3½ oz) firm tofu, pressed
(see note)
60 ml (2 fl oz/¼ cup) teriyaki
sauce
1 tablespoon sesame seeds
100 g (3½ oz) tri-coloured
quinoa, washed
1 teaspoon rice vinegar
1 teaspoon maple syrup
2 nori sheets
4 asparagus spears, blanched
1 tablespoon pickled ginger
tamari, to serve

Preheat the oven to 180°C (350°F). Line a baking tray with baking paper.

Slice the pressed tofu into batons and toss these in a bowl with 2 tablespoons of the teriyaki sauce and the sesame seeds. Cover, set aside and allow to marinate for 20 minutes, then transfer to the baking tray and bake for 20 minutes, turning over after 15 minutes. Set aside to cool.

Meanwhile, combine the washed quinoa with 150 ml (5 fl oz) water in a small saucepan. Bring to the boil then reduce the heat to low and cover with a lid. Simmer the quinoa for 15 minutes, or until all the water has been absorbed and the quinoa has puffed up. Remove the pan from the heat and stir through the vinegar and maple syrup.

Spread the cooked quinoa on a baking tray and refrigerate to cool.

Place one of the nori sheets on a bamboo mat (or a plate if you don't have a mat). Spread half of the quinoa in an even layer over the nori, leaving a 2 cm (¾ inch) area free along the baseline. Arrange half of the tofu, asparagus and ginger in a straight line along the top.

Drizzle with half of the remaining teriyaki sauce then roll the sushi into a long, tight cylinder shape. Repeat the process with the other sheet of nori and the remaining filling.

Slice each roll into six portions and serve with tamari.

Note:

Pressing tofu before cooking draws the moisture out and this makes it firmer, and helps the flavours you cook it with to penetrate. To press the tofu, sandwich it between several sheets of paper towel (or a clean tea towel) and two plates. Weight down the top plate with a few tins and leave in the fridge for up to 1 hour, so the excess moisture is squeezed out.

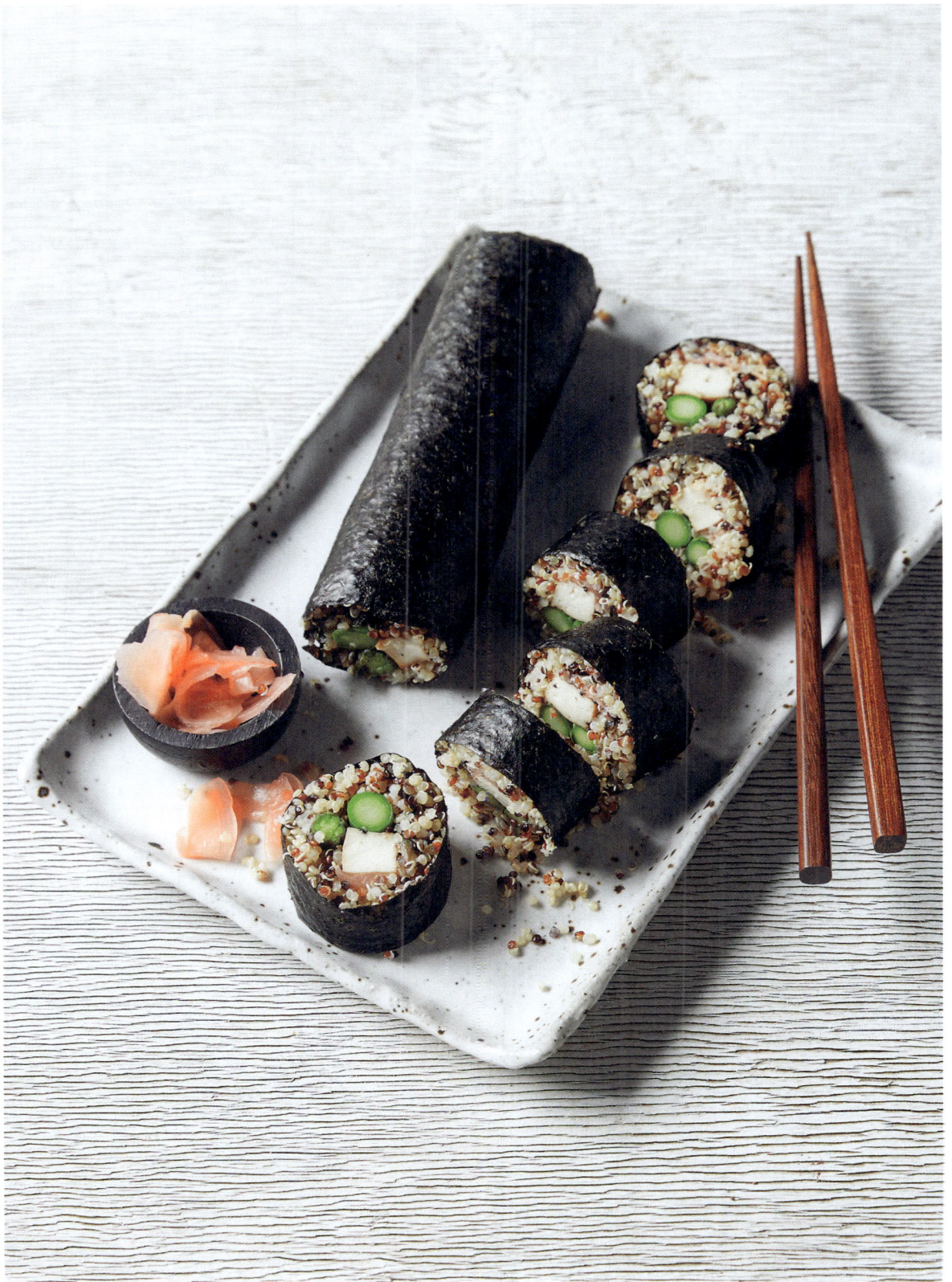

EDAMAME FALAFEL BITES

MAKES 20 (2 per snack) **PREP TIME** 20 minutes + chilling time **COOK TIME** 15 minutes

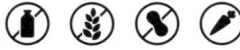

- **250 g (9 oz) dried chickpeas, soaked overnight**
- **80 g (2¾ oz/½ cup) edamame (soya beans), podded (thawed and drained if frozen)**
- **½ onion, coarsely chopped**
- **1 garlic clove, peeled**
- **1 tablespoon chickpea flour (besan)**
- **2 teaspoons ground cumin**
- **1 teaspoon ground coriander**
- **1 teaspoon salt**
- **½ bunch flat-leaf (Italian) parsley, coarsely chopped**
- **60 ml (2 fl oz/¼ cup) olive oil, for frying**

Optional: if not dairy free or vegan, serve with Greek-style yoghurt

Combine the drained chickpeas in a food processor with the rest of the ingredients except the olive oil and pulse to a slightly coarse paste. Set aside in the fridge to firm up.

With damp hands, roll the mixture into 30 g (2 tablespoon) balls. If the balls are not holding together, return the mixture to the food processor and continue processing until it is more paste-like. After rolling, place on a tray and put in the fridge for 1 hour to firm up. This helps the falafel hold their shape while cooking.

Place the olive oil in a large frying pan over medium heat and shallow-fry the falafel in batches for 2–3 minutes on each side, or until golden and warmed through. Set aside to drain on paper towel before serving.

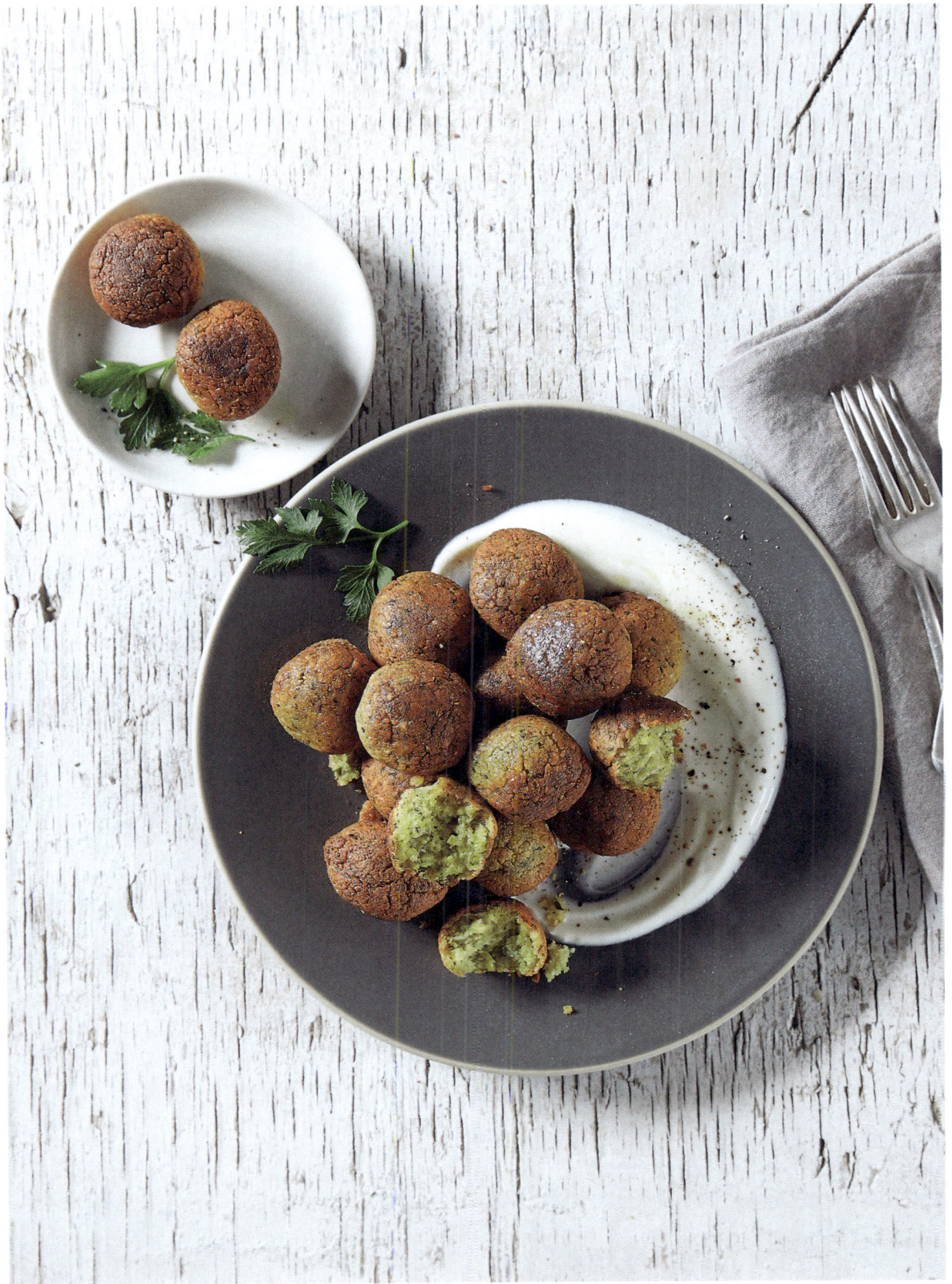

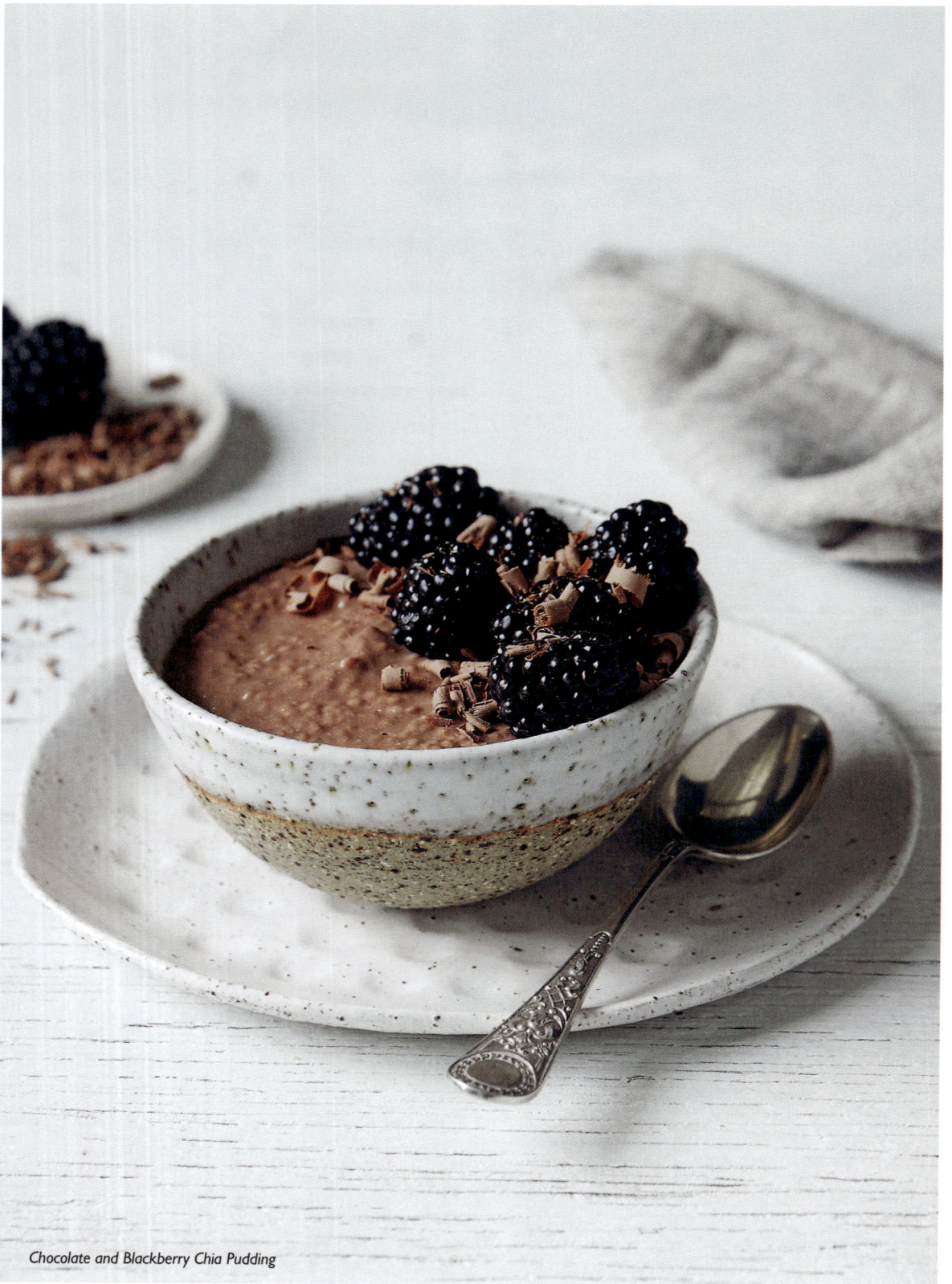

Chocolate and Blackberry Chia Pudding

CHOCOLATE AND BLACKBERRY CHIA PUDDING

SERVES 2
PREP TIME 40 minutes

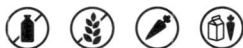

75 g (2⅔ oz/⅓ cup) coconut yoghurt
80 ml (2½ fl oz/⅓ cup) almond milk
2 tablespoons chia seeds
2 teaspoons maple syrup
½ teaspoon natural vanilla extract
2 teaspoons cocoa powder
30 g (1 oz/¼ cup) blackberries
10 g (¼ oz) vegan dark chocolate (70%), finely grated

Whisk the yoghurt, milk, chia seeds, maple syrup, vanilla and cocoa in a bowl until smooth.

Cover and refrigerate for 30 minutes or overnight

Divide the pudding between serving bowls, then top with blackberries and chocolate to serve.

APPLE AND HAZELNUT CHIA PUDDING

SERVES 1
PREP TIME 30 minutes

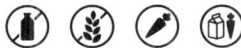

1 tablespoon chia seeds
¼ teaspoon ground cinnamon
½ teaspoon natural vanilla extract
80 ml (2½ fl oz/⅓ cup) almond milk
¼ apple, thinly sliced
15 g (½ oz) hazelnuts, chopped

Place the chia seeds, cinnamon, vanilla and milk in a small bowl or glass and mix well to combine. Place in the fridge for at least 30 minutes.

Remove the chia mixture from the fridge once all the liquid has been soaked up. Garnish with the apple slices and hazelnuts to serve.

ALMOND CHOCOLATE CHIP COOKIES

MAKES 10
PREP TIME 15 minutes
COOK TIME 20 minutes

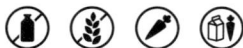

160 g (5⅔ oz) almond meal
1 tablespoon plain (all-purpose) flour
  (or gluten-free, if needed)
¼ teaspoon sea salt
55 g (2 oz/¼ cup) coconut oil, melted
2 tablespoons maple syrup
40 g (1½ oz) vegan dark chocolate chips

Preheat the oven to 160°C (320°F) and line a baking tray with baking paper.

Place all of the ingredients except the chocolate chips in a large bowl and mix until well combined, then stir through the chocolate chips.

Roll tablespoons of the mixture into 10 balls, place these on the baking tray and flatten gently with the back of a fork.

Bake for 10–12 minutes, or until lightly golden, then allow to cool for 10 minutes on the tray before transferring to a wire rack to cool completely.

UNBELIEVABLE CHOCOLATE BROWNIES

MAKES 18
PREP TIME 20 minutes
COOK TIME 35 minutes

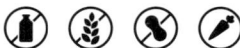

330 g (11⅔ oz/2 cups) gluten-free flour
½ teaspoon xanthan gum
100 g (3½ oz) cocoa powder
1 teaspoon baking powder
½ teaspoon sea salt flakes, crushed
1 tablespoon instant coffee granules
200 g (7 oz) bittersweet vegan chocolate,
  broken into chunks
250 ml (9 fl oz/1 cup) soy milk
1 tablespoon lemon juice
240 g (8½ oz/⅔ cup) rice malt syrup
250 ml (9 fl oz/1 cup) melted coconut oil
1 teaspoon natural vanilla extract

Preheat the oven to 180°C (350°F). Line a square 20 cm (8 inch) baking tin with baking paper then lightly spray it with cooking oil.

Sift the gluten-free flour, xanthan, cocoa powder and baking powder into a large mixing bowl. Stir through the salt and coffee granules and set aside.

Melt half of the chocolate in a heatproof bowl and microwave for 30 seconds at a time, stirring after each time, until melted and smooth. Alternatively, use the double-boiler method on page 73. Set aside.

Combine the soy milk and lemon juice in a jug to create a vegan buttermilk. Allow to curdle, then add to the dry ingredients along with the rice malt syrup, coconut oil and vanilla.

Roughly chop the remaining chocolate and fold this through the batter along with the melted chocolate. Pour the batter into the prepared tin, smoothing the top with the back of a spoon.

Bake for 35–40 minutes, or until fudgy and just cooked through. Allow the brownie to cool completely before portioning into 18. Store in an airtight container for up to 5 days.

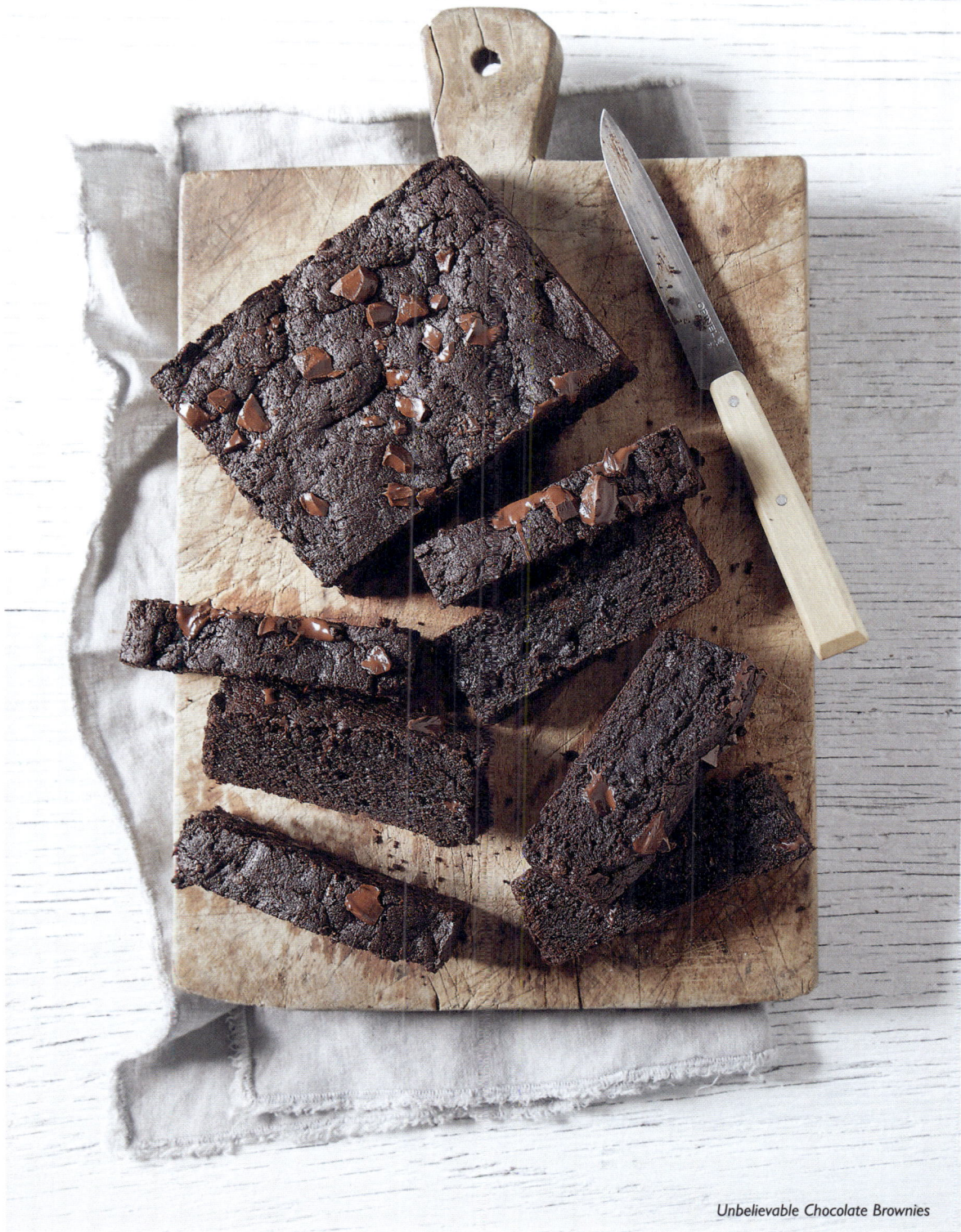

Unbelievable Chocolate Brownies

CHICKPEA AND CHOCOLATE BLONDIES

MAKES 12
PREP TIME 10 minutes
COOK TIME 25 minutes

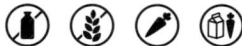

- 400 g (14 oz) tinned chickpeas, drained and rinsed
- 140 g (5 oz/½ cup) natural, crunchy peanut butter
- 25 g (1 oz/¼ cup) rolled (porridge) oats (use brown rice or quinoa flakes if gluten-free)
- ½ teaspoon ground cinnamon
- ½ teaspoon baking powder
- ¼ teaspoon bicarbonate of soda (baking soda)
- 80 ml (2½ fl oz/⅓ cup) maple syrup
- 1 teaspoon natural vanilla extract
- 90 g (3¼ oz/½ cup) vegan dark chocolate chips

Preheat the oven to 180°C (350°F) and line a square baking tin with baking paper.

Blitz all of the ingredients except the chocolate chips in a food processor and purée until smooth. Add 1–2 tablespoons water to help loosen the mixture a little, and scrape down the sides.

Pour the batter into the prepared tin, scatter over the chocolate chips, and press them gently into the batter.

Bake for 25 minutes, or until the blondie feels firm to the touch and is pulling away from the sides. Don't be tempted to overcook it! It will continue to set as it cools.

Once cool, cut into 12 squares. Store in an airtight container for up to 5 days.

APPLE RING 'DOUGHNUTS'

SERVES 2
PREP TIME 10 minutes

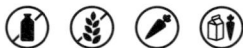

- 1 granny smith apple
- 1 teaspoon goji berries
- 1 teaspoon shredded coconut
- ¼ teaspoon salt

HAZELNUT BUTTER
- 2 tablespoons hazelnuts
- 2 teaspoon cocoa powder
- 1 teaspoon rice malt syrup
- 1 tablespoon coconut oil, melted
- 1 teaspoon natural vanilla extract

If the hazelnuts have skins on them, place them in a small frying pan over medium heat and dry fry for a few minutes, until their skin begins to loosen.

Remove the hazelnuts from the heat and tip them into a clean tea towel. Fold the tea towel over the nuts and gently rub to remove the papery skins.

Place the nuts in a food processor with the rest of the hazelnut butter ingredients and blitz until smooth, adding a little water if needed. Set aside.

Core the apple then cut it horizontally into slices about 1.5 cm (⅝ inch) thick (you should get four slices). Spread the hazelnut butter over the apple rings and sprinkle with goji berries, coconut and salt to serve.

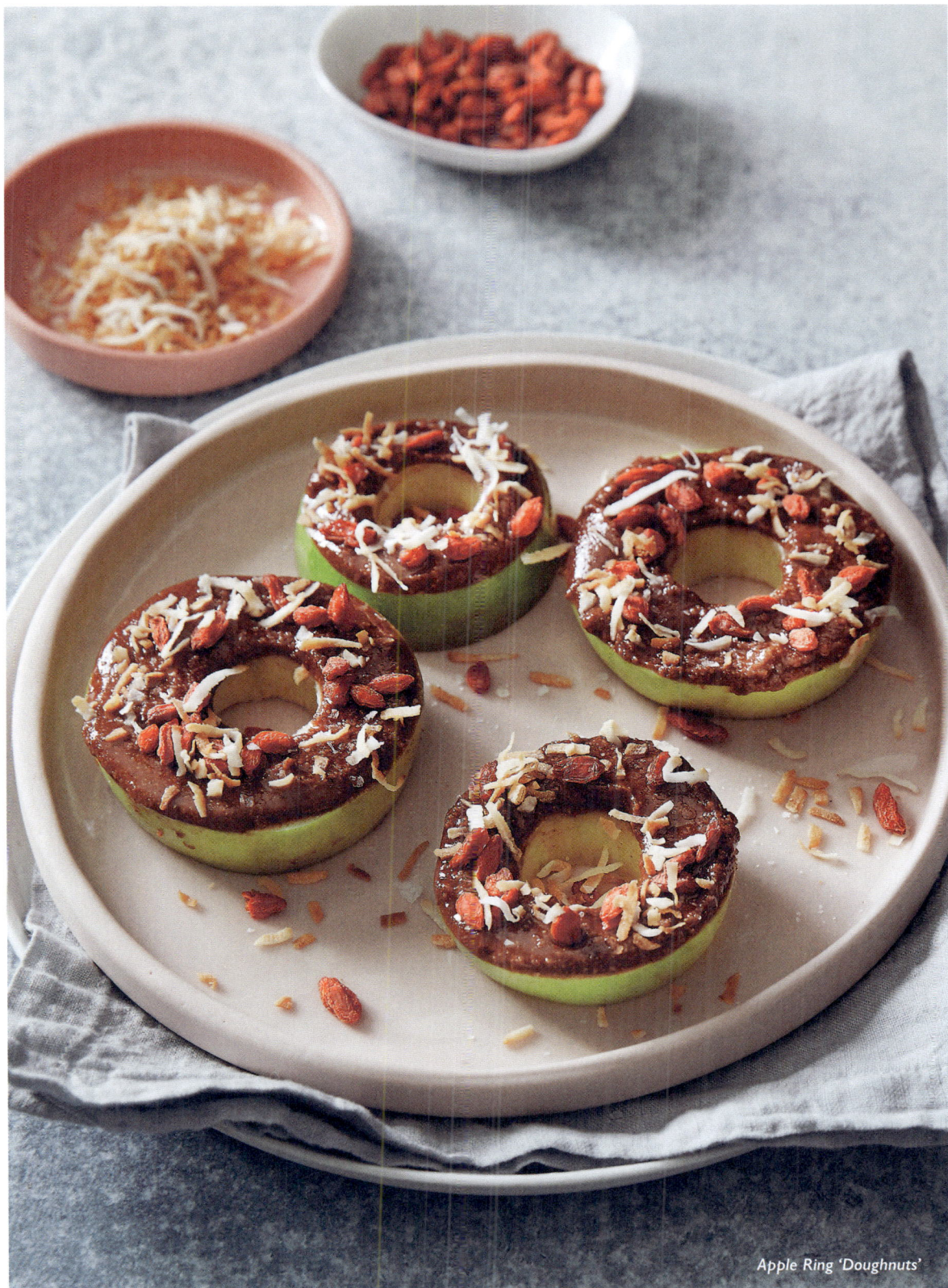

Apple Ring 'Doughnuts'

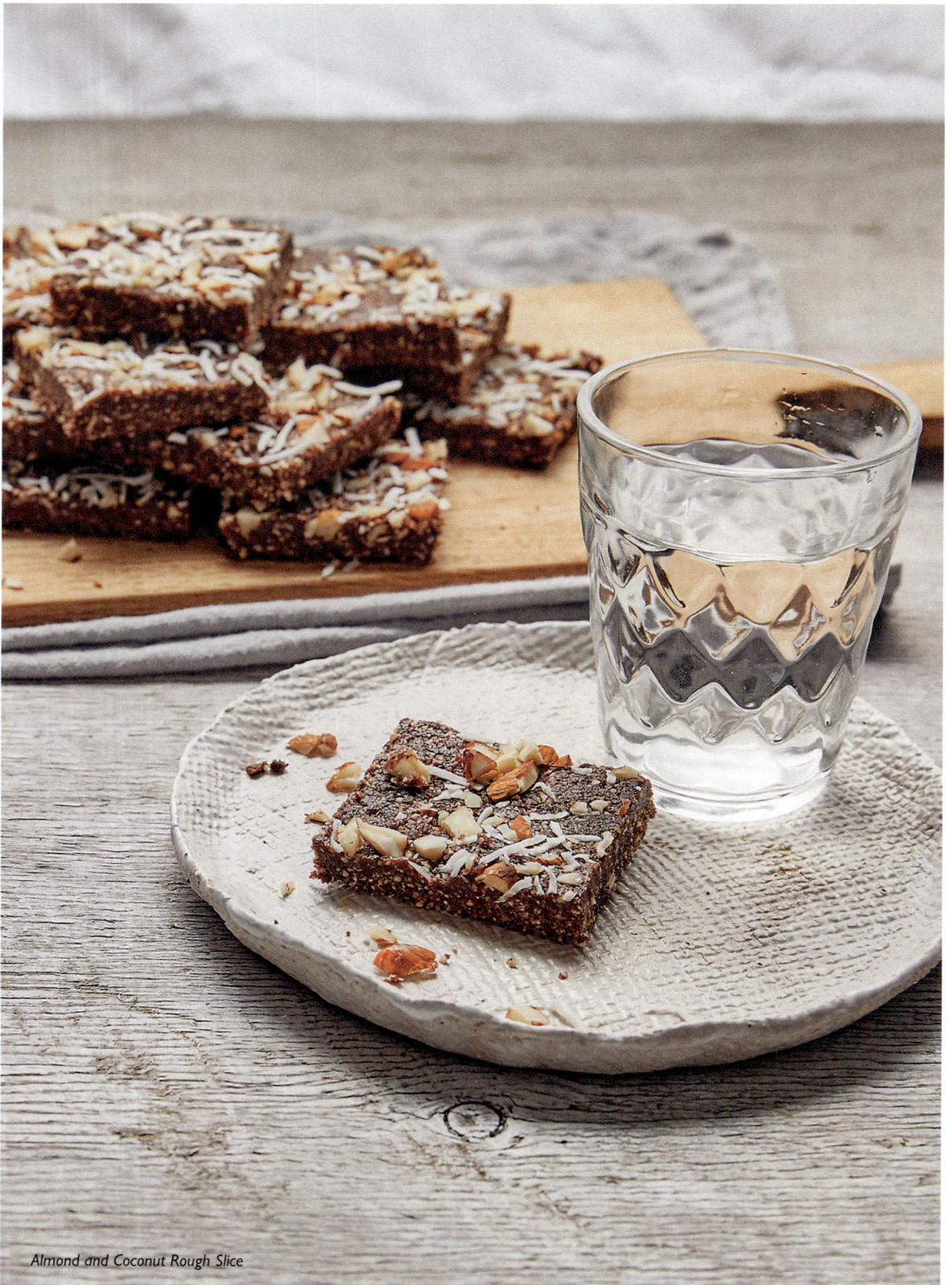

Almond and Coconut Rough Slice

ALMOND AND COCONUT ROUGH SLICE

MAKES 16
PREP TIME 10 minutes + chilling time

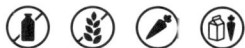

BASE
8 medjool dates, pitted
155 g (5½ oz/1 cup) chopped almonds
50 g (1¾ oz/½ cup) rolled (porridge) oats
    (use brown rice flakes or quinoa flakes if
    gluten free)
30 g (1 oz/¼ cup) raw cacao powder
1 teaspoon ground cinnamon
½ teaspoon salt
2 tablespoons melted coconut oil
2 tablespoons tahini
2 tablespoons rice malt syrup

TOPPING
2 teaspoons shredded coconut
1 tablespoon chopped almonds

Line a square 20 cm (8 inch) baking tin with baking paper.

Place all of the base ingredients in a food processor and pulse until all the mixture is a rough, sticky dough and is holding together.

Press this mixture firmly into the prepared tin, then gently press the coconut and almonds for the topping into the surface and freeze for 30 minutes.

Slice into 16 small portions. Store in an airtight container in the fridge for up to 5 days, or in the freezer for up to 3 months.

VEGAN BLUEBERRY SCONES

MAKES 12
PREP TIME 30 minutes + chilling time
COOK TIME 25 minutes

260 g (9¼ oz/1¾ cups) wholemeal
    (whole-wheat) flour, plus extra, for dusting
1 tablespoon baking powder
55 g (2 oz/¼ cup) coconut oil
250 ml (9 fl oz/1 cup) coconut milk
2 tablespoons maple syrup
125 g (4½ oz/1 cup) blueberries
zest from 1 lemon

Preheat the oven to 200°C (400°F). Line a baking tray with baking paper and set aside.

Combine the flour, baking powder and coconut oil in a large bowl. Rub the mixture between your fingers and thumbs until you have the texture of coarse breadcrumbs.

In a separate bowl, gently mix the coconut milk, 1 tablespoon of the maple syrup, the blueberries and lemon zest, then fold this mixture into the dry ingredients just until combined. Turn out onto a lightly floured surface.

Form the dough into a 20 cm (8 inch) disc then refrigerate for 30 minutes to firm up—this is a key step that ensures your scones don't spread too thin while baking.

Cut the dough into 12 wedges then place these on the baking tray. Bake for 25 minutes, or until puffed and golden brown. Brush with the remaining maple syrup and serve while warm.

STRAWBERRY AND CHIA JAM KISSES

MAKES 10 **PREP TIME** 15 minutes + chilling time **COOK TIME** 8 minutes

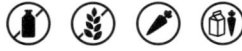

COOKIES
155 g (5½ oz/1 cup) raw cashew
    nuts
30 g (1 oz/¼ cup) coconut flour
3 tablespoons rice malt syrup
1 teaspoon coconut oil, melted
1 teaspoon natural vanilla
    extract
⅛ teaspoon salt

JAM
80 g (2¾ oz) strawberries, hulled
2 tablespoons chia seeds

Add the cashews and coconut flour to a food processor (or blender) and blitz to a fine crumb consistency. Add the remaining cookie ingredients and pulse until the mixture resembles a dough.

Shape the dough into a disc, cover tightly with plastic wrap and refrigerate for 30 minutes.

Preheat the oven to 180°C (350°F) and line a baking tray with baking paper.

Place the strawberries in a blender and blitz for a few seconds. Add the chia seeds and pulse again until combined. Set aside in the fridge for 20 minutes.

Roll the chilled dough out to about 5 mm (¼ inch) thick on a piece of baking paper. Use a 7 cm (2¾ inch) cookie cutter (or glass) to cut out cookies and place these on the prepared tray.

Using a 3 cm (1¼ inch) cookie cutter, cut out the centre of half the cookies. Re-roll any scraps of pastry and repeat the process. Make sure you have the same number of both cookies (those with and without holes in the middle). Bake for 5–8 minutes, or until golden.

Cool on the baking tray for a few minutes, then transfer to a wire rack to cool completely. Once cool, spread 1 teaspoon of the jam on a solid cookie and top with a cut-out cookie so the jam peeks through.

Store in an airtight container in the fridge for up to 5 days.

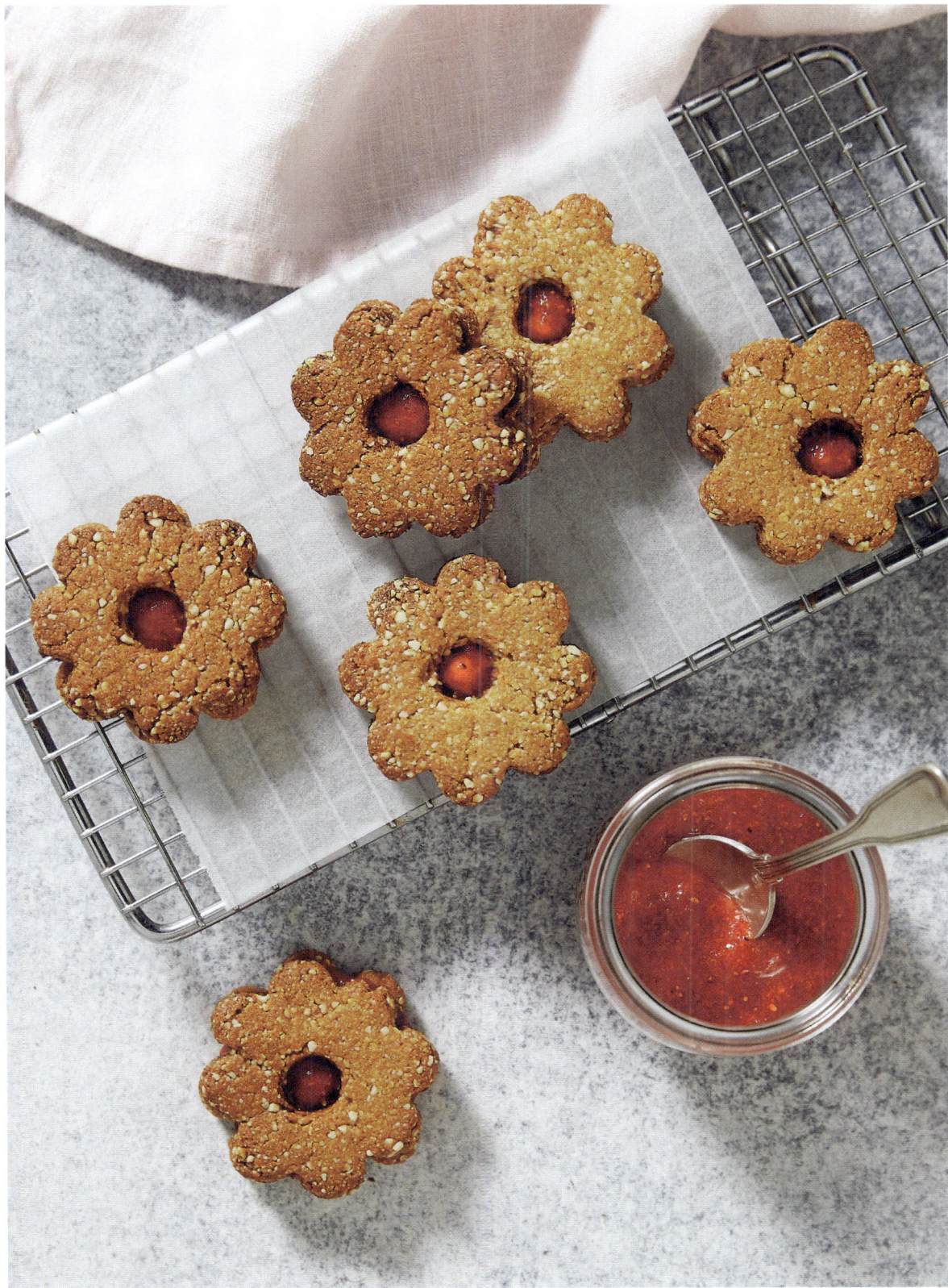

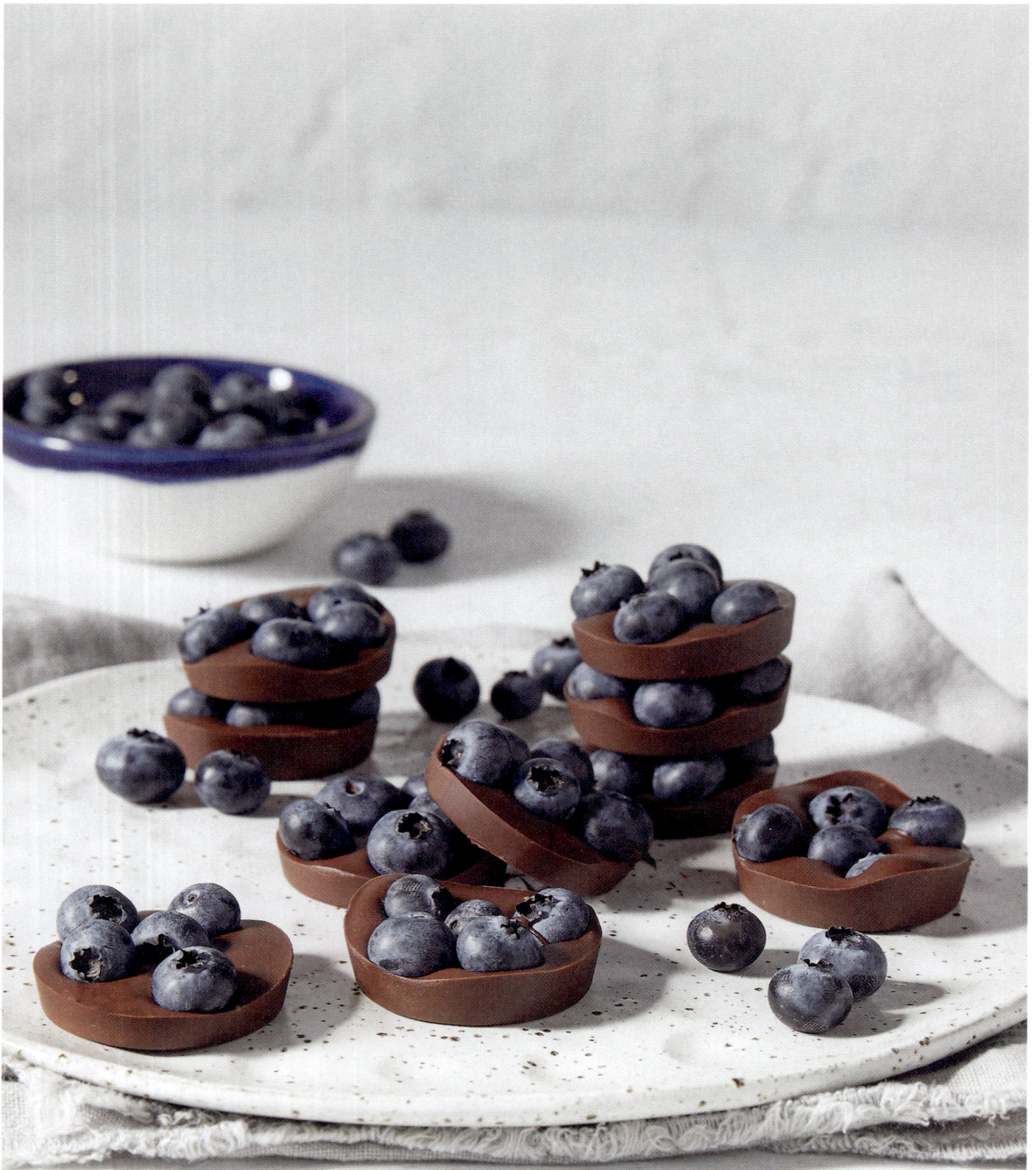

Dark Chocolate Blueberry Clusters

DARK CHOCOLATE BLUEBERRY CLUSTERS

MAKES 12
PREP TIME 20 minutes
COOK TIME 2 minutes

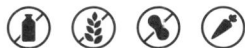

120 g (4¼ oz) vegan dark chocolate (70%),
   chopped
2 teaspoons coconut oil
120 g (4¼ oz) fresh blueberries

Combine the chocolate and coconut oil in a
small microwave-safe bowl and microwave for
30 seconds at a time, stirring after each time,
until melted and smooth. Alternatively, use the
double-boiler method on page 73.

Line a 12-hole mini-muffin tin with paper cases
(skip this step if using a silicone muffin mould).

Fill each hole with 2 teaspoons of the chocolate
mixture and top with blueberries.

Refrigerate for 2 hours, or until the chocolate has
set. Remove from the liners and serve.

RAW BLUEBERRY CHEESECAKE SLICE

SERVES 20
PREP TIME 30 minutes + overnight refrigeration

BASE
65 g (2⅓ oz/¾ cup) desiccated coconut
120 g (4¼ oz/¾ cup) almonds
6 medjool dates, pitted
3 tablespoons coconut oil
pinch of sea salt

FILLING
235 g (8½ oz /1½ cups) raw cashew nuts,
   soaked in water
250 ml (9 fl oz/1 cup) coconut milk
95 g (3¼ oz/½ cup) coconut oil
90 g (3¼ oz/¼ cup) rice malt syrup
250 g (9 oz) fresh blueberries
zest and juice of 1 lime

Line a 20 × 8 cm (8 × 3¼ inch) (or similar) loaf
(bar) tin with baking paper.

Place all of the ingredients for the base in a food
processor and pulse until the mixture comes
together and forms a ball.

Press the base mixture into the prepared tin and
refrigerate until firm.

Place all of the filling ingredients into a blender
and blitz for 5 minutes until very smooth. Pour
this mixture evenly over the chilled base, then
place in the fridge to set overnight.

Portion into twenty 1 cm (½ inch) thick slices
and serve.

ANZAC BISCUITS

MAKES 18 **PREP TIME** 10 minutes **COOK TIME** 25 minutes

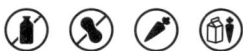

150 g (5½ oz/1 cup) wholemeal (whole-wheat) flour
100 g (3½ oz/1 cup) rolled (porridge) oats
35 g (1¼ oz/½ cup) shredded coconut
90 g (3¼ oz/¼ cup) rice malt syrup
2 tablespoons golden syrup
55 g (2 oz/¼ cup) coconut oil
1 teaspoon vanilla extract
½ teaspoon bicarbonate of soda (baking soda)
1 tablespoon hot water

Preheat the oven to 180°C (350°F). Line a baking tray with baking paper.

Mix the flour, oats and coconut together in a large bowl.

Put the rice malt syrup, golden syrup, coconut oil and vanilla in a saucepan over low heat and warm until all the ingredients are combined. Take the pan off the heat and set aside.

Mix the bicarb in a small jug with the hot water. Once combined, add to the wet ingredients, then mix the wet ingredients into the flour mixture. The mixture will be very firm—it's best to use your hands to 'massage' the ingredients together.

With damp hands, measure a packed tablespoon of mixture and roll it into a ball. If the mixture is too dry, just dampen your hands a little more.

Place the balls onto the baking tray and, using damp hands, press the cookies gently so they are about 6–7 cm (2½–2¾ inches) in diameter. You may need to dampen your fingers again if the mixture is sticky. (See tip.)

Bake for 20 minutes, or until golden, making sure they don't burn on the bottom.

Allow to cool on the tray for 5 minutes, then transfer to a wire rack to cool completely. Store in an airtight container for up to 5 days.

Tip:

Because these biscuits contain coconut oil rather than butter, they don't spread during the cooking process the way traditional ANZACs do, so you need to spread them a little yourself. If you leave them as smaller, thicker biscuits, they'll have a cakey centre; I prefer to squash them flat before baking for a crisp and crunchy biscuit.

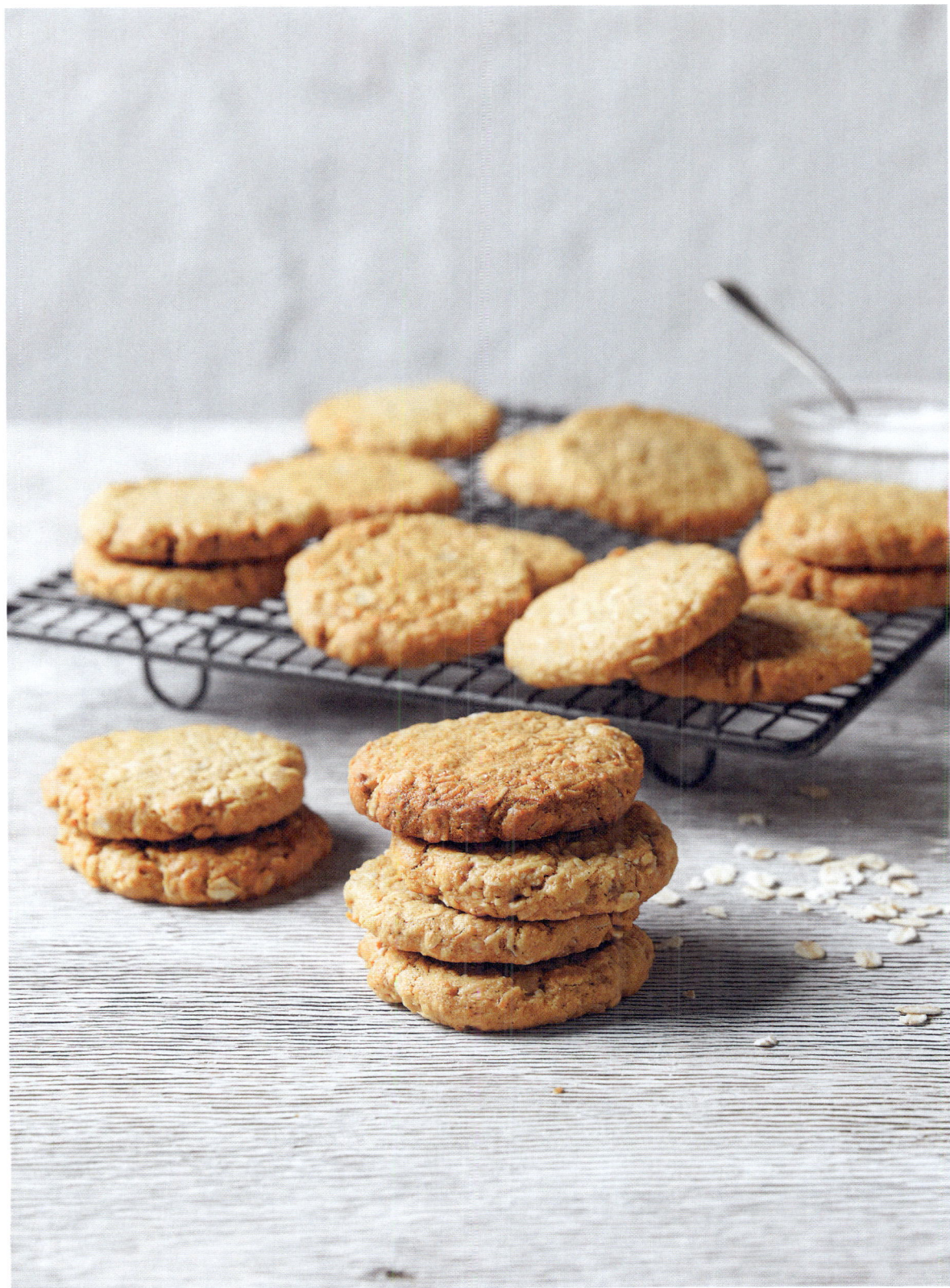

CHOCOLATE PEANUT BUTTER BALLS

MAKES 14
PREP TIME 20 minutes

30 g (1 oz/¼ cup) cocoa powder
215 g (7⅔ oz/¾ cup) natural, crunchy peanut butter
150 g (5½ oz) pitted medjool dates, coarsely chopped
75 g (2⅔ oz/¾ cup) rolled (porridge) oats
25 g (1 oz/¼ cup) desiccated coconut, for rolling

Place all of the ingredients except the desiccated coconut in a food processor and blitz until combined.

Form into 14 tablespoon-sized balls then roll in the coconut. Refrigerate for 1 hour before serving.

APRICOT AND COCONUT BLISS BALLS

MAKES 14
PREP TIME 15 minutes

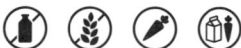

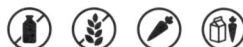

240 g (8½ oz/1½ cups) almonds
1 teaspoon vanilla extract
1 tablespoon coconut oil
2 tablespoons chia seeds
155 g (5½ oz/1 cup) dried apricots
115 g (4 oz/1¼ cups) desiccated coconut

Set aside 25 g (1 oz/¼ cup) of the desiccated coconut. Place all the other ingredients in a food processor and blitz on high until the mixture comes together.

Scoop tablespoons of the mixture from the food processor and roll into 14 balls. Roll those in the reserved coconut.

CRANBERRY, ALMOND AND OAT ENERGY BALLS

MAKES 10
PREP TIME 5 minutes

50 g (1¾ oz/½ cup) rolled (porridge) oats (use brown rice flakes or quinoa flakes if gluten free)
80 g (2¾ oz/½ cup) almonds
35 g (1¼ oz/¼ cup) dried cranberries
25 g (1 oz/¼ cup) desiccated coconut
1 tablespoon rice malt syrup
1 tablespoon natural crunchy peanut butter
½ teaspoon natural vanilla extract
¼ teaspoon ground cinnamon
pinch of salt

Place all of the ingredients in a food processor and blend with 1–1½ tablespoons water until a sticky mixture forms.

Roll into 10 tablespoon-sized balls and place on a tray in the freezer for 2 hours. Store in an airtight container in the fridge or freezer.

CACAO AND CHIA SNACK BALLS

MAKES 16 (2 balls per snack)
PREP TIME 15 minutes

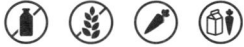

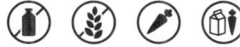

80 g (2¾ oz/½ cup) almonds
2 tablespoons chia seeds
45 g (1⅔ oz/½ cup) desiccated coconut
80 g (2¾ oz/½ cup) pitted medjool dates, coarsely chopped
1 tablespoon coconut oil, melted
2 tablespoons almond butter
2 tablespoons raw cacao powder

Place the almonds and chia seeds into a food processor with half of the coconut, and pulse until the nuts are coarsely chopped.

Add the dates, oil, almond butter and cacao powder to the food processor and blitz until well combined.

Using a tablespoon, scoop out the mixture and roll into 16 balls, then roll them in the remaining coconut and store in an airtight container in the fridge for up to 10 days.

CASHEW AND DATE BLISS BALLS

MAKES 12
PREP TIME 15 minutes

80 g (2¾ oz/½ cup) pitted medjool dates
235 g (8½ oz/1½ cups) raw cashew nuts
2 tablespoons almond butter
1 tablespoon chia seeds
2 tablespoons coconut oil, melted
2 tablespoons rice malt syrup
20 g (¾ oz/¼ cup) shredded coconut, to coat

Place the dates in a bowl, cover with boiling water and set aside to soften for 10 minutes. Drain.

Meanwhile, place the cashews in a food processor and blitz to a rough crumb.

Add the dates, almond butter, chia seeds, oil and rice malt syrup to the food processor and blitz until the ingredients come together.

Roll tablespoon-sized amounts of the mixture into 12 balls, then roll those in the shredded coconut. Store in an airtight container for up to 1 week.

VEGAN RASPBERRY CHOCOLATE FUDGE

MAKES 25
PREP TIME 10 minutes + chilling time
COOK TIME 45 minutes

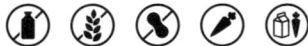

175 g (6 oz) coconut oil
200 g (7 oz) vegan dark chocolate (70%), broken into pieces
40 g (1½ oz/⅓ cup) cocoa powder, sifted, plus extra for dusting
120 g (4¼ oz/⅓ cup) rice malt syrup
1 teaspoon natural vanilla extract
100 g (3½ oz/½ cup) unsweetened apple sauce
110 g (3¾ oz/¾ cup) plain (all-purpose) flour (or gluten-free if required), sifted
125 g (4½ oz/1 cup) fresh raspberries (at room temperature)

Preheat the oven to 160°C (320°F). Lightly grease an 18 cm (7 inch) square cake tin and line the base with baking paper.

Melt the coconut oil and chocolate in a saucepan over low heat, and stir until combined and completely melted. Transfer to a large bowl and allow to cool slightly.

Add the cocoa, rice malt syrup and vanilla to the chocolate mixture and stir to combine.

Stir the apple sauce and flour into the batter, then gently fold in the raspberries. (Make sure the raspberries are at room temperature before doing this, especially if using frozen berries, or the coconut oil will solidify before you have time to stir them through.)

Pour the batter into the prepared tin and bake for about 40 minutes, or until the cake starts to come away from the sides of the tin then remove from the oven—the mixture will still be wobbly. Cool in the tin and then place in the fridge (still in the tin) for at least 1 hour before cutting into 25 squares. Dust with extra cocoa powder before serving. These are best kept in the fridge (or freezer).

CHOCOLATE FUDGE BALLS

MAKES 18
PREP TIME 15 minutes + chilling time

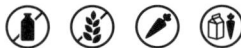

10 medjool dates, pitted
155 g (5½ oz/1 cup) macadamia nuts
90 g (3¼ oz/1 cup) desiccated coconut
2 tablespoons maple syrup
2 tablespoons coconut oil, melted
1 tablespoon cocoa powder
⅛ teaspoon salt
2 tablespoons cacao nibs

Place the dates in a bowl, cover with boiling water and set aside to soften for 10 minutes. Drain.

Put the dates in a food processor with all of the remaining ingredients and blitz until almost smooth and combined.

With damp hands, roll tablespoon-sized amounts of the mixture into 18 walnut-sized balls and refrigerate for 1 hour before serving. Refrigerate in an airtight container for up to 3 weeks.

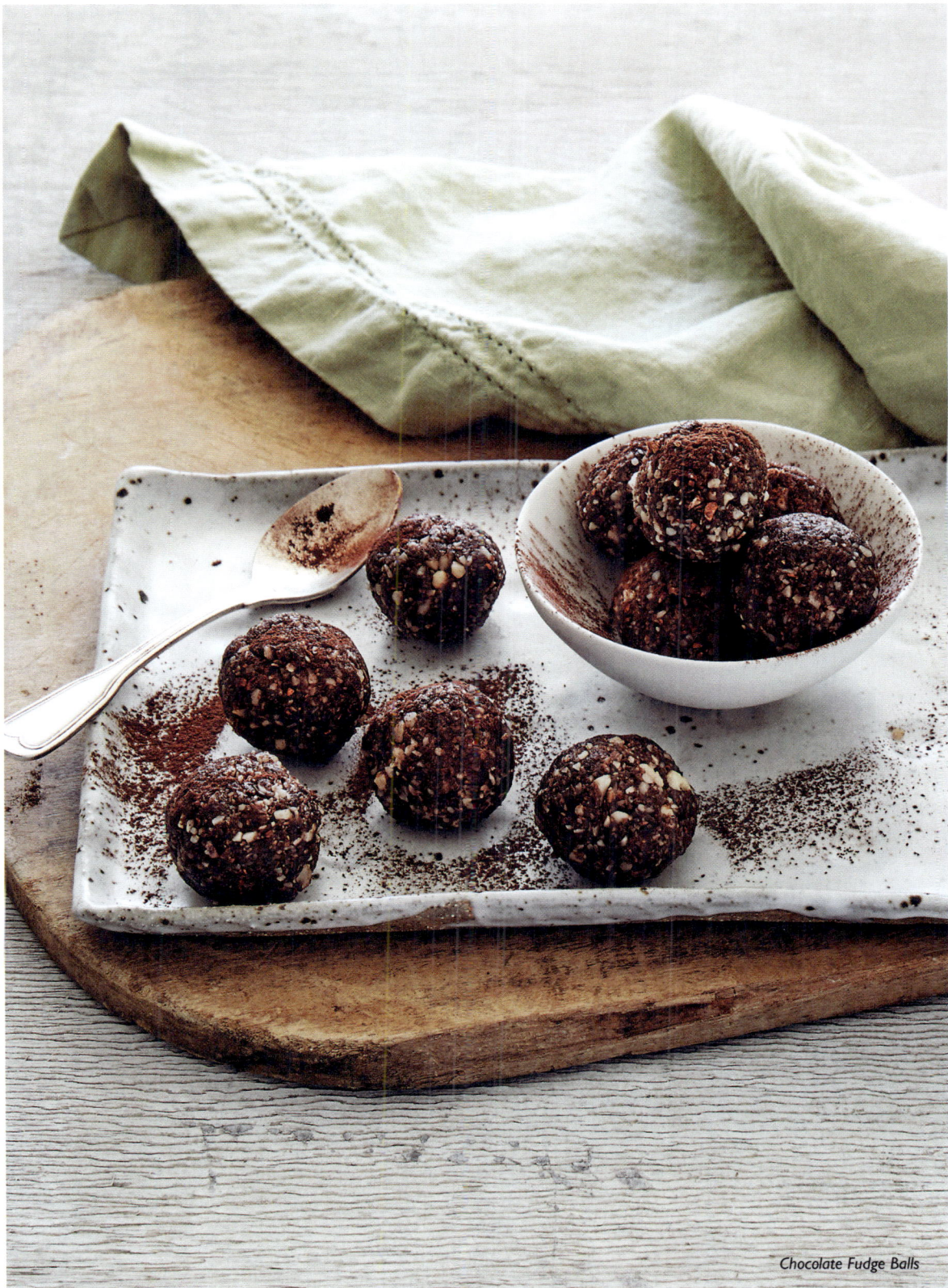

Chocolate Fudge Balls

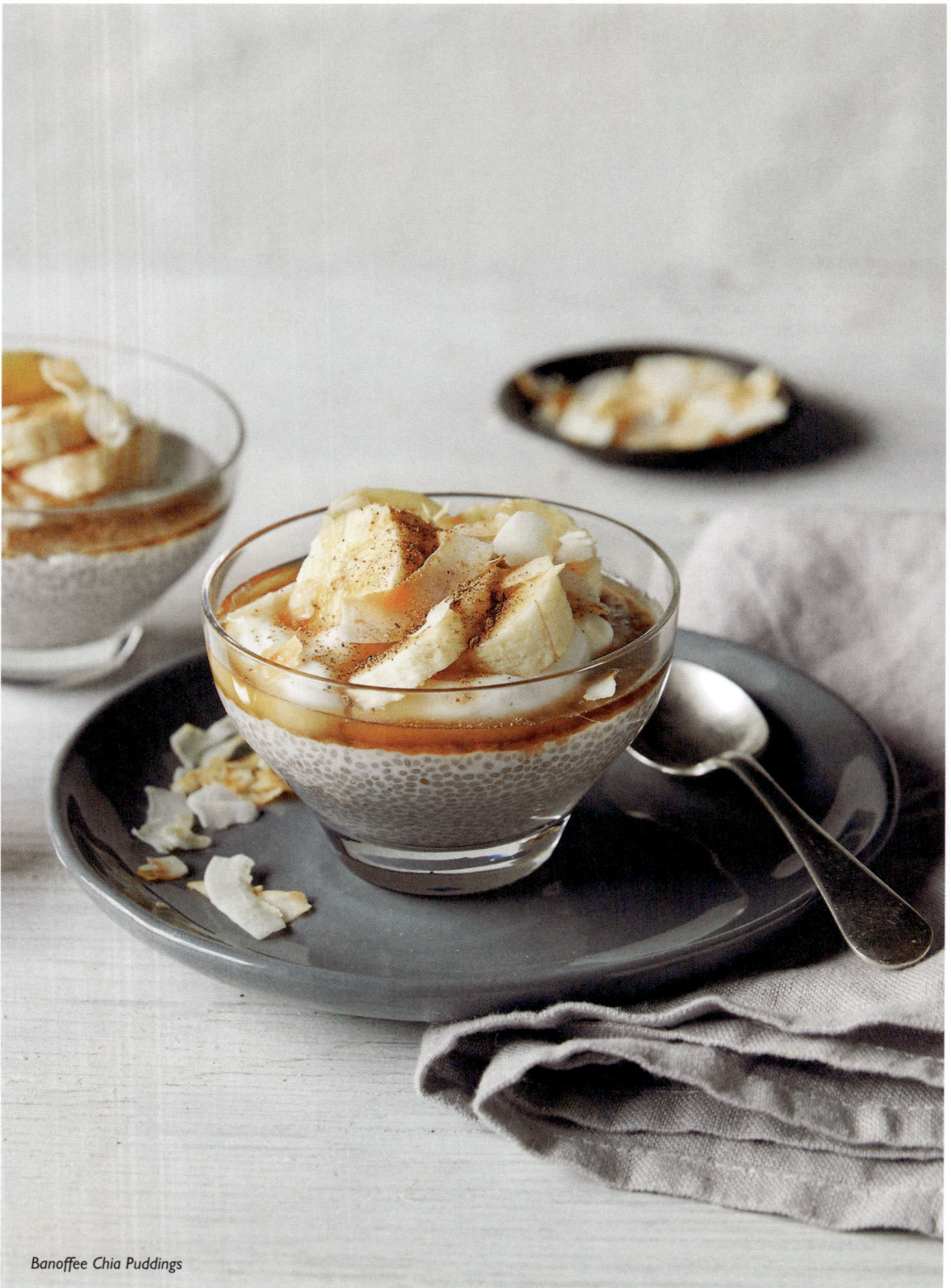

Banoffee Chia Puddings

BANOFFEE CHIA PUDDINGS

SERVES 4
PREP TIME 2 hours

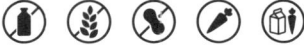

80 ml (2½ fl oz/⅓ cup) coconut milk
125 ml (4 fl oz/½ cup) water
35 g (1¼ oz/¼ cup) chia seeds
2 tablespoons coconut yoghurt
½ teaspoon vanilla extract
1 banana
2 teaspoons maple syrup
10 g (¼ oz) coconut flakes

Place the coconut milk, water and chia seeds in a small bowl and whisk to combine. Divide this mixture between four glasses and refrigerate for 2 hours, or overnight.

Mix together the yoghurt and vanilla, then spoon evenly over the puddings.

Right before serving, slice the banana and divide between the puddings, then drizzle with maple syrup and sprinkle with coconut flakes.

CHOCOLATE CHUNK COOKIES

MAKES 10
PREP TIME 5 minutes
COOK TIME 15 minutes

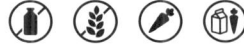

400 g (14 oz) tinned chickpeas, drained and rinsed
70 g (2½ oz/¼ cup) natural peanut butter
90 g (3¼ oz/¼ cup) rice malt syrup
1 teaspoon natural vanilla extract
2 tablespoons coconut oil, melted
25 g (1 oz/¼ cup) almond meal
90 g (3¼ oz/½ cup) vegan dark chocolate chips

Preheat the oven to 180°C (350°F). Lightly grease a baking tray then line it with baking paper.

Place the chickpeas between two sheets of paper towel and rub them to remove any excess liquid.

Place all of the ingredients except the almond meal and chocolate chips in a food processor and pulse for 1 minute, until all the ingredients are blended together into a dough.

Transfer the mixture to a bowl, and fold through the almond meal and chocolate chips.

Scoop out tablespoons of the mixture, roll these into balls and place on the baking tray. Flatten the balls out with the back of a spoon to form a cookie shape.

Bake for 10–12 minutes, or until golden.

Remove from the oven and allow to cool for a few minutes before transferring to a wire rack to cool completely. Keep in an airtight container for up to 5 days.

MINCE TARTS

MAKES 12
PREP TIME 30 minutes

CRUST
50 g (1¾ oz/½ cup) rolled (porridge) oats
35 g (1¼ oz/½ cup) shredded coconut
80 g (2¾ oz/½ cup) medjool dates, pitted

FRUIT MINCE FILLING
2 tablespoons dried cranberries
2 tablespoons currants
2 tablespoons dried apricots, chopped
2 tablespoons slivered almonds, toasted
½ granny smith apple, unpeeled and coarsely grated
zest of 1 orange
¼ teaspoon ground cinnamon
⅛ teaspoon ground nutmeg
⅛ teaspoon ground ginger

Line a 12-hole mini-muffin tin with paper cases (skip this step if you're using a silicone muffin mould).

Combine the crust ingredients in a food processor and blitz until the mixture forms a ball. Place two teaspoons of crust mixture into each muffin hole and press the mixture firmly into the base and up the sides. Roll the remaining crust into a ball and set aside.

Combine all the filling ingredients together in a medium bowl. Spoon 2 teaspoons of filling into each crust and set aside.

Roll out the remaining crust between two sheets of baking paper until it's 3 mm (⅛ inch) thick. Use a small (4 cm/1½ inch) star cutter to cut out 12 stars, then top each tart with them. Refrigerate for 2 hours to firm up before serving.

CHRISTMAS CHOCOLATE BARK

MAKES 10
PREP TIME 15 minutes + 20 minutes chilling time
COOK TIME 2 minutes

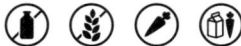

200 g (7 oz) vegan dark chocolate (70%), chopped
10 g (¼ oz) coconut flakes
20 g (¾ oz) pistachio nut kernels, chopped
20 g (¾ oz) dried cranberries

Melt the chocolate in a heatproof bowl and microwave for 30 seconds at a time, stirring after each time until melted and smooth. Alternatively, use the double-boiler method on page 73.

Place the coconut in a dry frying pan over medium heat. Toss for 1–2 minutes until lightly toasted. Transfer to a plate to cool.

Line a baking tray with baking paper and pour the chocolate onto the tray. Use a spatula to spread the chocolate out evenly so it's about 1 cm (½ inch) thick. Scatter over the pistachios, cranberries, and toasted coconut, then place in the freezer to set for 20 minutes.

Remove from the freezer and break into 10 pieces. Store in an airtight container in the fridge for up to 1 week, or wrap it up and gift it to friends for Christmas.

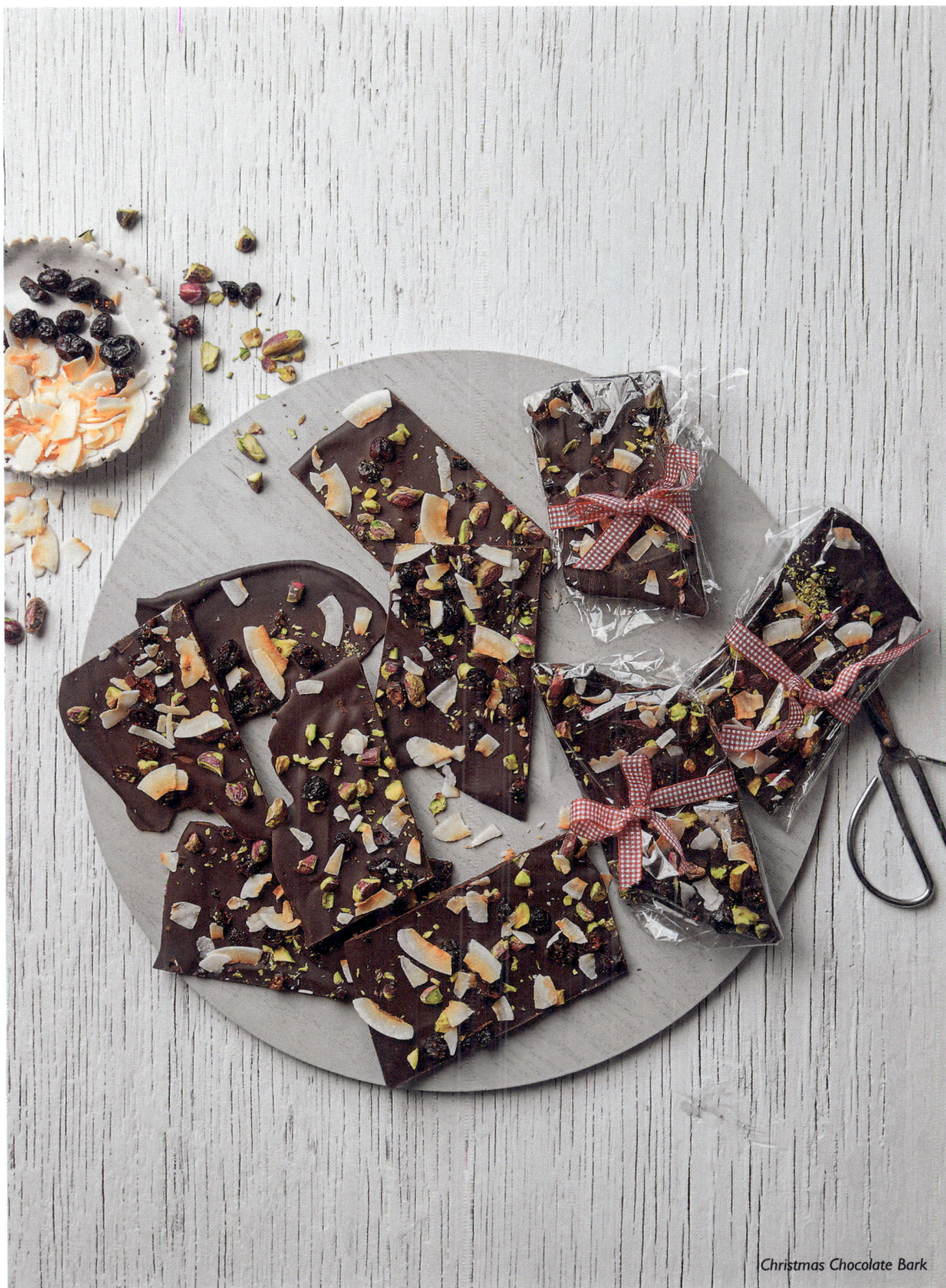

Christmas Chocolate Bark

REFERENCES

W Altorf-van der Kuil et al., 'Dietary protein and blood pressure: a systematic review', *PLoS One*, 2010 vol. 5, no. 8, doi: 10.1371/journal.pone.0012102

Jose Antonio et al., 'A high protein diet (3.4 g/kg/d) combined with a heavy resistance training program improves body composition in healthy trained men and women – a follow-up investigation', Journal of the International Society of Sports Nutrition, 2015, vol. 12, no. 1, doi: 10.1186/s12970-015-0100-0

Jose Antonio et al., 'The effects of consuming a high protein diet (4.4 g/kg/d) on body composition in resistance-trained individuals', *Journal of the International Society of Sports Nutrition*, 2014, vol. 11, no. 19, doi: 10.1186/1550-2783-11-19

Rachel L Batterham et al., 'Critical role for peptide YY in protein-mediated satiation and body-weight regulation', *Cell Metabolism*, 2006, vol. 4, no. 3, pp. 223–233, doi: 10.1016/j.cmet.2006.08.001

W A Blom, 'Effect of a high-protein breakfast on the postprandial ghrelin response', *American Journal of Clinical Nutrition*, 2006, vol. 83, no. 2, pp. 211–220, doi: 10.1093/ajcn/83.2.211

Lucy Chambers, Keri McCrickerd & Martin R.Yeomans, 'Optimising foods for satiety', *Trends in Food Science & Technology*, 2015, vol. 41, no. 2, doi: /10.1016/j.tifs.2014.10.007

J E Kerstetter, A M Kenny & K L Insogna, 'Dietary protein and skeletal health: a review of recent human research', *Curr Opin Lipidol*, 2011, vol. 2, no. 1, pp. 16–20, doi: 10.1097/MOL.0b013e3283419441

D K Layman, 'A reduced ratio of dietary carbohydrate to protein improves body composition and blood lipid profiles during weight loss in adult women', *Journal of Nutrition*, 2003, vol. 133, no. 2, pp. 411–417, doi: 10.1093/jn/133.2.411

D K Layman, 'Dietary protein and exercise have additive effects on body composition during weight loss in adult women', *Journal of Nutrition*, 2005, vol. 135, no. 8, pp. 1903–1910, doi: 10.1093/jn/135.8.1903

M P Lejeune et al., 'Ghrelin and glucagon-like peptide 1 concentrations, 24-h satiety, and energy and substrate metabolism during a high-protein diet and measured in a respiration chamber', *American Journal of Clinical Nutrition*, 2006, vol. 83, no. 1, pp. 89–94, doi: 10.1093/ajcn/83.1.89

Manny Noakes et al., 'Effect of an energy-restricted, high-protein, low-fat diet relative to a conventional high-carbohydrate, low-fat diet on weight loss, body composition, nutritional status, and markers of cardiovascular health in obese women', *The American Journal of Clinical Nutrition*, 2005, vol. 81, no. 6, pp. 1298–1306, doi: 10.1093/ajcn/81.6.1298

Susan Perry, 'The Neural Regulation of Thirst', *BrainFacts.org*, 2008, brainfacts.org/Archives/2008/The-Neural-Regulation-of-Thirst, accessed August 2019

S Soenen et al., 'Normal protein intake is required for body weight loss and weight maintenance, and elevated protein intake for additional preservation of resting energy expenditure and fat free mass', *Journal of Nutrition*, 2013, vol. 143, no. 5, pp. 591–596, doi: 10.3945/jn.112.167593

R Swaminathan et al., 'Thermic effect of feeding carbohydrate, fat, protein and mixed meal in lean and obese subjects', *The American Journal of Clinical Nutrition*, 1985, vol. 42, no. 2, pp. 177–181, doi: 10.1093/ajcn/42.2.177

David S Weigle et al., 'A high-protein diet induces sustained reductions in appetite, ad libitum caloric intake, and body weight despite compensatory changes in diurnal plasma leptin and ghrelin concentrations', The American Journal of Clinical Nutrition, 2005, vol. 82, no. 1, pp. 41–48, doi: 10.1093/ajcn/82.1.41

M S Westerterp–Plantenga et al., 'High protein intake sustains weight maintenance after body weight loss in humans', *International Journal of Obesity*, 2004, vol. 28, pp. 57–64, doi: 10.1038/sj.ijo.0802461

M S Westerterp-Plantenga et al., 'High protein intake sustains weight maintenance after body weight loss in humans', *The American Journal of Clinical Nutrition*, 1985, vol. 42, no. 2, pp. 177–181, doi: 10.1093/ajcn/42.2.177

Klaas R Westerterp, 'Diet induced thermogenesis', Nutrition & Metabolism 2004, vol. 1, no. 5, doi: 10.1186/1743-7075-1-5

INDEX

This edition published in 2026 by Murdoch Books,
an imprint of Allen & Unwin.
First published in 2020.

Murdoch Books Australia
83 Alexander Street
Crows Nest NSW 2065
Phone: +61 (0)2 8425 0100
murdochbooks.com.au
info@murdochbooks.com.au

Murdoch Books UK
Ormond House
26–27 Boswell Street
London WC1N 3JZ
Phone: +44 (0) 20 8785 5995
murdochbooks.co.uk
info@murdochbooks.co.uk

For corporate orders and custom publishing,
contact our business development team at
salesenquiries@murdochbooks.com.au

Publisher: Kelly Doust
Editorial Manager: Virginia Birch
Design Manager: Megan Pigott
Cover Designer: Sarah McCoy
Designer: Kirby Armstrong
Editor: Katie Bosher
Commissioning Editor (second edition): Justin Wolfers
Words & recipes: Tiffiny Hall, Barbara Macciolli, Karen McFarlane
and the TIFFXO team at Loup
Recipe photography: Brent Parker Jones, Loup, Ren Pidgeon
Recipe food stylist: Peta Gray
Recipe food preparation: Sarah Watson
Front cover photography: Jeremy Simons
Front cover food stylist: Jenn Tolhurst
Front cover home economist: Tammi Kwok
Hair and make-up: Paulie Bedggood
Production Manager: Natalie Crouch

Text © Tiffiny Hall 2020
The moral right of the author has been asserted.
Design © Murdoch Books 2020
Photography © Brent Parker Jones 2020, except for images on back cover (bottom)
and pages 2, 7, 37, 60, 90, 140 and 167 © Jeremy Simons 2020, and images on pages
136 and 174 © Ren Pidgeon

ISBN 978 1 76150 119 7

A catalogue record for this
book is available from the
National Library of Australia

A catalogue record for this book is available from the British Library

Colour reproduction by Splitting Image Colour Studio Pty Ltd, Clayton, Victoria
Printed by 1010 Printing International Limited, China

10 9 8 7 6 5 4 3 2 1

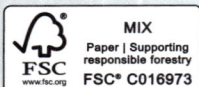

Acknowledgements

Thank you to my amazing community for being so
snacky and encouraging me to find a home for all my
delicious snacks in the one book. I'd also like to thank
the fabulous Murdoch Books team. Special thanks to my
publisher Kelly Doust and Barbara Macciolli for being as
passionate about snacks as I am, and for believing snacks may
be small but they are indeed mighty and deserve their own
book! To my husband, Ed Kavalee, this book wouldn't exist
without your ravenous appetite always inspiring me to
create fun and yum snacks.
And to my children, Arnold and Vada, who are
following in their hungry father's footsteps.

TIFF XO

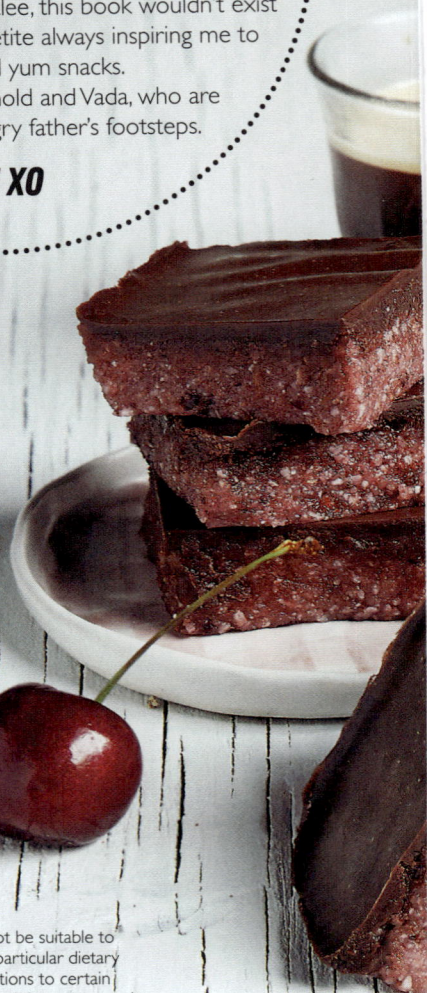